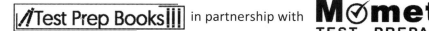 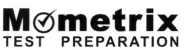

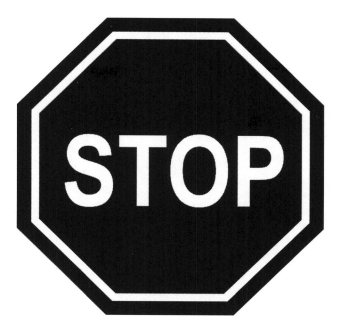

FREE Test Taking Tips Video/DVD Offer

To better serve you, we created videos covering test taking tips that we want to give you for FREE. **These videos cover world-class tips that will help you succeed on your test.**

We just ask that you send us feedback about this product. Please let us know what you thought about it—whether good, bad, or indifferent.

To get your **FREE videos**, you can use the QR code below or email freevideos@studyguideteam.com with "Free Videos" in the subject line and the following information in the body of the email:

a. The title of your product

b. Your product rating on a scale of 1-5, with 5 being the highest

c. Your feedback about the product

If you have any questions or concerns, please don't hesitate to contact us at info@studyguideteam.com.

Thank you!

Med Surg Certification Review Book

CMSRN Study Guide and Medical Surgical (RN-BC) Exam Prep with Practice Test Questions [5th Edition]

Joshua Rueda

Interested in buying more than 10 copies of our product? Contact us about bulk discounts:
bulkorders@studyguideteam.com

ISBN 13: 9781637754641
ISBN 10: 1637754647

Table of Contents

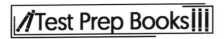

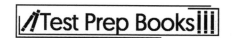

Welcome

Dear Reader,

Welcome to your new Test Prep Books study guide! We are pleased that you chose us to help you prepare for your exam. There are many study options to choose from, and we appreciate you choosing us. Studying can be a daunting task, but we have designed a smart, effective study guide to help prepare you for what lies ahead.

Whether you're a parent helping your child learn and grow, a high school student working hard to get into your dream college, or a nursing student studying for a complex exam, we want to help give you the tools you need to succeed. We hope this study guide gives you the skills and the confidence to thrive, and we can't thank you enough for allowing us to be part of your journey.

In an effort to continue to improve our products, we welcome feedback from our customers. We look forward to hearing from you. Suggestions, success stories, and criticisms can all be communicated by emailing us at info@studyguideteam.com.

Sincerely,
Test Prep Books Team

FREE Videos/DVD OFFER

Doing well on your exam requires both knowing the test content and understanding how to use that knowledge to do well on the test. We offer completely FREE test taking tip videos. **These videos cover world-class tips that you can use to succeed on your test.**

To get your **FREE videos**, you can use the QR code below or email freevideos@studyguideteam.com with "Free Videos" in the subject line and the following information in the body of the email:

- a. The title of your product
- b. Your product rating on a scale of 1-5, with 5 being the highest
- c. Your feedback about the product

If you have any questions or concerns, please don't hesitate to contact us at info@studyguideteam.com.

Quick Overview

As you draw closer to taking your exam, effective preparation becomes more and more important. Thankfully, you have this study guide to help you get ready. Use this guide to help keep your studying on track and refer to it often.

This study guide contains several key sections that will help you be successful on your exam. The guide contains tips for what you should do the night before and the day of the test. Also included are test-taking tips. Knowing the right information is not always enough. Many well-prepared test takers struggle with exams. These tips will help equip you to accurately read, assess, and answer test questions.

A large part of the guide is devoted to showing you what content to expect on the exam and to helping you better understand that content. In this guide are practice test questions so that you can see how well you have grasped the content. Then, answer explanations are provided so that you can understand why you missed certain questions.

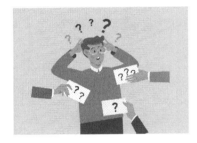

Don't try to cram the night before you take your exam. This is not a wise strategy for a few reasons. First, your retention of the information will be low. Your time would be better used by reviewing information you already know rather than trying to learn a lot of new information. Second, you will likely become stressed as you try to gain a large amount of knowledge in a short amount of time. Third, you will be depriving yourself of sleep. So be sure to go to bed at a reasonable time the night before. Being well-rested helps you focus and remain calm.

Be sure to eat a substantial breakfast the morning of the exam. If you are taking the exam in the afternoon, be sure to have a good lunch as well. Being hungry is distracting and can make it difficult to focus. You have hopefully spent lots of time preparing for the exam. Don't let an empty stomach get in the way of success!

When travelling to the testing center, leave earlier than needed. That way, you have a buffer in case you experience any delays. This will help you remain calm and will keep you from missing your appointment time at the testing center.

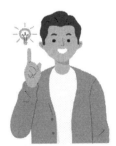

Be sure to pace yourself during the exam. Don't try to rush through the exam. There is no need to risk performing poorly on the exam just so you can leave the testing center early. Allow yourself to use all of the allotted time if needed.

Remain positive while taking the exam even if you feel like you are performing poorly. Thinking about the content you should have mastered will not help you perform better on the exam.

Once the exam is complete, take some time to relax. Even if you feel that you need to take the exam again, you will be well served by some down time before you begin studying again. It's often easier to convince yourself to study if you know that it will come with a reward!

Test-Taking Strategies

1. Predicting the Answer

When you feel confident in your preparation for a multiple-choice test, try predicting the answer before reading the answer choices. This is especially useful on questions that test objective factual knowledge. By predicting the answer before reading the available choices, you eliminate the possibility that you will be distracted or led astray by an incorrect answer choice. You will feel more confident in your selection if you read the question, predict the answer, and then find your prediction among the answer choices. After using this strategy, be sure to still read all of the answer choices carefully and completely. If you feel unprepared, you should not attempt to predict the answers. This would be a waste of time and an opportunity for your mind to wander in the wrong direction.

2. Reading the Whole Question

Too often, test takers scan a multiple-choice question, recognize a few familiar words, and immediately jump to the answer choices. Test authors are aware of this common impatience, and they will sometimes prey upon it. For instance, a test author might subtly turn the question into a negative, or he or she might redirect the focus of the question right at the end. The only way to avoid falling into these traps is to read the entirety of the question carefully before reading the answer choices.

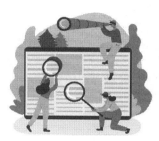

3. Looking for Wrong Answers

Long and complicated multiple-choice questions can be intimidating. One way to simplify a difficult multiple-choice question is to eliminate all of the answer choices that are clearly wrong. In most sets of answers, there will be at least one selection that can be dismissed right away. If the test is administered on paper, the test taker could draw a line through it to indicate that it may be ignored; otherwise, the test taker will have to perform this operation mentally or on scratch paper. In either case, once the obviously incorrect answers have been eliminated, the remaining choices may be considered. Sometimes identifying the clearly wrong answers will give the test taker some information about the correct answer. For instance, if one of the remaining answer choices is a direct opposite of one of the eliminated answer choices, it may well be the correct answer. The opposite of obviously wrong is obviously right! Of course, this is not always the case. Some answers are obviously incorrect simply because they are irrelevant to the question being asked. Still, identifying and eliminating some incorrect answer choices is a good way to simplify a multiple-choice question.

4. Don't Overanalyze

Anxious test takers often overanalyze questions. When you are nervous, your brain will often run wild, causing you to make associations and discover clues that don't actually exist. If you feel that this may be a problem for you, do whatever you can to slow down during the test. Try taking a deep breath or counting to ten. As you read and consider the question, restrict yourself to the particular words used by the author. Avoid thought tangents about what the author *really* meant, or what he or she was *trying* to say. The only things that matter on a multiple-choice test are the words that are actually in the question. You must avoid reading too much into a multiple-choice question, or supposing that the writer meant something other than what he or she wrote.

5. No Need for Panic

It is wise to learn as many strategies as possible before taking a multiple-choice test, but it is likely that you will come across a few questions for which you simply don't know the answer. In this situation, avoid panicking. Because

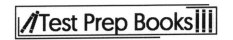
most multiple-choice tests include dozens of questions, the relative value of a single wrong answer is small. As much as possible, you should compartmentalize each question on a multiple-choice test. In other words, you should not allow your feelings about one question to affect your success on the others. When you find a question that you either don't understand or don't know how to answer, just take a deep breath and do your best. Read the entire question slowly and carefully. Try rephrasing the question a couple of different ways. Then, read all of the answer choices carefully. After eliminating obviously wrong answers, make a selection and move on to the next question.

6. Confusing Answer Choices

When working on a difficult multiple-choice question, there may be a tendency to focus on the answer choices that are the easiest to understand. Many people, whether consciously or not, gravitate to the answer choices that require the least concentration, knowledge, and memory. This is a mistake. When you come across an answer

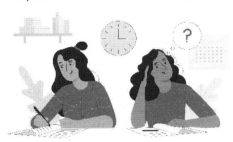

choice that is confusing, you should give it extra attention. A question might be confusing because you do not know the subject matter to which it refers. If this is the case, don't eliminate the answer before you have affirmatively settled on another. When you come across an answer choice of this type, set it aside as you look at the remaining choices. If you can confidently assert that one of the other choices is correct, you can leave the confusing answer aside. Otherwise, you will need to take a moment to try to better understand the confusing answer choice. Rephrasing is one way to tease out the sense of a confusing answer choice.

7. Your First Instinct

Many people struggle with multiple-choice tests because they overthink the questions. If you have studied sufficiently for the test, you should be prepared to trust your first instinct once you have carefully and completely read the question and all of the answer choices. There is a great deal of research suggesting that the mind can come to the correct conclusion very quickly once it has obtained all of the relevant information. At times, it may seem to you as if your intuition is working faster even than your reasoning mind. This may in fact be true. The knowledge you obtain while studying may be retrieved from your subconscious before you have a chance to work out the associations that support it. Verify your instinct by working out the reasons that it should be trusted.

8. Key Words

Many test takers struggle with multiple-choice questions because they have poor reading comprehension skills. Quickly reading and understanding a multiple-choice question requires a mixture of skill and experience. To help with this, try jotting down a few key words and phrases on a piece of scrap paper. Doing this concentrates the process of reading and forces the mind to weigh the relative importance of the question's parts. In selecting words and phrases to write down, the test taker thinks about the question more deeply and carefully. This is especially true for multiple-choice questions that are preceded by a long prompt.

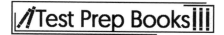
9. Subtle Negatives

One of the oldest tricks in the multiple-choice test writer's book is to subtly reverse the meaning of a question with a word like *not* or *except*. If you are not paying attention to each word in the question, you can easily be led astray by this trick. For instance, a common question format is, "Which of the following is...?" Obviously, if the question instead is, "Which of the following is not...?," then the answer will be quite different. Even worse, the test makers are aware of the potential for this mistake and will include one answer choice that would be correct if the question were not negated or reversed. A test taker who misses the reversal will find what he or she believes to be a correct answer and will be so confident that he or she will fail to reread the question and discover the original error. The only way to avoid this is to practice a wide variety of multiple-choice questions and to pay close attention to each and every word.

10. Reading Every Answer Choice

It may seem obvious, but you should always read every one of the answer choices! Too many test takers fall into the habit of scanning the question and assuming that they understand the question because they recognize a few key words. From there, they pick the first answer choice that answers the question they believe they have read. Test takers who read all of the answer choices might discover that one of the latter answer choices is actually *more* correct. Moreover, reading all of the answer choices can remind you of facts related to the question that can help you arrive at the correct answer. Sometimes, a misstatement or incorrect detail in one of the latter answer choices will trigger your memory of the subject and will enable you to find the right answer. Failing to read all of the answer choices is like not reading all of the items on a restaurant menu: you might miss out on the perfect choice.

11. Spot the Hedges

One of the keys to success on multiple-choice tests is paying close attention to every word. This is never truer than with words like *almost*, *most*, *some*, and *sometimes*. These words are called "hedges" because they indicate that a statement is not totally true or not true in every place and time. An absolute statement will contain no hedges, but

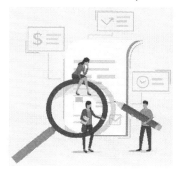

in many subjects, the answers are not always straightforward or absolute. There are always exceptions to the rules in these subjects. For this reason, you should favor those multiple-choice questions that contain hedging language. The presence of qualifying words indicates that the author is taking special care with his or her words, which is certainly important when composing the right answer. After all, there are many ways to be wrong, but there is only one way to be right! For this reason, it is wise to avoid answers that are absolute when taking a multiple-choice test. An absolute answer is one that says things are either all one way or all another. They often include words like *every*, *always*, *best*, and *never*. If you are taking a multiple-choice test in a subject that doesn't lend itself to absolute answers, be on your guard if you see any of these words.

12. Long Answers

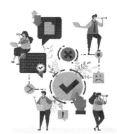

In many subject areas, the answers are not simple. As already mentioned, the right answer often requires hedges. Another common feature of the answers to a complex or subjective question are qualifying clauses, which are groups of words that subtly modify the meaning of the sentence. If the question or answer choice describes a rule to which there are exceptions or the subject matter is complicated, ambiguous, or confusing, the correct answer will require many words in order to be expressed clearly and accurately. In essence, you should not be deterred by answer choices that seem excessively long. Oftentimes, the author of the text will not be able to write the correct answer without offering some qualifications and

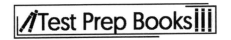

modifications. Your job is to read the answer choices thoroughly and completely and to select the one that most accurately and precisely answers the question.

13. Restating to Understand

Sometimes, a question on a multiple-choice test is difficult not because of what it asks but because of how it is written. If this is the case, restate the question or answer choice in different words. This process serves a couple of important purposes. First, it forces you to concentrate on the core of the question. In order to rephrase the question accurately, you have to understand it well. Rephrasing the question will concentrate your mind on the key words and ideas. Second, it will present the information to your mind in a fresh way. This process may trigger your memory and render some useful scrap of information picked up while studying.

14. True Statements

Sometimes an answer choice will be true in itself, but it does not answer the question. This is one of the main reasons why it is essential to read the question carefully and completely before proceeding to the answer choices. Too often, test takers skip ahead to the answer choices and look for true statements. Having found one of these, they are content to select it without reference to the question above. The savvy test taker will always read the entire question before turning to the answer choices. Then, having settled on a correct answer choice, he or she will refer to the original question and ensure that the selected answer is relevant. The mistake of choosing a correct-but-irrelevant answer choice is especially common on questions related to specific pieces of objective knowledge.

15. No Patterns

One of the more dangerous ideas that circulates about multiple-choice tests is that the correct answers tend to fall into patterns. These erroneous ideas range from a belief that B and C are the most common right answers, to the idea that an unprepared test-taker should answer "A-B-A-C-A-D-A-B-A." It cannot be emphasized enough that pattern-seeking of this type is exactly the WRONG way to approach a multiple-choice test. To begin with, it is highly unlikely that the test maker will plot the correct answers according to some predetermined pattern. The questions are scrambled and delivered in a random order. Furthermore, even if the test maker was following a pattern in the assignation of correct answers, there is no reason why the test taker would know which pattern he or she was using. Any attempt to discern a pattern in the answer choices is a waste of time and a distraction from the real work of taking the test. A test taker would be much better served by extra preparation before the test than by reliance on a pattern in the answers.

Bonus Content

We host multiple bonus items online, including all 3 practice tests in digital format. Scan the QR code or go to this link to access this content:

testprepbooks.com/bonus/medsurg

The first time you access the tests, you will need to register as a "new user" and verify your email address.

If you have any issues, please email support@testprepbooks.com.

Introduction

About this Guide

This study guide is intended for preparation for the following two exams:

- Certified Medical-Surgical Registered Nurse (CMSRN®) Exam produced by the Medical-Surgical Nursing Certification Board (MSNCB®)

- The Medical-Surgical Nursing Certification (MEDSURG-BC®) produced by the American Nurses Credentialing Center (ANCC)

The CMSRN® and MEDSURG-BC® outlines are structured differently but cover very similar material. The CMSRN® outline is structured around five knowledge domains: Patient/Care Management, Holistic Patient Care, Elements of Interprofessional Care, Professional Concepts, and Nursing Teamwork and Collaboration. The MEDSURG-BC® outline is structured around skill topics such as Assessment and Diagnosis; Planning, Implementation, and Evaluation; and Professional Role. The two outline structures are complementary as nursing knowledge and nursing skills must be paired together, and both are covered on each exam.

The developers of this guide have chosen to follow the CMSRN® outline heading structure, so each chapter title is that of a knowledge topic. The skill content, as emphasized in the MEDSURG-BC® outline, is then integrated into each concept that is discussed. Because the exams test such similar content, the two practice tests at the end can be used to prepare for either exam.

In summary, whether you are preparing for the CMSRN® or the MEDSURG-BC®, this the guide for you. It will educate you on the topics you need to know and then provide an opportunity to thoroughly test your knowledge. Be sure to take advantage of the detailed answer explanations as well.

We wish you the best on your exam!

Certified Medical-Surgical Registered Nurse (CMSRN®)

Function of the Test
The Certified Medical-Surgical Registered Nurse (CMSRN®) Exam is a test given by the Medical-Surgical Nursing Certification Board (MSNCB®) to those who hold a license as a registered nurse (RN), have accrued at least 2,000 hours of practice within the past three years, and have practiced two years as an RN in a medical-surgical setting.

The CMSRN® gives nurses the credential they need to work as Medical-Surgical Nurses. The CMSRN® certification is accredited by the Accreditation Board for Specialty Nursing Certification (ABSNC) and recognized for Magnet status.

*CMSRN® and MSNCB® are registered trademarks of the Medical-Surgical Nursing Certification Board, which neither sponsors nor endorses this product.

Test Administration
The CMSRN® is offered in computer-based format by Prometric. Candidates can either take the test at a testing center or take the test at home using remote proctoring. Before receiving the Authorization to Test (ATT), applications are reviewed by MSNCB. If the candidate applies through The FailSafe Certification Program, the application will be reviewed by the candidate's FailSafe organization. Candidates will receive an ATT email that provides a link for scheduling the exam. The exam must be taken within 90 days of receiving the email, and exams cannot be scheduled during the final 6 days of the 90-day exam window.

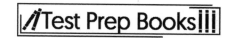
Test takers who do not pass the exam have the option of taking the exam again for a one-time discount, but only if it is considered their first retake. This is offered up to 12 months after the exam date. Those who require accommodations for a disability may submit an application to MSNCB® with the box for testing accommodations selected. Applicants must contact MSNCB® to receive the form needed to make the request for accommodations and then email the appropriate documentation to MSNCB. Test takers must bring a valid government ID with a photo and signature to their testing appointment.

Test Format

The exam includes 150 multiple-choice questions, of which 125 are scored. The other 25 are considered pretest questions and are used to assess their validity and utility as scored questions for future exams. The CMSRN® exam covers five different domains: Patient/Care Management, Holistic Patient Care, Elements of Interprofessional Care, Professional Concepts, and Nursing Teamwork and Collaboration. The table below breaks down the percentages of the content:

Domain	Percentage	Number of Questions
Patient/Care Management	32%	40
Holistic Patient Care	15%	19
Elements of Interprofessional Care	17%	21
Professional Concepts	15%	19
Nursing Teamwork and Collaboration	21%	26

Scoring

To pass the CMSRN®, a standard score of 95, or 71 percent correct, is required. Test takers' scores are not compared to each other, but rather are based on the Angoff procedure.

A scaled score for the CMSRN® will be given at the end of the exam. For those who do not pass the exam, the total score along with the subscores will highlight the areas that need work.

Recent Developments

The blueprint for the CMSRN® changed for the 2023 year, so please see the previous table or the recent blueprint on the website to get up-do-date information on the exam.

*CMSRN® and MSNCB® are registered trademarks of the Medical-Surgical Nursing Certification Board, which neither sponsors nor endorses this product.

The Medical-Surgical Nursing Certification (MEDSURG-BC®)

Function of the Test

The American Nurse Credential Center's Medical-Surgical Nursing Certification [Medical Surgical Nurse-Board Certified (MEDSURG-BC®)] exam is a competency-based exam for entry-level registered nurses in the medical-surgical specialty to demonstrate their clinical knowledge and skills. Successfully passing the exam earns the test taker the MEDSURG-BC® credential, which is then valid for five years. After this time, the credential can be maintained by keeping nursing license active and satisfying the requirements for renewal.

Candidates must meet eligibility criteria in order to register and sit for the exam. They must hold a current, active RN license. This license must be either from a state or territory of the United States or what is considered to be the legally-recognized, professional equivalent in another country. Candidates must have a minimum of two years of full-time professional experience as a registered nurse. Within the three years immediately prior to sitting for the

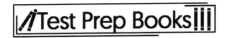

exam, a candidate must have accrued at least 2,000 hours of clinical practice specifically in the area of medical-surgical nursing, and completed 30 hours of continuing education in this specialty area.

Test Administration

The MEDSURG-BC® exam is administered via computer year-round at Prometric testing sites throughout the United States. Candidates must apply to take the test and provide proof of satisfying the eligibility requirements. Test takers are permitted to apply to retake the exam after 60 days if they do not pass. However, within a 12-month period, only three test attempts are permitted. Accommodations are available for test takers with documented disabilities. Candidates seeking accommodations must submit supporting paperwork and wait for confirmation or approval of the requested accommodations prior to registering for the exam.

Test Format

The exam includes 150 multiple-choice questions, of which 125 are scored. The other 25 are considered pretest questions and are used by the ANCC to assess their validity and utility as scored questions for future exams. Test takers have three hours to complete the exam. The major content areas and the number of questions and percentage of the test comprised by each is listed in the table below:

Content Area	Number of Questions	Percentage of Test
Assessment and Diagnosis	52	42%
Planning, Implementation, and Evaluation	58	46%
Professional Role	15	12%

Scoring

The MEDSURG-BC® exam is a pass-fail exam. Test takers must meet the minimum passing score to receive passing status and the MEDSURG-BC® credential. A test taker's raw score is determined by the number of questions answered correctly. Incorrect responses are not penalized, so test takers should guess, or complete all questions, if possible. The raw score is then converted to a scaled score from 0–500. The passing score is 350. Test takers earning at least 350 will receive the passing status. Those who score lower than 350 will receive their scaled score, the "fail" status, and diagnostic feedback pertaining to each of the three content areas on the exam.

Study Prep Plan

1 **Schedule** - Use one of our study schedules below or come up with one of your own.

2 **Relax** - Test anxiety can hurt even the best students. There are many ways to reduce stress. Find the one that works best for you.

3 **Execute** - Once you have a good plan in place, be sure to stick to it.

One Week Study Schedule		
Day 1	Patient/Care Management
Day 2	Infection Prevention and Control
Day 3	Holistic Patient Care
Day 4	Professional Concepts
Day 5	Practice Test #1
Day 6	Practice Tests #2 & #3
Day 7	Take Your Exam!

Two Week Study Schedule			
Day 1	Patient/Care Management	Day 8	Professional Concepts
Day 2	Cardiovascular/ Hematological	Day 9	Scope of Practice and Ethics
Day 3	Endocrine and Immunological	Day 10	Nursing Teamwork and Collaboration
Day 4	Infection Prevention and Control	Day 11	Practice Test #1
Day 5	Surgical/Procedural Nursing Management	Day 12	Practice Test #2
Day 6	Holistic Patient Care	Day 13	Practice Test #3
Day 7	Elements of Interprofessional Care	Day 14	Take Your Exam!

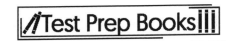

One Month Study Schedule					
Day 1	Patient/Care Management	Day 11	Surgical/Procedural Nursing Management	Day 21	Quality Management
Day 2	Pulmonary	Day 12	Perioperative Nursing Process	Day 22	Nursing Teamwork and Collaboration
Day 3	Cardiovascular/ Hematological	Day 13	Anesthesia	Day 23	Leadership
Day 4	Endocrine and Immunological	Day 14	Holistic Patient Care	Day 24	Practice Test #1
Day 5	Musculoskeletal/ Neurological/ Integumentary	Day 15	Health Promotion	Day 25	Answer Explanations #1
Day 6	Patient Safety Protocols	Day 16	Elements of Interprofessional Care	Day 26	Practice Test #2
Day 7	Infection Prevention and Control	Day 17	Documentation	Day 27	Answer Explanations #2
Day 8	Medication Management	Day 18	Professional Concepts	Day 28	Practice Test #3
Day 9	Medications	Day 19	Healthy Practice Environment	Day 29	Answer Explanations #3
Day 10	Pain Management	Day 20	Scope of Practice and Ethics	Day 30	Take Your Exam!

Build your own prep plan by visiting:

testprepbooks.com/prep

As you study for your test, we'd like to take the opportunity to remind you that you are capable of great things! With the right tools and dedication, you truly can do anything you set your mind to. The fact that you are holding this book right now shows how committed you are. In case no one has told you lately, you've got this! Our intention behind including this coloring page is to give you the chance to take some time to engage your creative side when you need a little brain-break from studying. As a company, we want to encourage people like you to achieve their dreams by providing good quality study materials for the tests and certifications that improve careers and change lives. As individuals, many of us have taken such tests in our careers, and we know how challenging this process can be. While we can't come alongside you and cheer you on personally, we can offer you the space to recall your purpose, reconnect with your passion, and refresh your brain through an artistic practice. We wish you every success, and happy studying!

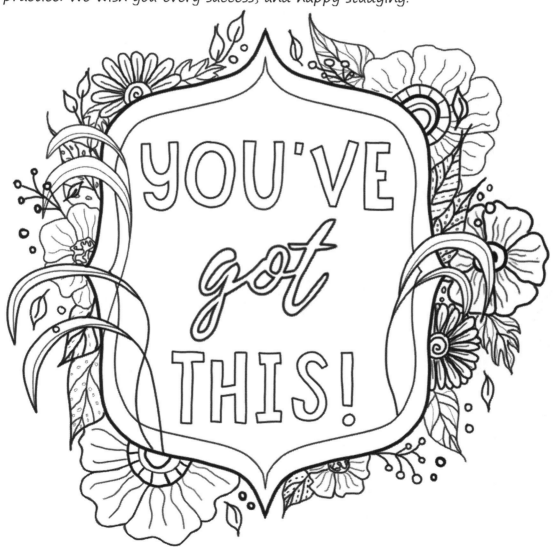

13

Patient/Care Management

Patient Safety

Nursing Process

Assessment

The **comprehensive history and a physical assessment** are essential first steps in establishing a therapeutic patient-provider relationship for a hospitalized patient or a patient who is new to a practice. The medical-surgical nurse has the opportunity to collect baseline data and to identify or eliminate physical assessment data that relate to the information provided by the patient in the interview portion of the assessment. As the nurse becomes familiar with the patient's condition, they can use this teachable moment to provide health promotion information. The nurse will develop and maintain expertise in conducting all phases of the history and physical assessment.

The seven elements of the comprehensive health history are as follows:

- Patient's identifying information
- Chief complaint
- History of the present illness
- Past history
- Family history
- Personal and social history
- Review of systems (ROS)

The **patient's identifying information** includes the date of the examination and the patient's name, gender, age, marital status, and occupation. This element also contains the identity and the reliability of the informant, who may be the patient, a family member, or an interpreter. The nurse will assess and document the veracity of the information that is provided. If the patient has been referred to the care of the nurse, any information recorded in the electronic health record (EHR) referencing the reason for the referral should be reviewed and documented in the comprehensive health history. The **chief complaint** is the patient's description of the problem or issue that prompted the visit. The patient's narrative may only vaguely describe the details of the current complaint, or the patient may prove to be an excellent historian. In either event, the nurse will document the information received from the patient using the patient's exact words whenever possible.

The **history of the present illness** is a chronological narrative that identifies the events from the onset of symptoms to the point at which the patient decides to access care for the problem. The nurse will also question the context in which the problem developed, all manifestations associated with the problem, and any treatments that have been used to address the problem.

The **seven cardinal elements** of each of the manifestations that are associated with the present illness must be identified and documented. The seven elements are location; quality; quantity or severity; the element of time, which includes onset, duration, and frequency; context; factors that alleviate or exacerbate the manifestations; and associated manifestations. This section will also identify the patient's assessment of how the current complaint has affected their ability to carry out activities of daily living (ADLs) and other activities. This section will also include the identification of "pertinent positives" or "pertinent negatives" among the manifestations associated with the present illness, which are signs that are either present or absent and may be associated with one of the conditions to be considered in the differential diagnosis for the present illness.

14

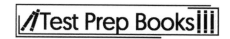

The nurse will also include the assessment of the patient's drugs, allergies, tobacco, alcohol, and recreational drug use. The review of the patient's drugs should include all prescription and nonprescription drugs as well as oral contraceptives and herbal supplements. Patients are often instructed to bring all of their drugs with the containers for review by the nurse. Specific details of any reaction to drugs, foods, insect bites, or environmental allergens must be reviewed and recorded. The patient's smoking history should be documented in the form of packs per day; for instance, a person who smoked 1.5 packs per day for ten years has a smoking history documented as a fifteen-pack-year history. If the patient has quit smoking, the length of time will be recorded. The use of and amounts of alcohol and recreational drugs are documented.

The **patient's past history** begins with the documentation of infectious childhood illnesses, chronic illnesses, and surgeries. There are four elements of the adult history, including the following:

- Medical
- Surgical
- Obstetric/Gynecologic
- Psychiatric

Medical issues should include documentation of chronic diseases including human immunodeficiency virus (HIV) status, sexual preference, and identification of high-risk sexual behaviors. Each surgical procedure should be documented with the identification of the purpose, recovery course, and surgical outcome. The obstetric/gynecologic history will document all pregnancies, induced and naturally occurring abortions, contraceptive use, and menstrual history. The psychiatric history includes specific disorders, hospitalizations, and treatments. This section should also include an assessment of the patient's age-specific immunization status and any screening tests that have been completed. Nurses should understand that many patients will not be able to identify each of these details; however, the information from the EHR or referral documentation can be used to prompt the patient's answers.

The **family history** is a comprehensive assessment of all members of the patient's family for the presence or absence of chronic and genetically linked conditions such as renal disease, hypertension (HTN), cardiovascular disease, arthritis, suicide, seizure disorders, breast cancer, ovarian cancer, and prostate cancer. The nurse will construct a chart that identifies the health status and age, or the age and health status at the time of death, for the patient's parents, grandparents, siblings, and grandchildren. The **personal and social history** identifies the patient's support structure, ways of coping, educational level, risk behaviors, and safety measures. The **review of systems (ROS)** can be completed during the physical examination; however, nurses should understand that the review of systems should be included with the comprehensive health history if there are multiple symptoms identified in the current complaint. Once each of these elements has been addressed, the nurse will complete the physical assessment in the following order:

- General assessment of appearance and weight change
- Skin
- Head and neck
- Breasts

The following systems are then assessed:

- Respiratory
- Cardiovascular
- Gastrointestinal
- Peripheral vascular
- Urinary

15

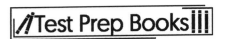
- Genital
- Musculoskeletal
- Psychiatric
- Neurologic
- Hematologic
- Endocrine

Diagnostic Test Selection

The medical-surgical nurse is responsible for selecting diagnostic tests that are accurate, necessary, and whenever possible, cost-effective. There is a large selection of evaluation measures, and they can be divided into screening tests and diagnostic tests. **Screening tests** are used to identify risk factors for a disease or the presence of early manifestations of the disease in asymptomatic individuals. **Diagnostic tests** are used to confirm the presence of the disease in a symptomatic patient or in an asymptomatic patient who has tested positive for the disease. Screening tests are used to identify common diseases in large numbers of people; therefore, the tests need to be inexpensive, generally less invasive than diagnostic tests, easy to administer, and highly sensitive.

The nurse will select those diagnostic tests that are most likely to provide the relevant information needed to support all clinical decisions. The appropriate selection of a diagnostic test also relies on the nurse's intuitive assessment skills. For instance, the context of the likelihood ratio is dependent on the identification of the pretest probability by the provider, and the pretest probability is derived from the physical assessment. The nurse also must remain current with recommendations related to the use of new assessment measures that might replace older measures that are more expensive, invasive, or less reliable. That being said, every new test should not automatically replace an existing test without careful consideration. The nurse will consider the possible benefits of the new versus the old before changing the diagnostic plan.

The patient's preferences should be reviewed by the medical-surgical nurse because the patient may have cultural concerns with invasive testing. Other common diagnostic tests such as magnetic resonance imaging (MRI) are not tolerated well by many patients, and if the MRI or any diagnostic test that is essential for appropriate patient care is refused by the patient, the nurse works with the patient to be certain that the needed information is collected. Anxious patients might need mild sedation in order to tolerate a procedure. However, if the patient does refuse to complete the test, the refusal should be well documented.

The medical-surgical nurse will use best practices to select the appropriate diagnostic tests to develop the patient's care plan. In making these choices, the nurse will consider the metrics of each test, the patient's preferences, and the cost effectiveness.

Plan of Care

In nursing, the nurse is instrumental in helping to carry out the developed plan of care. The plan of care begins with the nurse's assessment of the patient, followed by recommended nursing interventions. These interventions are then evaluated for their effectiveness and modified based on patient response, starting the entire care-planning process over again. An example of care performed according to a nursing care plan is when a patient is assessed by the nurse to be at risk for skin breakdown. Recommended interventions would include turning and repositioning the patient every two hours, providing regular perineal care and incontinence care, and ensuring that an adequate amount of the meal tray is consumed by the patient. The nurse assists with all these activities, and they document when the patient is turned, the intake and output record, and when baths and perineal care are performed.

Implementation and Evaluation

The outcomes set during the planning phase of the nursing process often require revisions. The revisions are based on the patient's inability to meet the stated goals or the patient's change in health status. The patient also has the

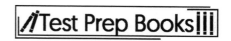

right to request revisions to the plan of care, and the nurse should work to ensure that the goals are patient-centered and realistic for each situation.

Updates to the plan of care can occur during the implementation or evaluation phase of the nursing process. When performing interventions, the nurse can determine if the patient can realistically perform the activities stated in the plan of care. The plan of care can be modified, or an attempt can be made to encourage the patient to meet the outcomes. The determination of a goal being met, not met, or partially met is achieved when the patient performs the interventions outlined in the plan of care. The nurse can then modify the care plan, if needed, to ensure that the outcomes align with the patient's current health status.

Modifications to the plan of care should be communicated to the patient, and education regarding the new expected outcomes should be provided. Revisions can include changing the nursing diagnosis, stating a more realistic outcome, adjusting the time criteria of goals, or changing the nursing interventions. The patient should be informed of the reason why the plan of care needs to be revised and how they will benefit from the modifications.

For example, an initial outcome for a patient undergoing abdominal surgery may be to tolerate fluids within the first 24 hours postoperatively. After the nurse provides a liquid diet, the patient becomes nauseated and vomits. The goal has not been met. At this point, the nurse would consider revising the time criteria or incorporating alternative interventions to help the patient achieve the expected outcome.

Gastrointestinal

Acute Abdomen Peritonitis and Appendicitis
An **acute abdomen** is defined as the presence of manifestations associated with nontraumatic intra-abdominal pathology that often requires surgical intervention.

Peritonitis
Peritonitis is an inflammatory process affecting the peritoneum, which is the serosal membrane that lines the abdominal cavity. The normally sterile environment of the peritoneum can become infected by a pathogen, irritated by bile from a perforated gallbladder or lacerated liver, or from secretions from the perforation of the stomach. The onset, severity, and course of the condition vary according to the precipitating event. Presenting manifestations may include abdominal pain, nausea and vomiting, diarrhea, fever and chills, altered peristalsis, abdominal distention, and possible encephalopathy. Diagnosis is based on the patient's history in addition to the results of routine lab studies and blood cultures; ultrasound, computerized tomography (CT), and x-ray studies of the abdomen; and paracentesis. Care of peritonitis is focused on eliminating the source of infection or irritation, controlling the infection and inflammatory process with aggressive antibiotic therapy as appropriate to prevent progression to generalized sepsis, and maintaining organ function of the abdominal organs.

Appendicitis
Appendicitis is defined as the inflammation of the vermiform appendix, which extends from the cecum at the terminal end of the ileum. The inflammation results from the obstruction of the lumen of the appendix by accumulated fecaliths, bacteria, or parasites. The condition presents a surgical emergency due to the risk of perforation of the wall of the structure with resulting peritonitis and sepsis. The classic presenting symptoms are anorexia and periumbilical pain that evolves to the right lower quadrant, followed by vomiting. The diagnosis is made by the results of the physical examination, routine lab studies, pregnancy testing to rule out ectopic pregnancy, and ultrasound imaging. Care includes antibiotic therapy and appendectomy.

Bleeding
Gastrointestinal (GI) bleeding is defined according to the area of the defect. Upper GI bleeding occurs superiorly to the junction of the duodenum and jejunum. Lower GI bleeding occurs in the large and small intestine. Conditions

17

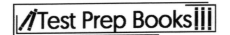

associated with upper GI bleeding include esophageal varices, gastric and duodenal ulcers, cancer, and Mallory-Weiss tears. Risk factors include age, history of gastroesophageal reflux disorder (GERD), use of nonsteroidal anti-inflammatory drugs (NSAIDs) and steroids, and alcoholism. Acute presenting manifestations include hematemesis, melena, hematochezia, and lightheadedness or fainting. Hematemesis, or bloody vomit, will appear with either a coffee ground (older blood) or bright red (new blood) appearance. The diagnosis is made by the patient's history and physical examination, routine lab studies including complete blood count (CBC) and coagulation tests, endoscopy, and chest films. Treatment is specific to the cause; e.g., peptic ulcer disease will be treated with the appropriate antibiotic and a proton-pump inhibitor (PPI).

Causative factors for GI bleeding of the lower intestine include anatomical defects such as diverticulosis, ischemic events of the vasculature related to radiation therapy or other embolic events, cancer, and infectious or noninfectious inflammatory conditions. Manifestations that are specific to the cause and location of the hemorrhage include melena, maroon stools or bright red blood, fever, dehydration, possible abdominal pain or distention, and hematochezia. Common diagnostic studies include routine lab studies, endoscopy, radionucleotide studies, and angiography. Treatment is focused on the identification and resolution of the source of the bleeding and correction of any hematologic deficits that resulted from the hemorrhage. Providers are aware that orthostatic hypotension defined as a decrease in diastolic blood pressure (BP) of 10 millimeters of mercury or more is associated with a blood loss of approximately 1000 milliliters. Therefore, the emergency care of massive GI bleeding requires aggressive fluid volume replacement with isotonic crystalloids while the exact source of the bleeding is being confirmed.

Cholecystitis
Cholecystitis is defined as an inflammation of the gallbladder. It is most often due to blockage of the cystic duct by gallstones. The condition may be complicated by the presence of perforation or gangrene of the gallbladder. Common risk factors include increasing age, female gender, obesity or rapid weight loss, and pregnancy. Symptoms include colicky epigastric pain that radiates to the right upper quadrant that may become constant, a palpable gallbladder, jaundice, nausea, vomiting, and fever. Providers understand that the elderly and chronically ill children may present with atypical manifestations of cholecystitis. Presenting symptoms in elderly patients may be limited to vague complaints of localized tenderness; however, the condition can rapidly progress to a more complicated form of cholecystitis due to infection, leading to gangrene or perforation of the gallbladder. This risk is increased in elderly patients with diabetes. Children with sickle cell disease, congenital biliary defects, or chronic illness requiring total parenteral nutrition (TPN) therapy may present with generalized abdominal pain and jaundice.

Diagnostic studies include routine lab tests, liver function tests, and abdominal ultrasounds. Additional imaging studies may be required; however, ultrasound is very sensitive for cholecystitis, does not expose the patient to radiation, and is readily available in hospitals. Treatment options depend on the severity of symptoms. Acalculous cholecystitis may progress quickly to perforation and gangrene of the gallbladder requiring emergency intervention, while uncomplicated cases of acute cholecystitis can be treated with bowel rest, intravenous (IV) fluids, and short-term antibiotic therapy. Providers understand that elective laparoscopic cholecystectomy is the procedure of choice, with the rate of conversion to open cholecystectomy at 5 percent; however, emergency laparoscopic cholecystectomy is associated with a 30 percent conversion rate.

Early recognition and intervention are required due to the rapid progression of acute acalculous cholecystitis to gangrene and perforation.

Cirrhosis
Cirrhosis of the liver is characterized by fibrotic changes that eventually accumulate as scar tissue that replaces functioning liver cells. The manifestations and onset of the disease, which may be gradual or rapid, depend on the exact etiology. Chronic hepatitis due to the hepatitis C virus has replaced alcoholic liver disease as the most common cause of cirrhosis in the United States. Although there are several additional conditions that are associated

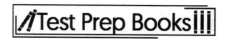

with the development of cirrhosis, as noted below, nonalcoholic fatty liver disease (NAFLD), which is common in patients with diabetes, obesity, and elevated triglyceride levels and is estimated to affect 33 percent of all individuals in the United States, is a growing concern for providers. Cirrhosis is characterized by the abnormal retention of lipids in the cells that worsens as the process of hepatic fibrosis progresses. Other contributing conditions to the development of cirrhosis include sarcoidosis, primary biliary cirrhosis, chronic right-sided heart failure, tricuspid regurgitation, autoimmune hepatitis, and alpha 1 antitrypsin deficiency.

Common symptoms include ascites; abdominal pain; portal hypertension; hepatic encephalopathy with the deterioration of the level of consciousness from normal to somnolence, drowsiness, and coma; hepatorenal disease; fever; anorexia; weight loss; spider angiomas; jaundice; and coagulopathy. Treatment is initially focused on preventing the progression of the precipitating conditions. Hepatitis C is treated with antiviral agents; cardiac conditions are treated with diuretics, beta-blockers, and digoxin; and autoimmune disorders are treated with immunosuppressant agents. Once the fibrotic changes have occurred, symptomatic interventions include treatment of pruritus, zinc deficiency, and osteoporosis. Patients with advanced cirrhosis may be candidates for a liver transplantation. The Model for End-Stage Liver Disease (MELD), which is used to allocate donor organs in the United States, calculates the projected patient survival rate following a liver transplant based on patient's age, serum bilirubin, creatinine, pro time international normalized ratio (INR), sodium level, and a history of current or recent renal dialysis.

Diverticulitis

Diverticulitis is the inflammation of the diverticula, which are described as outpouchings or defects in the wall, most commonly located in the rectosigmoid segment of the large intestine. The diverticula are common in people over fifty years old due to the increased pressure in the lumen of the bowel during defecation; however, most people do not experience diverticulitis. Inflammation of the diverticula occurs when fecaliths and other cellular debris become impacted in the outpouchings, initiating the changes in the mucous lining of the intestine.

Common manifestations of an acute episode include lower left quadrant pain, nausea, vomiting, chills, fever, and tachycardia. The condition must be differentiated from other inflammatory bowel diseases (IBDs), including Crohn's disease and ulcerative colitis, because the underlying pathology and treatment are different. Severe or prolonged manifestations will be treated with bowel rest, IV fluids, antibiotic therapy, and assessment of routine lab studies, including coagulation assay, blood cultures, and nasogastric decompression. More commonly, progressing from a clear liquid diet to a low-fiber diet until symptoms subside, followed by progression to a high-fiber diet, is successful in treating the disorder. Repeated episodes with increasingly severe manifestations are associated with possible thinning of the intestinal wall, which increases the risk of perforation of the bowel, resulting in hemorrhage and peritonitis.

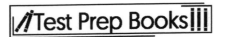
Decisions related to surgical intervention may be based on the Hinchey classification criteria, which stage the disease according to the extent of inflammatory changes and the integrity of the bowel wall. Surgical interventions may include colectomy, which is the resection of the diseased segment with anastomosis of the normal bowel segments, or the placement of a temporary or permanent colostomy depending on the dimensions of the damage. Postoperative risks include hemorrhage, altered fluid volume status, infection, delayed wound healing, impaired self-image, and repeated inflammatory attacks.

Diverticulosis and Diverticulitis

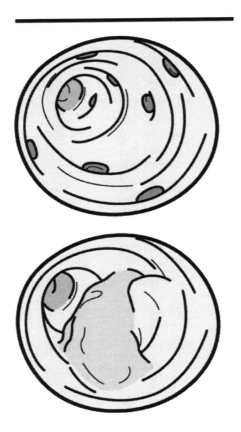

Esophageal Varices

Esophageal varices develop as a compensatory mechanism for the portal hypertension that occurs in liver disease. The superficial veins of the esophagus and the stomach function as a collateral circulation by diverting blood from the portal system to reduce pressure in the vasculature of the liver. Approximately 60 percent of patients with severe cirrhosis will develop esophageal varices at some point because portal hypertension is progressive in these patients. There may be no indication of the presence of esophageal varices until the vessels rupture, which means that all patients with cirrhosis require annual endoscopic screening for the assessment of the presence of varices.

Prophylactic treatment is recommended for varices that are 5 millimeters or more in diameter and/or exhibit longitudinal red streaks or wales along the varices, due to the significant risk of rupture and hemorrhage associated with these findings. Additional risk factors for hemorrhage include a patient history of constipation, vomiting,

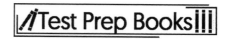
severe coughing, and alcohol abuse. Beta-blocker therapy is indicated for the prevention of hemorrhage; however, the medications are not effective in delaying the initial formation of the varices. The therapy is aimed at maintaining the heart at fifty-five beats per minute, and the therapy must be continued indefinitely because the risk of hemorrhage returns if the medication is stopped. Research indicates that as many as one-third of patients with esophageal varices will not respond to this therapy and instead report fatigue, dyspnea, and bradycardia.

Up to one-third of all patients with esophageal varices will suffer a hemorrhagic episode. The emergency care of this life-threatening condition includes endoscopy with ligation of the varices, vasopressin, placement of a transjugular intrahepatic shunt, surgery, and aggressive crystalloid and colloid fluid replacement.

Esophagitis

Esophagitis is defined as the inflammation of the mucosal lining of the esophagus that may be caused by chronic GERD, infectious agents such as Candida, cytomegalovirus (CMV), human immunodeficiency virus (HIV), herpes, or as the result of chemotherapy or radiation therapy. The condition may be asymptomatic or associated with common manifestations that include heartburn, dyspepsia, dysphagia, hoarseness, and retrosternal chest pain. Symptoms associated with infection may also include nausea, vomiting, fever, and sepsis. Diagnostic tests include CBC to identify signs of neutropenia or alterations in the hematocrit and hemoglobin, fecal occult blood exam, barium studies and endoscopy, ECG to rule out cardiac disease as the cause of the chest discomfort, and testing for autoimmune conditions.

Complications may include anorexia and weight loss, Barrett's esophagus, and rarely, perforation. With Barrett's esophagus, the cells that have been irritated by reflux disease undergo metaplastic transformation and exhibit an increased risk for the development of esophageal adenocarcinoma. Interventions include resolution of the causative agent or condition, pain management, histamine 2 receptor antagonists, PPIs, coating agents, blood component replacement as necessary, and lifestyle changes to alleviate the manifestations of chronic GERD. Corticosteroids may be necessary for esophagitis due to IBD or eosinophilic conditions. Emergency care of this condition involves treatment of bleeding or perforation and elimination of acute cardiac disease as the source of any reported chest pain.

Gastroenteritis

Gastroenteritis is a general term used to describe GI tract alterations. The characteristic manifestation is diarrhea; however, the exact characteristics of this manifestation are specific to the causative agent. These conditions may be related to osmotic, inflammatory, secretory, or motility alterations. The villi of the small intestine are most commonly affected by these alterations, resulting in fluid loss. Presenting symptoms may be mild to life-threatening, and outbreaks of these infectious conditions can rapidly reach epidemic proportions in susceptible populations. Prolonged diarrhea and vomiting result in severe fluid and electrolyte deficits, which may be associated with hypovolemic shock in high-risk individuals, including children and the elderly.

The norovirus is the causative agent for 50 to 70 percent of all cases of gastroenteritis. The virus is easily transmitted from person to person and is resistant to common cleaning agents. The attacks, manifested by diarrhea, fever, chills, and headache, usually last 36 hours. The rotavirus species may cause severe illness in children. The food-borne Salmonella infection is the second most common cause of gastroenteritis and is associated with fever, in addition to abdominal pain, nausea, vomiting, and diarrhea. Infection caused by *C. difficile* is the leading cause of hospital-acquired GI disease. The elderly population is more commonly affected; however, all patients are susceptible to this infection.

The organism exists in the feces and is spread by contact with contaminated surfaces. This condition is commonly associated with broad-spectrum antibiotic therapy that reduces the normal flora of the GI tract. Common manifestations include diarrhea, nausea, vomiting, and abdominal pain. This infection may be complicated by pseudomembranous colitis, toxic megacolon, perforation of the colon, and sepsis. Treatment is aimed at the agent-

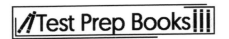

specific antibiotic therapy, supportive treatment of all manifestations, and possible surgical excision of compromised bowel segments. Emergency care requires restoration of fluid volume and electrolyte homeostasis.

Gastritis

Gastritis may be acute or chronic, and acute gastritis is further differentiated as erosive or nonerosive. Involvement of the entire stomach lining is termed pangastritis, while regional involvement is termed antral gastritis. Acute gastritis may be asymptomatic or may present with nonspecific abdominal pain, nausea, vomiting, anorexia, belching, and bloating. The most common causes of acute gastritis include use of NSAIDs and corticosteroids and infection by the *H. pylori* bacteria. Acute gastritis may also be associated with alcohol abuse. Double-contrast barium studies, endoscopy, and histological examination of biopsy samples most often confirm the diagnosis and the causative agent. Treatment includes normalization of fluid and electrolyte balance; discontinuance of causative agents such as NSAIDs; and corticosteroids, H^2 blockers, PPIs, and appropriate antibiotic therapy in the event of *H. pylori* infection.

Chronic gastritis is an inflammatory state that has not responded to therapy for acute gastritis. Chronic *H. pylori* infection is associated with the development of peptic ulcers, gastric adenocarcinoma, and mucosal-related lymphoid tissue (MALT) lymphoma. In addition to endoscopy and barium studies, gastric biopsy for assessment of antibiotic sensitivity is done because the initial antibiotic therapy was unsuccessful in eradicating the organism. Autoimmune gastritis is related to vitamin B-12 deficiency due to intrinsic factor deficiency and is associated with megaloblastic anemia and thrombocytopenia.

Chemical or reactive gastritis is due to chronic NSAID and steroid use and is manifested by mucosal epithelial erosion, ulcer formation, mucosal edema, and possible hemorrhage. Chronic gastritis is diagnosed by endoscopy, biopsy, and histological studies. Treatment is specific to the causative agent, and in the instance of *H. pylori* infection, a course of three antibiotics will be administered. *H. pylori* infection also requires long-term surveillance for reoccurrence of infection. Emergency care of the patient with acute or chronic gastritis is focused on the assessment for hemorrhage or other potential complications, restoration of fluid volume status, and pain management.

Hepatitis

Hepatitis is an inflammatory condition of the liver, which is further categorized as infectious or noninfectious. Causative infectious agents for hepatitis may be viral, fungal, or bacterial, while noninfectious causes include autoimmune disease, prescription and recreational drugs, alcohol abuse, and metabolic disorders. More than 50 percent of the cases of acute hepatitis in the United States are caused by a virus. Transmission routes include fecal-oral, parenteral, sexual contact, and perinatal transmission. There are four phases of the course of viral hepatitis. During phase 1, which is asymptomatic, the host is infected and the virus replicates; the onset of mild symptoms occurs in phase 2; progressive symptoms of liver dysfunction appear in phase 3; and recovery from the infection occurs in phase 4. These phases are specific to the causative agent and the individual.

The most common viral agents are hepatitis A (HAV), hepatitis B (HBV), and hepatitis C (HCV). Less commonly, hepatitis D (HDV), hepatitis E (HEV), CMV, Epstein-Barr virus, and adenovirus may cause hepatitis. HAV and HBV often present with nausea, jaundice, anorexia, right upper quadrant pain, fatigue, and malaise. HCV may be asymptomatic or, alternatively, may present with similar symptoms. Approximately 20 percent of acute infections with HBV and HCV result in chronic hepatitis, which is a risk factor for the development of cirrhosis and liver failure. The care of the patient with acute hepatitis due to HAV and HCV is focused on symptom relief, while the antiviral treatment for HBV is effective in decreasing the incidence of adenocarcinoma.

Chronic hepatitis is a complication of acute hepatitis and frequently progresses to hepatic failure, which is associated with deteriorating coagulation status and the onset of hepatic encephalopathy due to alterations in the blood-brain barrier that result in brain cell edema. Emergency care of the patient with hepatic failure is focused on fluid volume, homeostasis, and reduction of encephalopathy.

22

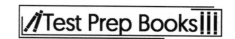

Hernia

A **hernia** is manifested by the displacement or protrusion of a segment of the bowel through an area of weakness in the abdominal wall. This weakness may be an anatomical site, such as the umbilicus, or acquired due to a surgical incision. Hernias are also defined as reversible or irreversible, depending on whether the protruding bowel segment can be repositioned with gentle pressure. An irreversible hernia may become incarcerated or strangulated if the blood supply is compromised for any period of time. Either of these conditions represents a surgical emergency and may be associated with necrosis and perforation of the bowel loop and possible intestinal obstruction.

Manifestations include possible visible protrusion or fullness at the site that increases with any increase in intrabdominal pressure and diffuse pain radiating to the site. Risk factors include male gender, advanced age, increased intra-abdominal pressure related to pregnancy and obesity, and genetic defects. Inguinal hernias in the male account for 75 percent of the 800,000 hernia repairs performed annually in the United States.

CT scans and ultrasonography may be used to identify hernias that are not readily identified by the physical examination. A flat plate of the abdomen is useful for identifying free air that may result from bowel perforation secondary to a strangulated hernia. Conservative management of reducible hernias includes modified activity such as no lifting or straining and prevention of constipation. If the manifestations worsen or the protrusion becomes irreversible, surgery is required to prevent incarceration and/or strangulation. Emergency care of the patient with a strangulated hernia is focused on restoration of the blood segment to the bowel segment and prevention of perforation and obstruction.

Inflammatory Bowel Disease

Inflammatory bowel disease (IBD) is an idiopathic disease that results from a harmful immune response to normal intestinal flora. Two types of IBD include Crohn's disease and ulcerative colitis (UC). Crohn's disease is characterized by inflammatory changes in all layers of the bowel. Although the entire length of the GI tract may be involved, the ileum and colon are affected most often. The inflamed areas are commonly interrupted by segments of normal bowel. Endoscopic views reveal the cobblestone appearance of these affected segments. UC is characterized by inflammatory changes of the mucosa and submucosa of the bowel that affect only the colon. There is a genetic predisposition for Crohn's disease, and there is also an increased incidence of cancer in patients with either form of IBD. Additional risk factors include a family history of IBD or colorectal cancer, NSAID and antibiotic use, smoking, and psychiatric disorders. IBD is diagnosed by a patient's history, including details of any recent foreign travel or hospitalization to rule out tuberculosis or *C. difficile* as the precipitating cause, in addition to endoscopy, CT and magnetic resonance imaging (MRI), serum and stool studies, and histologic studies.

Manifestations are nonspecific and are most often associated with the affected bowel segment. Common manifestations of IBD include diarrhea with blood and mucus and possible incontinence; constipation primarily with UC that is associated with progression to obstipation and bowel obstruction; rectal pain with associated urgency and tenesmus; and abdominal pain and cramping in the right lower quadrant with Crohn's disease and in the umbilical area or left lower quadrant with UC. In addition, anemia, fatigue, and arthritis may be present.

The treatment of IBD focuses on attaining periods of remission and preventing recurrent attacks by modifying the inflammatory response. The stepwise treatment protocol begins with aminosalicylates and progresses to antibiotics, corticosteroids, and immunomodulators. Emergency care of the patient with IBD is focused on assessment and treatment of possible hemorrhage, megacolon, or bowel obstruction.

Intussusception

Intussusception is the abnormal movement of one portion of the bowel that is folded back into the subsequent segment. Adhesions, tumor formation, effects of bariatric surgery, and inflammatory changes due to IBD are possible causes of intussusception in older children and adults. Surgical treatment is appropriate for older children and adults. A laparoscopic approach is used to manually reduce the intussusception. If reduction is not possible or if

23

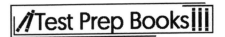

there is additional bowel damage such as perforation present, surgical resection and anastomosis of the affected bowel segment are necessary. Emergency care is focused on the identification and immediate intervention of the condition.

Obstructions

There are three anatomical areas of the GI system that are prone to obstruction: the gastric outlet at the pylorus, the small intestine, and the bowel. The small intestine is the most commonly affected site, and adhesions are responsible for more than 60 percent of all obstructions. These conditions may also be categorized as mechanical or nonmechanical depending on the cause, where mechanical obstructions are due to some extrinsic source such as adhesions, tumor formation, intussusception, or hernias, and nonmechanical obstructions are due to decreased peristalsis, neurogenic disorders, vascular insufficiency, or electrolyte imbalance. The mechanical obstruction of the biliary tract is due to effects of cirrhosis and hepatitis.

The manifestations are specific to the anatomical site of obstruction. The gastric outlet obstruction occurs most commonly in the pylorus and is associated with upper abdominal distention, nausea, vomiting, weight loss, and anorexia. Diagnostic tests include endoscopy and assessment of nutritional deficits in addition to testing to eliminate *H. pylori* or diabetic gastric paresis as the cause. Obstruction of the small bowel is associated with severe fluid and electrolyte losses, metabolic acidosis, nausea and vomiting, fever, and tachycardia and may lead to strangulation of the affected bowel segment. Bowel obstruction, most frequently due to tumor formation or stricture resulting from diverticular disease, is manifested by lower abdominal distention, possible metabolic acidosis, cramping abdominal pain, and minimal fluid and electrolyte losses. Common diagnostic studies include endoscopy, common lab studies, flat plate of the abdomen to assess for free air, and CT imaging.

Treatments are specific to the cause and may include tumor excision, antibiotic therapy for *H. pylori*, colectomy to remove the affected bowel segment, and/or colostomy placement. Although some obstructions may be treated with gastric or enteric decompression, bowel rest, and fluids, emergency intervention is usually necessary to prevent complications such as peritonitis and hemorrhage.

Pancreatitis

Pancreatitis has a rapid onset and progression to a critical illness, which is manifested by characteristic abdominal pain, nausea, vomiting, and diarrhea. In addition, fever, tachycardia, hypotension, and abdominal distention and rebound tenderness may be present. The exocrine function of the pancreas is the production and secretion of digestive enzymes. Pancreatitis exists when one of the causative agents inhibits the homeostatic suppression of the enzyme secretion, resulting in excessive amounts of the enzymes in the pancreas.

This excess of enzymes precipitates the inflammatory response, which results in increased pancreatic vascular permeability, which, in turn, leads to edema, hemorrhage, and eventual necrosis of the pancreas. The inflammatory mediators can result in systemic complications that may include sepsis, respiratory distress syndrome, renal failure, and GI hemorrhage. Chronic alcoholism and biliary tract obstruction are the most common causes of pancreatitis; however, as many as 35 percent of the cases of pancreatitis are idiopathic. Pancreatitis can also occur after endoscopic retrograde cholangiopancreatography (ERCP) due to defects in the sphincter of Oddi. Aggressive pre-procedure hydration and rectal indomethacin post procedure are employed to prevent this complication. Less common causes include some antibiotics and chemotherapy agents.

Diagnosis is based on the patient's presenting history and routine lab studies that include amylase P, lipase, metabolic panel, liver panel, C-reactive protein, CBC, and arterial blood gases (ABGs). Imaging studies may be used, if the diagnosis is unclear, to rule out gallbladder disease. Nonsurgical treatment includes bowel rest with nasogastric decompression, analgesics, and IV fluid administration. Surgical procedures may be open or minimally invasive and are aimed at removing diseased tissue to limit the progression to systemic complications, to repair the pancreatic duct, or to repair defects in the biliary tree. The emergency care of pancreatitis focuses on prompt

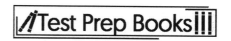
diagnosis, aggressive fluid management, and treatment of the cause because the disease is associated with the rapid onset of systemic complications.

Trauma

The GI system may be traumatized by blunt or penetrating forces. Penetrating trauma is most commonly due to gunshot or stabbing injuries and usually results in a predictable pattern of injury; however, careful assessment for occult injuries is necessary to prevent catastrophic damage. Presenting manifestations depend on the degree of penetration and the site of the damage but commonly include visible hemorrhage, alterations in level of consciousness, tachycardia, and hypotension. Diagnosis requires a detailed inquiry into all of the facts of the incident, including a description of the weapon, the number of times the patient was stabbed, and an estimation of blood loss at the scene, in addition to the progression of the patient's manifestations during resuscitation and transport. Treatment is aimed at restoring and maintaining fluid volume status with colloids and crystalloids, assessment for and treatment of hemorrhage, prevention of infection, and surgical repair of the damaged structures.

GI injuries due to blunt force trauma often are not immediately apparent, which means that assessment for progression of the original insult is ongoing. Abdominal pain and tenderness and hypotension may be the only signs of massive internal injuries. Trauma related to automobile accidents may present with a characteristic seatbelt or steering wheel pattern, Cullen's sign due to periumbilical trauma, or an abdominal bruit that may be associated with comorbid vascular disease or acute vascular trauma. Domestic violence must be considered in the event of abdominal blunt force trauma. Diagnosis is based on the history of the event, routine lab studies, ultrasound and CT scanning, peritoneal lavage, and possible exploratory laparotomy. The goals of treatment for blunt trauma are similar to penetrating trauma and include restoring and maintaining fluid volume status with colloids and crystalloids, assessment for and treatment of hemorrhage, prevention of infection, and surgical repair of the damaged structures.

Ulcers

Ulcers of the GI tract are categorized as to the anatomical site of injury. Gastric ulcers are located in the body of the stomach, and peptic ulcers are located in the duodenum. The presenting symptom is abdominal pain 2 to 4 hours after eating for duodenal ulcers, in addition to hematemesis and melena. The defect is due to erosion of the mucosal lining by infectious agents, most commonly *H. pylori*; extreme systemic stress such as burns or head trauma; ETOH abuse; chronic kidney and respiratory disease; and psychological stress. Untreated, the mucosal erosion can progress to perforation, hemorrhage, and peritonitis.

Laboratory studies include examination of endoscopic tissue samples for the presence of the *H. pylori* organism, urea breath test, CBC, stool samples, and metabolic panel. Endoscopy (which is used to obtain tissue samples and achieve hemostasis) and double barium imaging studies may be obtained. The treatment depends on the extent of the erosion and will be focused on healing the ulcerated tissue and preventing additional damage. The treatment protocol for *H. pylori* infection includes the use of a PPI, amoxicillin, and clarithromycin for a minimum of seven to fourteen days. Subsequent testing will be necessary to ensure that the organism has been eradicated. Patients infected with *H. pylori* also must discontinue the use of NSAIDs or continue the long-term use of PPIs. Surgery may be indicated for significant areas of hemorrhage that were not successfully treated by ultrasound, and the procedure will be specific to the anatomical area of ulceration. Emergency care is focused on prompt management of bleeding and identification of the causative agent to guide treatment.

Fecal Incontinence

Evacuation of waste products in the form of stool is a voluntary action controlled by the anal sphincter. Loss of sphincter control leads to fecal incontinence. **Fecal incontinence** is the involuntary evacuation of stool or gas from the rectum. There are numerous reasons why patients develop fecal incontinence. The external voluntary anal

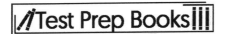

sphincter is aided by abdominal skeletal and intestinal smooth muscle contractions to produce the act of defecation. Muscle weakness or damage can cause a decrease in the ability to control these muscles. One cause of muscle damage occurs in females during childbirth as the result of overstretching or tearing. Nerve endings line the rectal wall and are activated when stool is present. Nerve damage does not allow for the sensation to defecate. Spinal cord injuries, trauma, surgery, and constant pressure to the rectal area can cause nerve damage. Stool that does not move along the intestinal tract causes a blockage, also known as an **intestinal obstruction**.

Obstructions lead to constipation. **Constipation** is the inability to pass or empty out stool. When an obstruction is present, pressure is exerted on the intestinal wall and the muscles are weakened. This can lead to water seeping out through the sides of the obstruction and cause fecal incontinence. **Diarrhea** is described as watery stool. In the normal process of digestion, excess water is absorbed in the large intestine. An increase in peristalsis does not allow for complete water absorption in the colon. Watery stool is not as easily retained as formed stool and can lead to fecal incontinence. Age is a common risk factor for fecal incontinence. Aging leads to a decrease in muscle tone and tissue elasticity. Defecating is part of toileting. Patients who have physical disabilities may not be able to walk to a restroom. Chronic illnesses, such as multiple sclerosis (MS), Parkinson's disease (PD), and diabetes, may affect muscle tone and nerve activity that can cause fecal incontinence. Patients with cognitive disorders, such as late-stage Alzheimer's, are at risk for fecal incontinence. The inability of patients with cognitive disorders to communicate self-care needs and recognize surroundings can result in fecal incontinence.

Pulmonary

Aspiration
There are four types of respiratory aspiration that can result in aspiration pneumonitis, pneumonia, or an acute respiratory emergency. The aspiration of gastric contents often causes chemical pneumonitis. Infective organisms from the oropharynx can result in aspiration pneumonia. Depending on its size and composition, the aspiration of a foreign body can result in a respiratory emergency or bacterial pneumonia. Rarely, aspiration of mineral or vegetable oil can cause an exogenous lipoid pneumonia.

Aspiration Pneumonitis/Pneumonia
Respiratory aspiration is the abnormal entry of foreign substances (such as food, drink, saliva, or vomitus) into the lungs as a person swallows. This is normally prevented by the epiglottis, a flap of cartilage that pulls forward and forces substances into the esophagus and digestive tract. If inoculum is inhaled into the lungs, it can (depending on the amount) lead to aspiration pneumonitis/pneumonia. Aspiration pneumonia often results from a primary bacterial infection, while aspiration pneumonitis (which is non-infectious) results from aspiration of the acidic gastric contents.

Risk factors for aspiration pneumonitis/pneumonia are altered or reduced consciousness and a poor gag reflex. These risk factors are associated with the following conditions:

- Excessive alcohol and/or drugs
- Stroke
- Seizures
- Dysphagia
- Head trauma
- General anesthesia
- Critical illness
- Dementia
- Intracranial mass lesion
- Multiple sclerosis
- Pseudobulbar palsy

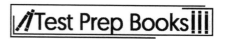

- Myasthenia gravis
- Gastroesophageal reflux disease (GERD)
- Use of H_2 agonists, H_2 blockers, or proton pump inhibitors
- Bronchoscopy
- Endotracheal intubation
- Tracheostomy
- Upper endoscopy
- Nasogastric (NG) tube
- Feeding tubes

Signs and symptoms of aspiration pneumonitis/pneumonia include the following:

- Fever
- Cyanosis
- Wheezing
- Dyspnea
- Tachypnea
- Tachycardia
- Rales
- Hypoxia
- Altered mental status
- Hypotension
- Decreased breath sounds
- Fatigue
- Cough with discolored phlegm
- Chest pain
- Hypothermia (possible in older patients)
- Pleuritic chest pain

The diagnosis of aspiration pneumonitis/pneumonia is based upon a chest X-ray revealing pulmonary infiltrates, an arterial blood gas (ABG) analysis consistent with hypoxemia, a complete blood count (CBC) with an elevated white blood cell count (WBC) with neutrophils predominating, and other clinical findings. Infiltrates are most commonly found in the right, lower lobe of the lung, but can be found in other lobes, depending on an individual's position at the time of aspiration. If possible, a sputum specimen for culture, sensitivity, and gram stain should be collected before beginning antibiotic therapy. In addition, blood cultures should be obtained, as indicated.

Treatment of aspiration pneumonitis/pneumonia includes the following:

- Suctioning of the upper airway as needed to remove the aspirate
- Oxygen supplementation
- Pulse oximetry
- Cardiac monitoring
- Antibiotics (only if symptoms fail to resolve within 48 hours)
- Supportive care with intravenous fluids (IVFs) and electrolyte replacement
- For those with severe respiratory distress, possible intubation and mechanical ventilation
- NG drainage to avoid gastric distention (in the ventilated patient)

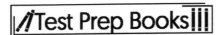
Foreign Body Aspiration

Foreign body aspiration is a respiratory emergency. A foreign body can lodge in the larynx or trachea causing varying degrees of airway obstruction. Complete airway obstruction can quickly lead to asphyxia and death. The most commonly aspirated object is food. Other frequently aspirated objects include nuts, nails, seeds, coins, pins, small toys, needles, bone fragments, and dental appliances. In children and adolescents, aspirated foreign bodies are found with equal frequency on either side of the lungs. In adults, they are most often found in the right lung because of the acute angle of the right mainstem bronchus.

Signs and symptoms of foreign body aspiration include the following:

- Coughing
- Wheezing
- Decreased breath sounds
- Dyspnea
- Choking
- Cyanosis
- Hemoptysis
- Chest pain
- Asphyxia (with complete airway obstruction)
- Inability to speak (with complete airway obstruction)

As more time elapses, local inflammation and edema can worsen the airway obstruction. This also makes removing the foreign body more difficult and the lung more likely to bleed with manipulation.

Foreign body aspiration can be diagnosed using a chest x-ray or a computed tomography (CT) scan. Less than 20 percent of all aspirated foreign bodies are radiopaque. A CT scan can provide information about the anatomic location, composition, shape, size, and extent of edema associated with the aspirated foreign body. ABG analysis can reveal hypoxemia. Bronchoscopy (rigid or flexible) can be diagnostic as well as therapeutic.

Treatment of foreign body aspiration can include the following:

- Heimlich maneuver for acute choking with total airway obstruction by foreign body
- Foreign body extraction via bronchoscopy (rigid or flexible)
- Surgical bronchotomy or segmental lung resection (rarely required)
- Antibiotics for secondary pneumonia or other respiratory infection
- Oxygen supplementation
- Symptomatic respiratory support

Since the likelihood of complications increases after 24 to 48 hours, prompt extraction of the foreign body is critical. Complications can include mediastinitis, atelectasis, pneumonia, tracheoesophageal fistulas, or bronchiectasis.

Asthma

Status Asthmaticus

Status asthmaticus is an acute episode of worsening asthma that's unresponsive to treatment with bronchodilators. Even after increasing their bronchodilator use to every few minutes, individuals still experience no relief. Status asthmaticus represents a respiratory emergency that can lead to respiratory failure. Airway inflammation, bronchospasm, and mucus plugging highlight the condition. Common triggers include exposure to an allergen or irritant, viral respiratory illness, and exercise in cold weather. Status asthmaticus is more common among individuals of low socioeconomic status, regardless of race.

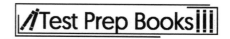
The main symptoms of status asthmaticus are wheezing, cough, and dyspnea; however, severe airway obstruction can result in a "silent chest" without audible wheezes. This can be a sign of impending respiratory failure. Other signs and symptoms of status asthmaticus include the following:

- Chest tightness or pain
- Tachypnea
- Tachycardia
- Cyanosis
- Use of accessory respiratory muscles
- Inability to speak more than one or two words at a time
- Altered mental status
- Pulsus paradoxus >20mm Hg
- Syncope
- Hypoxemia
- Hypercapnia
- Retractions and the use of abdominal muscles to breathe
- Hypertension
- Seizures (late sign)
- Bradycardia (late sign)
- Hypotension (late sign)
- Agitation (late sign)

Useful tests for the diagnosis of status asthmaticus include the following:

- Chest x-ray (for the exclusion of pneumonia, pneumothorax, and CHF)

- ABG analysis can be diagnostic as well as therapeutic (tracking response to treatment measures). Assess cost/benefit for children due to pain associated with ABG sampling.

- CBC with differential can reveal an elevated WBC count with left shift (possible indication of a microbial infection)

- Peak flow measurement can be diagnostic as well as therapeutic (tracking response to treatment measures)

- Pulse oximetry provides continuous measurement of O_2 saturation. Reading is affected by decreased peripheral perfusion, anemia, and movement.

- Blood glucose levels, stress, and therapeutic medications can lead to hyperglycemia. Younger children may exhibit hypoglycemia.

- Blood electrolyte levels (therapeutic medications can lead to hypokalemia)

Intubation and mechanical ventilation should be used with extreme caution in individuals with status asthmaticus. It's usually considered a therapy of last resort due to its inherent dangers: air trapping leading to an increased risk for barotrauma (especially pneumothorax); decreased cardiac output; and increasing bronchospasm. Mechanical ventilation of individuals with status asthmaticus often requires controlled hypoventilation with low tidal volumes, prolonged exhalation times, low respiratory rates, and tolerance of permissive hypercapnia. The majority of individuals needing mechanical ventilation can be extubated within 72 hours.

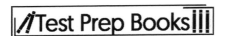
Supportive Treatment

- O_2 therapy to maintain O_2 saturation > 92%; non-rebreathing mask can deliver 98% O_2
- Hydration
- Correction of electrolyte abnormalities
- Antibiotics only with evidence of concurrent infective process

Pharmacological Agents Used for Acute Asthma

Various classes of pharmacological agents are used for the treatment and control of status asthmaticus. The following discussion concentrates on pharmacological agents to treat and control acute asthma rather than chronic asthma. Urgent care of asthma can include the following:

Beta-2 Adrenergic Agonists (Beta-2 Agonists)

Short-acting preparations of Beta-2 agonists are the first line of therapy for the treatment of status asthmaticus. These medications relax the muscles in the airways, resulting in bronchodilation (expanding of the bronchial air passages) and increased airflow to the lungs. It is important to remember that one of the underlying factors in asthma is bronchoconstriction. Albuterol is the most commonly used short-acting Beta-2 agonist. Dosing for acute asthma is 2.5 mg to 5 mg once, then 2.5 mg every twenty minutes for 3 doses via nebulizer, and finally 2.5 mg to 10 mg every one to four hours as needed. Adverse effects of albuterol include tachycardia, tremors, and anxiety. Another short-acting Beta-2 agonist used to treat acute asthma is levalbuterol (Xopenex®). This medication is related to albuterol and has the same result, but without the adverse effects. Dosage for acute asthma is 1.25 mg to 2.5 mg every twenty minutes for 3 doses, then 1.25 mg to 5 mg every one to four hours as needed. However, it must be noted that the frequent use of adrenergic agents prior to receiving emergency care can decrease a patient's response to these medications in a hospital setting.

Anticholinergics

These medications block the action of the neurotransmitter acetylcholine which, in turn, causes bronchodilation. Anticholinergics can also increase the bronchodilating effects of short-acting Beta-2 agonists. The most commonly used anticholinergic is ipratroprium (Atrovent®), which is used in combination with short-acting Beta-2 agonists for the treatment of status asthmaticus. Dosing for acute asthma is 2.5 mL (500 mcg) every twenty minutes for 3 doses via nebulizer, then as needed. Adverse effects can include dry mouth, blurred vision, and constipation.

Corticosteroids

Corticosteroids are potent anti-inflammatory medications that fight the inflammation accompanying asthma. Corticosteroids commonly used in the treatment of status asthmaticus include prednisone, prednisolone, and methylprednisolone. Methylprednisolone (Solu-Medrol®) is administered once in doses of 60 mg to 125 mg intravenously (IV) in cases of status asthmaticus and then followed by a taper of oral prednisone over seven to ten days. The intravenous administration of corticosteroids is equal in effectiveness to oral corticosteroid administration. Corticosteroids have numerous adverse effects, and they should not be used for more than two weeks. Adverse effects of long-term corticosteroid use can include weight gain, osteoporosis, thinning of skin, cataracts, easy bruising, and diabetes. Therefore, it is necessary to monitor blood glucose routinely and use regular insulin on a sliding scale. Electrolytes (particularly potassium) must also be monitored.

Methylxanthines

These medications are used as bronchodilators and as adjuncts to Beta-2 agonists and corticosteroids in treating status asthmaticus. The primary methylxanthines are theophylline and aminophylline. At therapeutic doses, methylxanthines are much weaker bronchodilators than Beta-2 agonists. The adverse effects of methylxanthines can include nausea, vomiting, tachycardia, headaches, and seizures. As a result, therapeutic monitoring is mandatory. Therapeutic levels of theophylline range from 10 mcg/mL to 20 mcg/mL. Dosing of theophylline is a loading dose of 6 mg/kg, followed by a maintenance dose of 1 mg/kg/h IV. Methylxanthines aren't frequently used

30

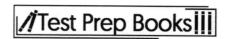
to treat status asthmaticus because of their possible adverse effects and the need for close monitoring of drug blood levels.

Magnesium Sulfate

Magnesium sulfate is a calcium antagonist that relaxes smooth muscle in the lung passages leading to bronchodilation. Clinical studies indicate it can be used as an adjunct to Beta-2 agonist therapy during status asthmaticus. A dose of 30 mg/kg to 70 mg/kg is administered by IV over 20 to 30 minutes. It is given slowly to prevent adverse effects such as bradycardia and hypotension. The use of magnesium sulfate is controversial.

Leukotriene Inhibitors

These medications target inflammation related to asthma. Typically used for the long-term control of asthma, a minority of individuals with status asthmaticus may respond to this class of medication. The primary leukotriene inhibitors used in the treatment of asthma are zafirlukast (Accolate®) and zileuton (Zyflo®). Zafirlukast can be administered orally in doses of 10 mg to 20 mg twice daily. Zileuton can be administered in a dose of 600 mg four times daily. Adverse effects of leukotriene inhibitors include headache, rash, fatigue, dizziness, and abdominal pain.

Heliox

Heliox, administered via face mask, is a mixture of helium and oxygen that can help relieve airway obstruction associated with status asthmaticus. Benefits of heliox include decreased work of breathing, decreased carbon dioxide production, and decreased muscle fatigue. It can only be used in individuals able to take a deep breath or while on mechanical ventilation. The 80/20 mixture of helium to oxygen has been the most effective in clinical trials. One limitation to using heliox is the amount of supplemental oxygen required by an individual suffering from status asthmaticus. Heliox loses its clinical efficacy when the fraction of inspired oxygen (FiO_2) is greater than 40 percent. No significant adverse effects have been reported with heliox.

COPD

Chronic Obstructive Pulmonary Disease (COPD) is characterized by an airflow obstruction that's not fully reversible. It's usually progressive and is associated with an abnormal inflammatory response in the lungs. The primary cause of COPD is exposure to tobacco smoke and is one of the leading causes of death in the United States. COPD includes chronic bronchitis, emphysema, or a combination of both. Though asthma is part of the classic triad of obstructive lung diseases, it is not part of COPD. However, someone with COPD can have an asthma component to their disease. Chronic bronchitis is described as a chronic productive cough for three or more months during each of two consecutive years. Emphysema is the abnormal enlargement of alveoli (air sacs) with accompanying destruction of their walls. Signs and symptoms of COPD can include the following:

- Dyspnea
- Wheezing
- Cough (usually worse in the morning and that produces sputum/phlegm)
- Cyanosis
- Chest tightness
- Fever
- Tachypnea
- Orthopnea
- Use of accessory respiratory muscles
- Elevated jugular venous pressure (JVP)
- Barrel chest
- Pursed lip breathing
- Altered mental status

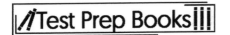
A diagnosis of COPD can be made through pulmonary function tests (PFTs), a chest x-ray, blood chemistries, ABG analysis, or a CT scan. A formal diagnosis of COPD can be made through a PFT known as spirometry, which measures lung function. PFTs measure the ratio of forced expiratory volume in one second over forced vital capacity (FEV_1/FVC) and should normally be between 60 percent and 90 percent. Values below 60 percent usually indicate a problem. The other diagnostic tests mentioned are useful in determining the acuity and severity of exacerbations of the disease. In acute exacerbations of COPD, ABG analysis can reveal respiratory acidosis, hypoxemia, and hypercapnia. Generally, a pH less than 7.3 indicates acute respiratory compromise. Compensatory metabolic alkalosis may develop in response to chronic respiratory acidosis. A chest x-ray can show flattening of the diaphragm and increased retrosternal air space (both indicative of hyperinflation), cardiomegaly, and increased bronchovascular markings. Blood chemistries can suggest sodium retention or hypokalemia. A CT scan is more sensitive and specific than a standard chest x-ray for diagnosing emphysema.

Treatment for acute exacerbations of COPD can include oxygen supplementation, short-acting Beta-2 agonists, anticholinergics, corticosteroids, and antibiotics. Oxygen should be titrated to achieve an oxygen saturation of at least 90 percent. Short-acting Beta-2 agonists (albuterol or levalbuterol) administered via nebulizer can improve dyspnea associated with COPD. The anticholinergic medication ipratroprium, administered via nebulizer, can be added as an adjunct to Beta-2 agonists. Short courses of corticosteroids can be given orally or intravenously. In clinical trials, the administration of oral corticosteroids in the early stage of COPD exacerbation decreased the need for hospitalization. Also in clinical trials, the use of antibiotics was found to decrease the risk of treatment failure and death in individuals with a moderate to severe exacerbation of COPD.

Acute Respiratory Tract Infections

Acute Bronchitis

Acute bronchitis is inflammation of the bronchial tubes (bronchi), which extend from the trachea to the lungs. It is one of the top five reasons for visits to healthcare providers and can take from ten days to three weeks to resolve. Common causes of acute bronchitis include respiratory viruses (such as influenza A and B), RSV, parainfluenza, adenovirus, rhinovirus, and coronavirus. Bacterial causes include Mycoplasma species, Streptococcus pneumoniae, Chlamydia pneumoniae, Haemophilus influenzae, and Moraxella catarrhalis. Other causes of acute bronchitis are irritants such as chemicals, pollution, and tobacco smoke.

Signs and symptoms of acute bronchitis can include the following:

- Cough (most common symptom) with or without sputum
- Fever
- Sore throat
- Headache
- Nasal congestion
- Rhinorrhea
- Dyspnea
- Fatigue
- Myalgia
- Chest pain
- Wheezing

Acute bronchitis is typically diagnosed by exclusion, which means tests are used to exclude more serious conditions such as pneumonia, epiglottitis, or COPD. Useful diagnostic tests include a CBC with differential, a chest x-ray, respiratory and blood cultures, PFTs, bronchoscopy, laryngoscopy, and a procalcitonin (PCT) test to determine if the infection is bacterial.

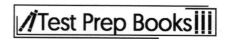

Treatment of acute bronchitis is primarily supportive and can include the following:

- Bedrest
- Cough suppressants, such as codeine or dextromethorphan
- Beta-2 agonists, such as albuterol for wheezing
- Nonsteroidal anti-inflammatory drugs (NSAIDs) for pain
- Expectorants, such as guaifenesin

Although acute bronchitis should not be routinely treated with antibiotics, there are exceptions to this rule. It's reasonable to use an antibiotic when an existing medical condition poses a risk of serious complications. Antibiotic use is also reasonable for treating acute bronchitis in elderly patients who have been hospitalized in the past year, have been diagnosed with congestive heart failure (CHF) or diabetes, or are currently being treated with a steroid.

Acute Epiglottitis

Acute epiglottitis (also known as supraglottitis) is inflammation of the epiglottis. The epiglottis is the small piece of cartilage that's pulled forward to cover the windpipe when a person swallows. The cause of the condition is usually bacterial, with *Haemophilus influenzae* type B being the most common. Other bacterial causes include *Streptococcus pneumoniae*, *Streptococcus* groups A, B, and C, and non-typeable *Haemophilus influenzae*. The disease is most commonly diagnosed in children but can be seen in adolescents and adults. A decline in the number of cases of acute epiglottitis has been noted since the introduction of the *Haemophilus influenzae* type B (Hib) vaccine in the 1980s.

Acute epiglottitis is usually accompanied by the classic triad of symptoms: dysphagia, drooling, and respiratory distress. Other signs and symptoms can include the following:

- Fever
- Sore throat
- Inability to lay flat
- Voice changes (can be muffled or hoarse)
- Tripod breathing position (a position said to optimize the mechanics of breathing where an individual sits up on their hands, head leaning forward, and tongue protruding)
- Tachypnea
- Hypoxia
- Agitation
- Cyanosis

Direct visualization of the epiglottis via a nasopharyngoscopy/laryngoscopy is the gold standard for diagnosing acute epiglottitis since an infected epiglottis has a cherry red appearance.

Acute epiglottitis is a potentially life-threatening medical emergency and should be treated promptly. It can quickly progress to total obstruction of the airway and death. Treatment of the condition can include the following:

- IV antibiotics (after blood and epiglottic cultures have been obtained)

- Analgesic-antipyretic agents such as aspirin, acetaminophen, and nonsteroidal anti-inflammatory drugs (NSAIDs), such as ibuprofen

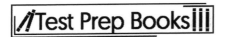

- Intubation with mechanical ventilation, tracheostomy, or needle-jet insufflation (options for immediate airway management, if needed)

- Racemic epinephrine, corticosteroids, and Beta-2 agonists are also sometimes used; however, they have yet to be proven as useful treatments

Acute Tracheitis

A rare condition, **acute tracheitis**, is the inflammation and infection of the trachea (windpipe). The majority of cases occur in children under the age of sixteen. The etiology of acute tracheitis is predominantly bacterial, with Staphylococcus aureus being the leading cause. Community-associated, methicillin-resistant Staphylococcus aureus (CA-MRSA) has recently emerged as an important causative agent. Other bacterial causes of acute tracheitis include Streptococcus pneumoniae, Haemophilus influenzae, and Moraxella catarrhalis.

Acute tracheitis is often preceded by an upper respiratory infection (URI). Signs and symptoms of acute tracheitis can include the following:

- Bark-like cough
- Dyspnea
- Fever
- Tachypnea
- Respiratory distress
- Stridor
- Wheezing
- Hoarseness
- Nasal flaring
- Cyanosis

The only definitive means of diagnosis is the use of a laryngotracheobronchoscopy to directly visualize mucopurulent membranes lining the mucosa of the trachea. Additional tests can include pulse oximetry, blood cultures, nasopharyngeal and tracheal cultures, and neck x-rays.

Treatment of acute tracheitis should be prompt because of the increased likelihood of complete airway obstruction leading to respiratory arrest and death. Treatment can include the following:

- IV antibiotics (if living in an area with high or increasing rates of CA-MRSA, the addition of vancomycin should be considered)

- Intubation and mechanical ventilation or tracheostomy (rarely needed) are options if immediate airway management is needed

- Fever reducers

Pneumonia

Pneumonia is an infection that affects the functional tissue of the lung. Microscopically, it is characterized by consolidating lung tissue with exudate, fibrin, and inflammatory cells filling the alveoli (air sacs). Pneumonia can represent a primary disease or a secondary disease (e.g., post-obstructive pneumonia due to lung cancer), and the most common causes of pneumonia are bacteria and viruses. Other causes of pneumonia include fungi and parasites.

Pneumonia can be categorized according to its anatomic distribution on a chest x-ray or the setting in which it is acquired. Pneumonia categorized according to its anatomic distribution on chest x-ray can be:

34

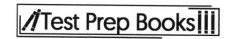

- Lobar: Limited to one lobe of the lungs. It can affect more than one lobe on the same side (multilobar pneumonia) or bilateral lobes ("double" pneumonia).

- Bronchopneumonia: Scattered diffusely throughout the lungs

- Interstitial: Involving areas between the alveoli

Pneumonia categorized according to the setting in which it is acquired can be:

- Community-Acquired Pneumonia (CAP): Pneumonia in an individual who hasn't been recently hospitalized, or its occurrence in less than 48 hours after admission to a hospital.

- Hospital-Acquired (Nosocomial) Pneumonia: Pneumonia acquired during or after hospitalization for another ailment with onset at least 48 hours or more after admission.

- Aspiration Pneumonia: Pneumonia resulting from the inhalation of gastric or oropharyngeal secretions.

CAP

Common causes of community-acquired pneumonia (CAP) include the following:

- Streptococcus pneumoniae
- Haemophilus influenzae
- Moraxella catarrhalis
- Atypical organisms (such as Legionella species, Mycoplasma pneumoniae, and Chlamydia pneumonia)
- Staphylococcus aureus
- Respiratory viruses

Streptococcus Pneumoniae

Streptococcus pneumonia (also known as S. pneumonia or pneumococcus) is a gram-positive bacterium and the most common cause of CAP. Due to the introduction of a pneumococcal vaccine in 2000, cases of pneumococcal pneumonia have decreased. However, medical providers should be aware there is now evidence of emerging, antibiotic-resistant strains of the organism. Signs and symptoms of pneumococcal pneumonia can include the following:

- Cough productive of rust-colored sputum (mucus)
- Fever with or without chills
- Dyspnea
- Wheezing
- Chest pain
- Tachypnea
- Altered mental status
- Tachycardia
- Rales over involved lung
- Increase in tactile fremitus
- E to A change
- Hypotension
- Lung consolidation

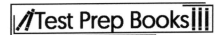

Diagnosis of pneumococcal pneumonia can include the following:

- CBC with differential
- Chest x-ray
- CT scan (if underlying lung cancer is suspected)
- Sputum gram stain and/or culture
- Blood cultures
- Procalcitonin and C-reactive protein blood level tests
- Sputum, serum, and/or urinary antigen tests
- Immunoglobulin studies
- Bronchoscopy with bronchoalveolar lavage (BAL)

Treatment of pneumococcal pneumonia can include the following:

- Antibiotics, such as ceftriaxone plus doxycycline, or azithromycin
- Respiratory quinolones, such as levofloxacin (Levaquin®), moxifloxacin (Avelox®), or Gemifloxacin (Factive®)
- Supplemental oxygen
- Beta-2 agonists, such as albuterol via nebulizer or metered-dose inhaler (MDI), as needed for wheezing
- Analgesics and antipyretics
- Chest physiotherapy
- Active suctioning of respiratory secretions
- Intubation and mechanical ventilation

Mycoplasma Pneumoniae

Mycoplasma pneumonia, also known as M. pneumoniae, is a bacterium that causes atypical CAP. It is one of the most common causes of CAP in healthy individuals under the age of forty. The most common symptom of mycoplasma pneumonia is a dry, nonproductive cough. Other signs and symptoms can include diarrhea, earache, fever (usually $\leq$ 102 °F), sore throat, myalgias, nasal congestion, skin rash, and general malaise. Chest x-rays of individuals with mycoplasma pneumonia reveal a pattern of bronchopneumonia. Cold agglutinin titers in the blood can be significantly elevated (> 1:64). Polymerase chain reaction (PCR) is becoming the standard confirmatory test for mycoplasma pneumonia, though currently it is not used in most clinical settings. Other diagnostic tests for M. pneumoniae are usually nonspecific and therefore do not aid in its diagnosis.

Treatments for mycoplasma pneumonia are no different than for CAP, except for antibiotic choices, which include the following:

- Macrolide antibiotics, such as erythromycin, azithromycin (Zithromax®), clarithromycin (Biaxin®, Biaxin XL®)
- Doxycycline (a tetracycline antibiotic derivative)

Methicillin-Resistant Staphylococcus Aureus

Community-Acquired Methicillin-Resistant Staphylococcus Aureus (CA-MRSA) has emerged as a significant cause of CAP over the past twenty years. It also remains a significant cause of hospital-acquired pneumonia. The majority (up to 75 percent) of those diagnosed with CA-MRSA pneumonia are young, previously healthy individuals with influenza as a preceding illness. Symptoms are usually identical to those seen with other causes of CAP. Chest x-ray typically reveals multilobar involvement with or without cavitation/necrosis. Gram staining of sputum and/or blood can reveal gram-positive bacteria in clusters. Other diagnostic tests are nonspecific and do not aid in the diagnosis of CA-MRSA pneumonia.

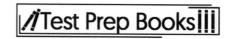

Treatment of CA-MRSA should be prompt as it has a high mortality rate. Supportive measures are needed as in other cases of CAP. CA-MRSA is notoriously resistant to most antibiotics with the exception of the following:

- Vancomycin: The mainstay and only treatment for CA-MRSA pneumonia for many years (unfortunately with a disappointing cure rate). A loading dose of 25 mg/kg (max 2,000 mg) is needed with a maintenance dose based on creatinine clearance and body weight (in kg). Vancomycin trough should be drawn prior to fourth dose with a target goal of 15-20 mcg/mL (mg/L).

- Linezolid: An alternative to vancomycin and quickly becoming the agent of choice for the treatment of CA-MRSA pneumonia. It is administered 600 mg PO/IV every twelve hours.

Viral Pneumonia

Viral pneumonia is more common at the extremes of age (young children and the elderly). It accounts for the majority of cases of childhood pneumonia. Cases of viral pneumonia have been increasing over the past decade, mostly as a result of immunosuppression (weakened immune system). Common causes of viral pneumonia in children, the elderly, and the immunocompromised are the influenza viruses (most common), RSV, parainfluenza virus, and adenovirus.

Signs and symptoms of viral pneumonia largely overlap those of bacterial pneumonia and can include the following:

- Cough (nonproductive)
- Fever/chills
- Myalgias
- Fatigue
- Headache
- Dyspnea
- Tachypnea
- Tachycardia
- Wheezing
- Cyanosis
- Hypoxia
- Decreased breath sounds
- Respiratory distress

Viral pneumonia is diagnosed via a chest x-ray and viral cultures. The chest x-ray usually reveals bilateral lung infiltrates instead of the lobar involvement commonly seen in bacterial causes. Viral cultures can take up to two weeks to confirm the diagnosis. Rapid antigen testing and gene amplification via polymerase chain reaction (PCR) have been recently incorporated into the diagnostic mix to shorten the diagnosis lag.

Treatment of viral pneumonia is usually supportive and can include the following:

- Supplemental oxygen
- Rest
- Antipyretics
- Analgesics
- Intravenous fluids
- Parenteral nutrition
- Intubation and mechanical ventilation

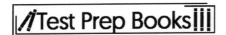

Specific causes of viral pneumonia can benefit from treatment with antiviral medications. Influenza pneumonia can be treated with oseltamivir (Tamiflu®) or zanamivir (Relenza®). Ribavirin® is the only effective antiviral agent for the treatment of RSV pneumonia.

Inhalation Injuries

Gases and vapors are the most common causes of lung inhalation injuries. This is because inhaled substances cause direct injury to respiratory epithelium. Exposure to accidental chemical spills, fires, and explosions can all lead to lung inhalation injuries. Some of the more common pulmonary irritants and gases include smoke, ozone, chlorine (Cl_2), hydrogen chloride (HCl), ammonia (NH_3), hydrogen fluoride (HF), sulfur dioxide (SO_2), and nitrogen oxides. The degree of inhalation injury is dependent on such factors as:

- specific gas or substance inhaled.
- presence of soot.
- degree of exposure.
- presence of underlying lung disease.
- inability to flee the area.

Inhalation injuries can even occur when there are no skin burns or other visible, external signs of exposure. Therefore, medical professionals should maintain a high level of suspicion when it comes to inhalation injuries, watching for signs and symptoms that can include the following:

- Tachypnea
- Dyspnea
- Facial burns
- Cough productive of carbonaceous sputum
- Wheezing
- Rhinitis
- Retractions
- Decreased breath sounds
- Hoarseness
- Blistering or swelling involving the mouth
- Singed nasal hairs
- Headache
- Vomiting
- Dizziness
- Change in mental status
- Coma

The best diagnostic tools for inhalation injuries are clinical presentation and findings from a bronchoscopy (the gold standard for diagnosing inhalation injuries). Other useful tests include the following:

- Chest x-ray
- CT scan
- Pulse oximetry
- ABG analysis
- Blood carboxyhemoglobin levels (for all fire and explosion victims)
- Pulmonary function tests (PFTs)

Inhalation injuries have an excellent prognosis since more than 90 percent of those affected make complete recoveries with no long-term pulmonary complications. However, depending on the injury source, medical providers

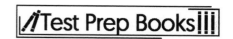
should be aware that respiratory function can deteriorate up to 36 hours post-injury. Treatment of inhalation injuries is largely supportive care, which can include the following:

- Supplemental oxygen (usually 100 percent humidified oxygen)
- IV fluids, especially in individuals with burns
- Inhaled bronchdilators for bronchospasm, such as albuterol
- Gentle respiratory suctioning
- Close observation of developing edema around the head and neck
- Mucolytic agents such as N-acetylcysteine (NAC)
- Hyperbaric oxygen therapy (specifically for carbon monoxide poisoning)
- Hydroxocobalamin (Cyanokit®) (preferred agent), sodium thiosulfate, or sodium nitrite for hydrogen cyanide (HCN) poisoning/toxicity
- Intubation and mechanical ventilation, tidal volume of 6 mL/kg recommended to reduce likelihood of barotrauma
- Monitoring for the onset of secondary pneumonia (commonly caused by Staphylococcus aureus and Pseudomonas aeruginosa)

Obstruction

Obstruction is a blockage in any part of the respiratory tract. The upper respiratory tract consists of the nose, paranasal sinuses, throat, and larynx. The lower respiratory tract consists of the trachea, bronchi, and lungs. Obstructions can be categorized as upper airway obstructions or lower airway obstructions. Obstructions can be partial (allowing some air to pass) or complete (not allowing any air to pass), and they can also be acute or chronic. This discussion focuses on acute upper airway obstruction.

The most common causes of acute upper airway obstruction are anaphylaxis, croup, epiglottitis, and foreign objects. These are all considered respiratory emergencies. Anaphylaxis is a severe allergic reaction usually occurring within minutes of exposure to an allergen. During anaphylaxis, the airways swell and become blocked. Bee stings, penicillin (an antibiotic), and peanuts are the most common allergens that cause anaphylaxis.

Signs and symptoms of acute upper airway obstruction can include the following:

- Dyspnea
- Agitation/panic
- Wheezing
- Cyanosis
- Drooling
- Decreased breath sounds
- Tachypnea
- Tachycardia
- Swelling of the face and tongue
- Choking
- Confusion
- Unconsciousness

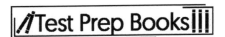

Diagnosis of acute upper airway obstruction can entail imaging studies (x-rays of the neck and chest; CT scans of the head, neck, or chest), pulse oximetry, blood tests and cultures, and bronchoscopy/laryngoscopy. Treatment depends on the etiology of the obstruction and can include the following:

- Heimlich maneuver (if choking on a foreign object)
- Epinephrine, antihistamines, and anti-inflammatory medications (for anaphylaxis)
- Supplemental oxygen
- Tracheostomy or cricothyrotomy (to bypass a total obstruction)
- CPR (if unconscious and unable to breathe)

Pleural Effusion

A **pleural effusion** is an abnormal accumulation of fluid in the pleural space. The pleural space is located between the parietal and visceral pleurae of each lung. The parietal pleura covers the inner surface of the chest cavity, while the visceral pleura surrounds the lungs. Approximately 10 milliliters of pleural fluid is maintained by oncotic and hydrostatic pressures and lymphatic drainage and is necessary for normal respiratory function. Pleural effusions can be categorized as transudates or exudates. Transudates result from an imbalance between oncotic and hydrostatic pressures, so they are characterized by low protein content. The transudates are often the result of congestive heart failure (CHF), cirrhosis, low albumin blood levels, nephrotic syndrome, and peritoneal dialysis. Exudates result from decreased lymphatic drainage or inflammation of the pleura, so they are characterized by high protein content. The exudates are often the result of malignancy, pancreatitis, pulmonary embolism, uremia, infection, and certain medications.

The main symptoms of a pleural effusion include dyspnea, cough, and chest pain. Diagnosis of a pleural effusion can include chest x-ray, chest CT scan, ultrasonography, and thoracentesis. Thoracentesis can provide pleural fluid for analysis such as LDH, glucose, pH, cell count and differential, culture, and cytology. Pleural fluid should be distinguished as either transudate or exudate. Exudative pleural effusions are characterized by:

- ratio of pleural fluid to serum protein > 0.5
- ratio of pleural fluid to serum LDH > 0.6
- pleural fluid LDH > 2/3 of the upper limit of normal blood value.

Treatment of a pleural effusion is usually dictated by the underlying etiology; however, the treatment of a very large pleural effusion can include the following:

- Thoracentesis

- Chest tube (also known as tube thoracostomy)

- Pleurodesis (instillation of an irritant to cause inflammation and subsequent fibrosis to obliterate the pleural space)

- Indwelling tunneled pleural catheters

Pneumothorax

Pneumothorax is the abnormal presence of air in the pleural cavity, which is the space between the parietal and visceral pleurae. Pneumothorax can be categorized as:

- Spontaneous Pneumothorax: This can be classified as either primary or secondary. Primary spontaneous pneumothorax (PSP) occurs in individuals with no history of lung disease or inciting event. Those at risk for PSP are typically eighteen to forty years old, tall, thin, and smokers. There's also a familial tendency for

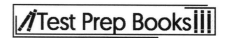

primary spontaneous pneumothorax. Secondary spontaneous pneumothorax occurs in individuals with an underlying lung disease such as COPD, cystic fibrosis, asthma, tuberculosis (TB), or lung cancer.

- Traumatic Pneumothorax: This occurs as a result of blunt or penetrating trauma to the chest wall. The trauma disrupts the parietal and/or visceral pleura(e). Examples of inciting events include gunshot or stab wounds; air bag deployment in a motor vehicle accident; acute respiratory distress syndrome (ARDS); and medical procedures such as mechanical ventilation, lung biopsy, thoracentesis, needle biopsy, and chest surgery.

- Tension Pneumothorax: This is the trapping of air in the pleural space under positive pressure. It causes a mediastinal shift toward the unaffected lung and a depression of the hemidiaphragm on the side of the affected lung. Shortly after, the event is followed by severe cardiopulmonary compromise. Tension pneumothorax can result from any of the conditions or procedures listed for spontaneous and traumatic pneumothorax.

Signs and symptoms of pneumothorax depend on the degree of lung collapse (partial or total) and can include the following:

- Chest pain
- Dyspnea
- Cyanosis
- Tachypnea
- Tachycardia
- Hypotension
- Hypoxia
- Anxiety
- Adventitious breath sounds
- Unilateral distant or absent breath sounds
- Jugular venous distention (JVD)
- Tracheal deviation away from the affected side (with tension pneumothorax)

Diagnosis of pneumothorax is primarily clinical (based on signs and symptoms), but can involve an upright posteroanterior chest x-ray, chest CT scan (the most reliable imaging for diagnosis), ABG analysis, and ultrasonography of the chest. Treatment of a pneumothorax depends on the severity of the condition and can include the following:

- Supplemental oxygen

- The standard of treatment for all large, symptomatic pneumothoraces is a tube thoracostomy (chest tube).

- Observation (a reasonable option for small asymptomatic pneumothorax; multiple series of chest X-rays are needed until resolution)

- Simple needle aspiration (an option for small, primary spontaneous pneumothorax)

- Because they can quickly cause life-threatening cardiopulmonary compromise, the standard of treatment for all tension pneumothoraces is an emergent needle thoracostomy.

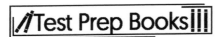

Noncardiogenic Pulmonary Edema

Pulmonary edema can be categorized as cardiogenic or noncardiogenic in origin. Cardiogenic pulmonary edema is the most common type, while noncardiogenic pulmonary edema is the least common. This discussion focuses on noncardiogenic pulmonary edema. Direct injury to the lungs, followed by subsequent inflammation, leads to the development of noncardiogenic pulmonary edema. The inflammation causes lung capillaries in the alveoli to leak and fill with fluid, resulting in impaired oxygenation. Common causes of noncardiogenic pulmonary edema include the following:

- Acute respiratory distress syndrome (ARDS)
- High altitudes
- Nervous system conditions (especially head trauma, seizures, or subarachnoid hemorrhage)
- Pulmonary embolism
- Kidney failure
- Illicit drug use (especially cocaine and heroin)
- Medication side effects (such as aspirin overdose or chemotherapy)
- Inhaled toxins (such as ammonia, chlorine, or smoke)
- Pneumonia
- Near drowning

Signs and symptoms of noncardiogenic pulmonary edema can include the following:

- Dyspnea (most common symptom)
- Wheezing
- Respiratory distress
- Cough
- Anxiety
- Hypoxia
- Tachypnea
- Altered mental status
- Fatigue
- Lung crackles
- Headache
- Cyanosis

There is no single test to determine whether the cause of the pulmonary edema is cardiogenic or noncardiogenic. Diagnosis of noncardiogenic pulmonary edema can include chest x-ray, blood tests, pulse oximetry, ABG analysis, electrocardiogram (ECG), echocardiogram, cardiac catheterization with coronary angiogram, and pulmonary artery catheterization. For pulmonary artery catheterization, a pulmonary artery wedge pressure <18 mmHg is consistent with pulmonary edema of noncardiogenic origin. Most of these tests help to differentiate between cardiogenic and noncardiogenic causes of pulmonary edema.

Treatment of noncardiogenic pulmonary edema is directed toward its underlying cause and can include the following:

- Supplemental oxygen (first-line treatment)
- Hyperbaric oxygen chamber
- Intubation and mechanical ventilation
- Morphine (can be used to allay anxiety)

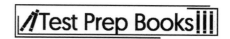
Pulmonary Embolism

A **pulmonary embolism** (PE) is the abnormal presence of a blood clot, or thrombus, causing a blockage in one of the lungs' pulmonary arteries. It is not a specific disease, but rather a complication due to thrombus formation in the venous system of one of the lower extremities, which is termed *deep venous thrombosis* (DVT). Other rarer causes of PEs are thrombi arising in the veins of the kidneys, pelvis, upper extremities, or the right atrium of the heart. Occasionally, other matter besides blood clots can cause pulmonary emboli, such as fat, air, and septic (infected with bacteria) emboli. PE is a common and potentially fatal condition.

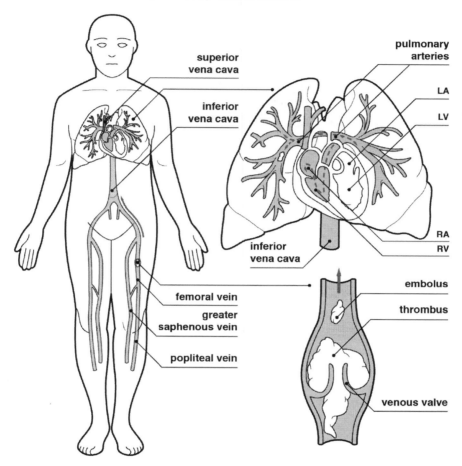

43

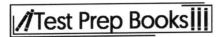
The primary influences on the development of DVT and PE are shown in Virchow's triad: blood hypercoagulability, endothelial (vessel wall) injury/dysfunction, and stasis of blood.

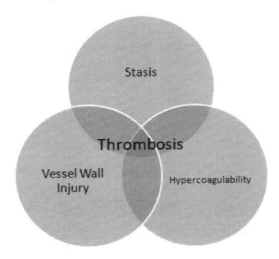

Risk factors for DVT and PE include the following:

- Cancer
- Heart disease, especially congestive heart failure (CHF)
- Prolonged immobility (such as prolonged bedrest or lengthy trips in planes or cars)
- Surgery (one of the leading risk factors, accounting for up to 15 percent of all postoperative deaths)
- Obesity/being overweight
- Smoking
- Pregnancy
- Supplemental estrogen from birth control pills or estrogen replacement therapy (ERT)

The signs and symptoms of PE are nonspecific, which often presents a diagnostic dilemma and a delay in diagnosis. Nearly half of all individuals with PE are asymptomatic. The signs and symptoms of PE can vary greatly depending on the size of the blood clots, how much lung tissue is involved, and an individual's overall health. Signs and symptoms of PE can include the following:

- Pleuritic chest pain
- Dyspnea
- Cough
- Tachypnea
- Hypoxia
- Fever
- Diaphoresis
- Rales
- Cyanosis
- Unilateral lower extremity edema (symptom of DVT)

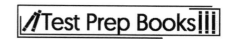

The diagnosis of PE can be a difficult task. Many clinicians support determining the clinical probability of PE before proceeding with diagnostic testing. This process involves assessing the presence or absence of the following manifestations:

- Pulmonary Signs: Tachypnea, rales, and cyanosis

- Cardiac Signs: Tachycardia, S_3 - S_4 gallop, attenuated second heart sound, and cardiac murmur

- Constitutional Signs: Fever, diaphoresis, signs and symptoms of thrombophlebitis, and lower extremity edema

Once the clinical probability of PE has been determined, diagnostic testing ensues. Duplex ultrasonography is the standard for diagnosing a DVT. A spiral computed tomography (CT) scan with or without contrast has replaced pulmonary angiography as the standard for diagnosing a PE. If spiral CT scanning is unavailable or if individuals have a contraindication to the administration of intravenous contrast material, ventilation-perfusion (V/Q) scanning is often selected. Magnetic resonance imaging (MRI) is usually reserved for pregnant women and individuals with a contraindication to the administration of intravenous contrast material. A D-dimer blood test is most useful for individuals with a low or moderate pretest probability of PE, since levels are typically elevated with PE. Arterial blood gas (ABG) analysis usually reveals hypoxemia, hypocapnia, and respiratory alkalosis.

A chest x-ray, though not diagnostic for PE since its findings are typically nonspecific, can exclude diseases that mimic PE, as can an echocardiography. Electrocardiography is also useful because it can assess right ventricular heart function and be prognostic, since there is a 10 percent death rate from PE with right ventricular dysfunction. Lastly, transesophageal echocardiography (TEE) can reveal central PE.

Treatment of PE should begin immediately to prevent complications or death. PE treatment is focused on preventing an increase in size of the current blood clots and the formation of new blood clots. Supportive care treatment of PE can include the following:

- Supplemental oxygen to ease hypoxia/hypoxemia
- Dopamine (Inotropin®) or dobutamine (Dobutrex®) administered via IV for related hypotension
- Cardiac monitoring in the case of associated arrhythmias or right ventricular dysfunction
- Intubation and mechanical ventilation

Medications involved in treatment can include: thrombolytics or clot dissolvers (such as tissue plasminogen activator (tPA), alteplase, urokinase, streptokinase, or reteplase). These medications are reserved for individuals with a diagnosis of acute PE and associated hypotension (systolic BP < 90 mm Hg). They are not given concurrently with anticoagulants. Anticoagulants or blood thinners may also be used. The historical standard for the initial treatment of PE was unfractionated heparin (UFH) administered via IV or subcutaneous (SC) injection, which requires frequent blood monitoring. Current treatment guidelines recommend low-molecular weight heparin (LMWH) administered via SC injection over UFH IV or SC as it has greater bioavailability than UFH and blood monitoring is not necessary. Fondaparinux (Arixtra®) administered via SC injection is also recommended over UFH IV or SC; blood monitoring is not necessary.

Warfarin (Coumadin®), an oral anticoagulant, was the historical standard for the outpatient prevention and treatment of PE. It is initiated the same day as treatment with UFH, LMWH, or fondaparinux. It is recommended INR of 2-3 with frequent blood monitoring, at which time IV or SC anticoagulant is discontinued. Alternatives to warfarin include oral factor Xa inhibitor anticoagulants such as apixaban (Eliquis®), rivaroxaban (Xarelto®), and edoxaban (Savaysa®), or the oral direct thrombin inhibitor anticoagulant dabigatran (Pradaxa®). Blood monitoring is not necessary with these medications. The most significant adverse effect of both thrombolytics and anticoagulants is bleeding.

45

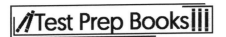
- An embolectomy (removal of emboli via catheter or surgery) is reserved for individuals with a massive PE and contraindications to thrombolytics or anticoagulants. Vena cava filters (also called inferior vena cava [IVC] filters or Greenfield filters) are only indicated in individuals with an absolute contraindication to anticoagulants, a massive PE who have survived and for whom recurrent PE will be fatal, or documented recurrent PE.

ARDS

Acute respiratory distress syndrome (ARDS) is the widespread inflammation of the lungs and capillaries of the alveoli and results in the rapid development of pulmonary system failure. It can occur in both adults and children and is considered the most severe form of acute lung injury. Presence of the syndrome is determined by the following:

- Timing: Onset of symptoms within one week of inciting incident
- Chest X-ray: Bilateral lung infiltrates not explained by consolidation, atelectasis, or effusions
- Origin of Edema: Not explained by heart failure or fluid overload
- Severity of Hypoxemia

It should be noted that the severity of hypoxemia is based on PaO_2/FiO_2 ratio while on 5 cm of continuous positive airway pressure (CPAP). PaO_2 is the partial pressure of oxygen, while FiO_2 is the fraction of inspired oxygen. Categories are as follows:

- Mild (PaO_2/FiO_2 = 200-300)
- Moderate (PaO_2/FiO_2 = 100-200)
- Severe ($PaO_2/FiO_2 \leq 100$)

ARDS has a high mortality rate (30–40 percent), which increases with advancing age. It also leads to significant morbidity because of its association with extended hospital stays, frequent nosocomial (hospital-acquired) infections, muscle weakness, significant weight loss, and functional impairment. The most common cause of ARDS is sepsis, a life-threatening bacterial infection of the blood. Other common causes include the following:

- Severe pneumonia
- Inhalation of toxic fumes
- Trauma (such as falls, bone fractures, motor vehicle accidents, near drowning, and burns)
- Massive blood transfusion

It should also be noted that for one in five patients with ARDS there will be no identifiable risk factors. Therefore, the cause of ARDS may not be evident.

The onset of ARDS symptoms is fairly rapid, occurring 12 to 48 hours after the inciting incident. Many of the signs and symptoms of ARDS are nonspecific. Signs and symptoms of ARDS can include the following:

- Dyspnea (initially with exertion, but rapidly progressing to occurring even at rest)
- Hypoxia
- Tachypnea
- Tachycardia
- Fever
- Bilateral rales
- Cyanosis
- Hypotension
- Fatigue

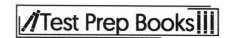

The diagnosis of ARDS is clinical since there's no specific test for the condition. Diagnosing ARDS is done by exclusion, ruling out other diseases that mimic its signs and symptoms. Tests used to diagnose ARDS can include the following:

- Chest x-ray, which, by definition, should reveal bilateral lung infiltrates
- ABG analysis (usually reveals extreme hypoxemia and respiratory alkalosis or metabolic acidosis)
- CBC with differential (can reveal leukocytosis, leukopenia, and/or thrombocytopenia)
- Plasma *B*-type natriuretic peptide (BNP), a level < 100 pg/mL favors ARDS rather than CHF
- CT scan
- Echocardiography, which is helpful in excluding CHF (cardiogenic pulmonary edema)
- Bronchoscopy with bronchoalveolar lavage (BAL), which is helpful in excluding lung infections

Numerous medications, such as corticosteroids, synthetic surfactant, antibody to endotoxin, ketoconazole, simvastatin, ibuprofen, and inhaled nitric oxide, have been used for the treatment of ARDS, but none have proven effective. Therefore, treating the underlying symptoms of ARDS and providing supportive care are the most crucial components of therapy. The only therapy found to improve survival in ARDS is intubation and mechanical ventilation using low tidal volumes (6 mL/kg of ideal body weight). Because sepsis, an infection, is the most common etiology of ARDS, early administration of a broad-spectrum antibiotic is crucial.

Treatment also includes fluid management and nutritional support. For individuals with shock secondary to sepsis, initial aggressive fluid resuscitation is administered, followed by a conservative fluid management strategy. It is best to institute nutritional support within 48 to 72 hours of initiation of mechanical ventilation.

Important preventative measures include DVT prophylaxis with enoxaparin, stress ulcer prophylaxis with sucralfate or omeprazole, turning and skin care to prevent decubitus ulcers, and elevating the head of the bed and using a subglottic suction device to help prevent ventilator-associated pneumonia.

Trauma

Chest trauma is a significant factor in all trauma deaths. There are two general categories of chest traumas: blunt chest traumas and penetrating chest traumas.

Pulmonary Contusion

A **pulmonary contusion** is a deep bruise of the lung secondary to chest trauma. Associated swelling and blood collecting in the alveoli of the lung lead to loss of structure and function. It is estimated that 50–60 percent of individuals with pulmonary contusions develop ARDS. Motor vehicle accidents, sports injuries, explosive blast injuries, work injuries, serious falls, or crush injuries can cause blunt chest trauma. Signs and symptoms of a pulmonary contusion typically develop 24 to 48 hours after the inciting event. Signs and symptoms can include the following:

- Dyspnea
- Hypoxia
- Cyanosis
- Tachypnea
- Tachycardia
- Hemoptysis
- Chest pain
- Hypotension

Diagnosis of a pulmonary contusion relies on physical examination and diagnostic tests. A chest x-ray is useful in the diagnosis of most significant pulmonary contusions; however, it often underestimates the extent of the injury,

47

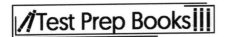
which is sometimes not apparent for 24 to 48 hours after the event. CT scans are more accurate than chest x-rays for identifying a pulmonary contusion; they can also accurately assess and reflect the extent of lung injury. ABG analysis is used to assess the extent of hypoxemia, and pulse oximetry is used to assess the extent of hypoxia.

Treatment for a pulmonary contusion is primarily supportive, and no treatment is known to accelerate its resolution. These treatments can include the following:

- Supplemental oxygen to relieve hypoxia
- Analgesics (as needed for pain)
- Conservative fluid management to reduce the likelihood of fluid overload and PE
- Aggressive suction of pulmonary secretions to reduce likelihood of pneumonia
- Incentive spirometry to reduce the likelihood of atelectasis, which can lead to pneumonia
- Intubation and mechanical ventilation (in severe cases)

Hemothorax

Hemothorax, the presence of blood in the pleural space, is most commonly the result of blunt or penetrating chest trauma. The pleural space lies between the parietal pleura of the chest wall and the visceral pleura of the lungs. A large accumulation of blood in the pleural space can restrict normal lung movement and lead to hemodynamic compromise. Common signs and symptoms of hemothorax include chest pain, dyspnea, and tachypnea. When there is substantial systemic blood loss, tachycardia and hypotension can also be present.

Diagnosis of hemothorax primarily involves a chest x-ray, which reveals blunting at the costophrenic angle on the affected side of the lung. A helical CT scan has a complementary role in the management of hemothorax, and it can localize and quantify the retention of blood or clots within the pleural space.

Small hemothoraces usually require no treatment but need close observation to ensure resolution. Tube thoracostomy drainage is the mainstay of treatment for significant hemothoraces. Needle aspiration has no place in the management of hemothorax. Blood transfusions can be necessary for those with significant blood loss or hemodynamic compromise. Complications from hemothorax can include empyema (secondary bacterial infection of a retained clot) or fibrothorax (fibrosis of the pleural space which can trap lung tissue and lead to decreased pulmonary function).

Flail Chest

Flail chest is clinically defined as the paradoxical movement of a segment of the chest wall caused by at least two fractures per rib (usually anteriorly and posteriorly) in three or more ribs while breathing. The ribs are then free to float away from the chest wall and produce paradoxical breathing, which is the flail area contracting on inspiration and relaxing on expiration. The flail area of the chest disrupts the normal mechanics of breathing. Variations include anterior flail segments, posterior flail segments, and flail affecting the sternum and fractures of the ribs bilaterally. Flail chest requires a tremendous amount of blunt force trauma to the thorax in order to fracture multiple ribs in multiple places. This type of trauma can be produced by motor vehicle accidents, serious falls, crush injuries, rollover injuries, and physical assaults.

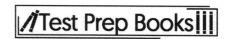
The diagnosis of flail chest is visual. It is seen in individuals with a history of blunt chest trauma by the presence of paradoxical chest wall motion while spontaneously breathing. The rib fractures can be verified with chest x-ray. A CT scan of the chest provides very little additional information and isn't usually indicated in the initial assessment of a chest wall injury. In flail chest, the lungs cannot expand properly, which can lead to varying degrees of respiratory compromise. Treatment of flail chest can include the following:

- Supplemental oxygen (to relieve hypoxia, if present)

- Analgesia (for relief of pain secondary to multiple rib fractures, usually via patient-controlled administration (PCA) or continuous epidural infusion)

- External fixation and stabilization of rib fractures (once the historical standard for treatment, it has been replaced by intubation and mechanical ventilation)

- Intubation and mechanical ventilation (usually needed for the treatment of an underlying disease such as pulmonary contusion; addition of positive pressure provides stabilization of the chest wall and helps improve oxygenation and ventilation)

- Operative fixation of ribs (reserved for individuals requiring a thoracotomy for underlying lung injuries)

Common complications of flail chest include hemothorax, pneumothorax, pulmonary contusion, and pneumonia. Hemothorax or pneumothorax would require concomitant tube thoracostomy drainage. Chest physiotherapy and aggressive pulmonary hygiene should be implemented to reduce the likelihood of complicating pneumonia.

Fractured Ribs

A **fracture** is a crack or splinter in a bone. Simple rib fractures are the most common injury after sustaining blunt chest trauma. Only 10 percent of individuals admitted with a diagnosis of blunt chest trauma have multiple rib fractures. Causes of rib fractures include falls from an elevation or from standing (most common in the elderly), motor vehicle accidents (most common in adults), and recreational and athletic activities (most common in children). Rib fractures can also be pathologic or related to cancers that have undergone metastasis such as prostate, renal, and breast.

Ribs four through nine (4–9) are the most commonly fractured ribs. Other rib fractures and possible underlying injuries are as follows:

- Ribs 1–2: Tracheal, bronchus, or great vessels can be injured
- Right-sided $\geq$ rib 8: Liver trauma
- Left-sided $\geq$ rib 8: Spleen trauma

Common signs and symptoms of rib fractures include tenderness on palpation, chest wall deformities, and crepitus. Other signs and symptoms can include cyanosis, dyspnea, tachycardia, agitation, tachypnea, retractions, and use of accessory respiratory muscles.

Laboratory blood tests are of no use in the diagnosis of fractured ribs. A chest x-ray can be used to diagnose rib fractures and other underlying injuries such as hemothorax, lung contusion, pneumothorax, atelectasis, and pneumonia. A chest CT scan is more sensitive than a chest x-ray for the detection of rib fractures. A bone scan of the chest wall is the preferred diagnostic imaging study for the diagnosis of rib stress fractures.

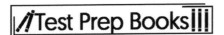

The treatment of rib fractures is primarily supportive. Younger individuals with rib fractures have a better prognosis than older individuals (age ≥ 65 years) who have higher rates of serious lung complications. Therapies for rib fractures can include the following:

- Supplemental oxygen
- Incentive spirometry (to avoid complications such as atelectasis and pneumonia)
- Pain control, which is essential and usually provided by NSAIDs and/or other analgesics

Tracheal Perforation/Injury

Tracheal perforation/injury is a tear in the trachea or bronchial tubes, which are major airways leading to the lungs. Common causes of tracheal perforation/injury include trauma (gunshot wounds and motor vehicle accidents), infections, and ulcerations secondary to foreign objects. Common signs and symptoms of tracheal perforation/injury can include hemoptysis, dyspnea, subcutaneous emphysema, and respiratory distress. Diagnosis may include chest x-rays, a chest CT scan, and MRI. A CT scan is the preferred imaging method for diagnosing a tracheal perforation/injury. Treatment should be prompt and depends on the etiology and the extent of the damage to the area. Surgical repair of the tear is often needed, and other measures to manage a tracheal perforation/injury include the following:

- Intubation and mechanical ventilation
- Tube thoracostomy drainage
- Rigid or fiberoptic bronchoscopy (to extract foreign objects)
- Antibiotics (as indicated)

Ruptured Diaphragm

The diaphragm separates the thoracic (chest) cavity and the abdominal cavity. Rupture of the diaphragm is rare and usually the result of a blunt or penetrating trauma. The majority of blunt traumas causing ruptures of the diaphragm are the result of motor vehicle accidents. Gunshot and knife injuries are the most common causes of a traumatic diaphragmatic rupture. A ruptured diaphragm can lead to significant ventilatory compromise, and difficulty breathing is a common symptom. A chest x-ray is the most important diagnostic tool in diagnosing a ruptured diaphragm. It can reveal elevation of a hemidiaphragm, a nasogastric (NG) tube being present in chest (rather than in the abdomen), or the abnormal presence of bowel in the chest. Abnormalities such as widening of the mediastinum can also be observed on a chest x-ray. Treatment of a ruptured diaphragm requires surgical repair. The prognosis is excellent with the emergent repair of the diaphragmatic rupture.

Cardiovascular/Hematological

Cardiovascular emergencies are life-threatening conditions. Any condition that impedes circulation has the potential to damage the myocardium, or heart muscle. A damaged myocardium may be unable to meet the oxygen demands of the body. It is important to quickly identify any patient exhibiting symptoms indicative of such emergencies so that they can receive prompt treatment to prevent further cardiovascular injury or death. Every patient presenting with possible cardiovascular symptoms should immediately be given a focused assessment. Simultaneously, an intravenous (IV) line should be established and an electrocardiogram (ECG) and laboratory and radiographic studies should be performed. The assessment, diagnostics, and treatment of such patients must be prioritized to preserve cardiac function and, ultimately, life.

Acute Coronary Syndrome

Acute coronary syndrome (ACS) is the term used to describe the clinical symptoms caused by the sudden reduction in blood flow to the heart, but it is also known as **acute myocardial ischemia**. The causes of the ischemia include stable and unstable angina (UA), non-ST elevation myocardial infarction (NSTEMI), and ST elevation myocardial infarction (STEMI), which are shown in the figure below:

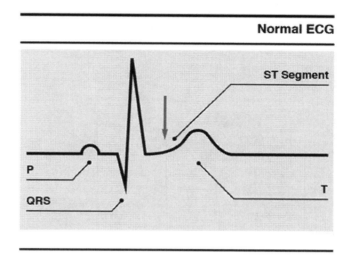

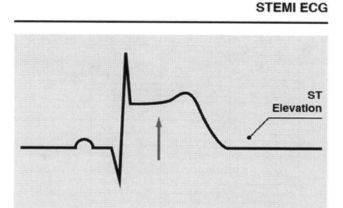

51

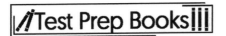

Common symptoms of a patient presenting with ACS include the following:

- Chest pain or discomfort in the upper body that radiates to the arms, back, neck, jaw, or stomach, as shown in the image below

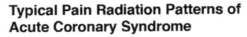

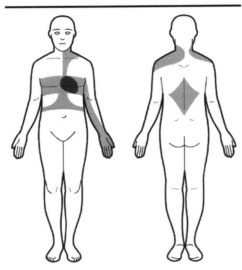

- Dizziness, syncope, or changes in the level of consciousness (LOC)

- Nausea or vomiting

- Palpitations or tachycardia

- Shortness of breath (SOB) or dyspnea

- Unusual fatigue

Angina

Angina is the term used to describe chest pain caused by decreased blood flow to the myocardium. The two primary categories of angina are stable or unstable, with stable angina being more common. It presents in a predictable pattern for patients, responds quickly to cessation of exertion or medication, and while it increases the likelihood of a future heart attack, it is not necessarily indicative of such an event occurring imminently. Unstable angina is often more frequent and severe. It may occur without physical exertion and be unresponsive to medication or activity cessation. It should be treated as an emergency and can signal an imminent heart attack.

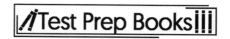

Treatment for angina depends on the severity of the symptoms and can range from lifestyle modifications to surgical intervention. Pharmacological treatments for angina include beta-blockers, calcium channel blockers (CCBs), angiotensin-converting enzyme (ACE) inhibitors, statins, and antiplatelet and anticoagulant medications. These medications treat the symptoms related to angina by lowering blood pressure (BP), slowing heart rate (HR), relaxing blood vessels, reducing strain on the heart, lowering cholesterol levels, and preventing blood clot formation. Generally, the risk factors for the development of angina include the following:

- Diabetes
- Dietary deficiency (fruits and vegetables)
- Excessive alcohol consumption
- Family history of early coronary heart disease
- Hypertension (HTN)
- High LDL (low-density lipoprotein)
- Low HDL (high-density lipoprotein)
- Males
- Obesity
- Old age
- Sedentary lifestyle
- Smoking

Stable Angina

Atherosclerotic buildup generally occurs slowly over time. Because the buildup is gradual, the heart can usually continue to meet the body's oxygen demands despite the narrowing lumen of the vessel. However, in situations with increased oxygen demand, such as exercise or stress, the myocardium may not be able to meet the increased demands, thereby causing angina. The angina subsides with rest. Stable angina is predictable; it occurs in association with stress or certain activities. It does not increase in intensity or worsen over time. Nitroglycerine is effective in the treatment of stable angina because it dilates the blood vessels, reducing the resistance to blood flow, which decreases the demand on the myocardium. Lifestyle modifications such as smoking cessation and a regular exercise program are needed to slow atherosclerotic buildup.

Unstable Angina

Unstable angina (UA) is a more severe form of heart disease than stable angina. The angina associated with UA is generally related to small pieces of atherosclerotic plaque that break off and cause occlusions. The occlusions suddenly decrease blood flow to the myocardium, resulting in angina, without causing an actual MI. The pain symptomatic of UA occurs suddenly without a direct cause, worsens over a short period of time, and may last 15 to 20 minutes. Dyspnea (shortness of breath) and decreased blood pressure are also common. Because the angina is related to an acute decrease in blood flow, rest does not alleviate symptoms. Generally, UA does not respond to the vasodilatory effect of nitroglycerine. Laboratory values are typically negative for cardiac enzymes related to cardiac damage, but they can be slightly elevated. Therefore, a comprehensive history and physical exam that properly identify pertinent risk factors are critical for early diagnosis and treatment.

Depending on the severity of symptom presentation, pharmacological treatment for UA will include one or more antiplatelet medications and a cholesterol medication. In addition, medications to treat hypertension, arrhythmias, and anxiety may be necessary. The recommended intervention is angioplasty with coronary artery stenting. A coronary artery bypass grafting (CABG) surgery may be necessary in the case of extensive occlusion of one or more of the coronary arteries.

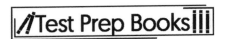

NSTEMI

The **NSTEMI** does not produce changes in the ST segment of the EKG cycle. However, troponin levels are positive. Patients with a confirmed NSTEMI are hospitalized. Morphine, oxygen, nitroglycerin, and aspirin (MONA protocol) is administered. Additional pharmacological agents for treatment are beta-blockers, ACE inhibitors, statins, and antiplatelet medications. Coronary angiography and revascularization may be necessary.

The primary difference between UA and an NSTEMI is whether the ischemia is severe enough to damage the myocardium to the extent that cardiac markers indicative of injury are released and detectable through laboratory analysis. A patient is diagnosed with an NSTEMI when the ischemia is severe enough to cause myocardial damage and the release of a myocardial necrosis biomarker into the circulation (usually cardiac-specific troponins T or I). In contrast, a patient is diagnosed with UA if such a biomarker is undetectable in their bloodstream hours after the ischemic chest pain's initial onset.

STEMI

The **STEMI** is the most serious form of MI. It occurs when a coronary artery is completely blocked and unable to receive blood flow. Emergent revascularization is needed either through angioplasty or a thrombolytic medication.

UA and NSTEMIs generally indicate a partial-thickness injury to the myocardium, but a STEMI indicates injury across the full thickness of the myocardium, as shown in the image below. The etiology behind ischemia is partial or full occlusion of coronary arteries.

Differentiation Between Non-ST and ST MIs

Transverse section of the heart

Partial thickness damage

Full thickness damage

Treatment and Risk Scoring for UA and NSTEMI

Treatment for UA and NSTEMI is planned according to a risk score using the Thrombolysis in Myocardial Infarction (TIMI) tool. In the presence of UA or an NSTEMI, seven categories are scored: age, risk factors, a prior coronary artery stenosis, ST deviation on ECG, prior aspirin intake, presence and number of angina episodes, and elevated creatinine kinase (CK-MB) or troponins. In the presence of a STEMI, the TIMI tool scores eleven categories: age, angina history, hypertension, diabetes, systolic BP, heart rate, Killip class, weight, anterior MI in an ECG, left bundle

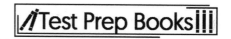

branch block (LBBB) in an ECG, and a treatment delay after an attack. The Global Registry of Acute Coronary Events (GRACE), or ACS risk calculator, is a common tool used to predict death during admission and six months, as well as three years after a diagnosis of Acute Coronary Syndrome (ACS).

ACS can be life threatening. Treatment and survival are time-dependent. Quick recognition by the nurse followed by a thorough focused assessment that includes evaluation of pain type, location, characteristic, and onset is essential. The MONA protocol is implemented immediately. The nurse should obtain a family, social, and lifestyle assessment to identify high-risk patients. An evaluation of recent medical history is imperative, since most ACS patients experience prodromal symptoms a month or more prior to the acute event. Establishing IV access is paramount for rapid administration of medications. Obtaining and reviewing an ECG and drawing and reviewing labs including troponins, CK-MB, complete blood count (CBC), C-reactive protein (CRP), electrolytes, and renal function will provide critical diagnostic data. A chest x-ray and echocardiogram will also add to the differential diagnosis. Immediate and long-term complications of ACS are cardiac dysrhythmia, heart failure (HF), and cardiogenic shock. Education should be provided to each patient about the diagnosis, risk factors, lifestyle modifications, and medications once the acute event has stabilized.

Aneurysm/Dissection

An **aneurysm** is an abnormal bulge or ballooning that can form on an artery wall, as seen in the image below. Depending on the location, the rupture of an aneurysm can result in hemorrhage, stroke, or death. The most common places for the formation of an aneurysm are the left ventricle (LV) of the heart, the aorta, the brain, and the spleen.

Blood Vessel with an Aneurysm and Rupture

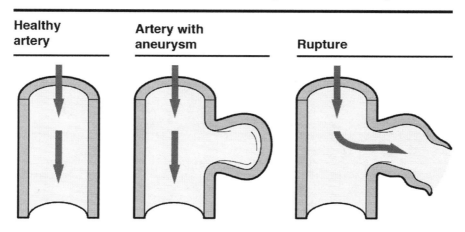

55

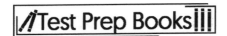
Anatomical Review

Generally, arteries carry oxygenated blood away from the heart to the organs and tissues of the body. The largest artery is the aorta, which receives blood directly from the LV of the heart. Oxygen-carrying blood continues to travel down the arterial system through successively smaller arteries that supply organs, ending with the arterioles that empty into the capillary bed.

Pulmonary and Systemic Circulation

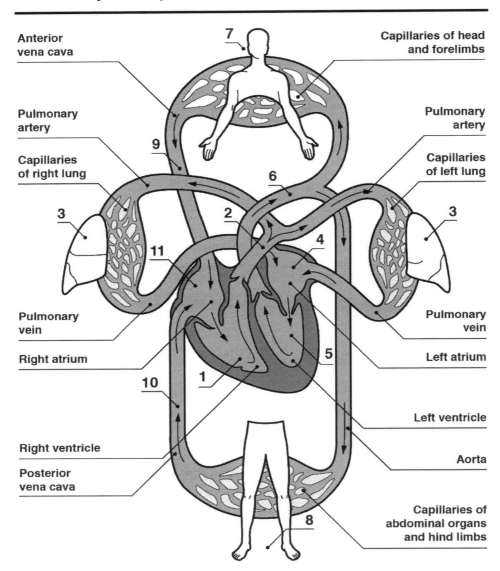

The capillary beds are drained on their opposite side by the venules, which return the now-deoxygenated blood back to the right atrium through progressively larger veins, ending in the great veins of the heart, known as the superior and inferior vena cava. The deoxygenated blood from the great veins moves into the right atrium, then the right ventricle, which pumps the blood to the lungs via the pulmonary artery to become oxygenated once again. The

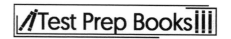
oxygenated blood flows from the pulmonary vein into the left atrium, then the LV, and into the aorta to repeat the cycle.

Arteries and Veins

There are three tissue layers in the structure of arteries and veins. The endothelium, or tunica intima, forms the inner layer. The middle layer, the tunica media, contains elastin and smooth muscle fibers. Connective tissue forms the outside coating called the tunica externa.

Arteries have a thicker elastin middle layer that enables them to withstand the fluctuations in pressure that result from the high-pressure contractions of the LV. Arterioles regulate blood flow into the capillary bed through constriction and dilation, so they are the primary control structures for blood pressure regulation. Meanwhile, the venous side of circulation operates under very low pressures, so veins have no elastin in their structure; instead, they use valves to prevent backflow in those vessels working against gravity, as shown in the image below:

Structure of an Artery and Vein

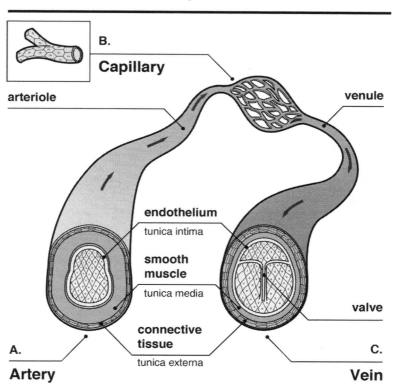

Left Ventricular Aneurysm

A **left ventricular aneurysm** (LVA) is a bulge or ballooning of a weakened area of the LV, generally caused by an MI. There are no symptoms of an LVA, which should be diagnosed with an echocardiogram and angiogram. Small LVAs usually do not require treatment. Clot formation is a common occurrence with LVAs. In the body's attempt to repair the aneurysm, the inflammatory process and the clotting cascade are initiated, both of which increase the propensity for clot formation. Patients are most likely prescribed anticoagulants. Rapid treatment for an MI reduces the incidence of LVA formation.

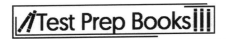

Aorta

The **aorta** stretches from the LV through the diaphragm into the abdomen and pelvis. In the groin, the aorta separates into two main arteries that supply blood to the lower trunk and the legs. An aneurysm can occur anywhere along the aorta; an abdominal aortic aneurysm (AAA) is the most common. Atherosclerosis, hypertension, diabetes, infection, inflammation, and injury such as from a fall or auto accident are frequent causes. The most common presenting symptoms with an AAA are chest pain and back pain. The clinician may be able to palpate a pulsating bulge in the abdomen. Nausea and vomiting may be present. Other symptoms include lightheadedness, confusion, dyspnea, rapid heartbeat, sweating, numbness, and tingling. When an AAA develops slowly over a period of years, it is less likely to rupture, in which case the patient should be regularly monitored with ultrasound imaging. Aneurysms greater than 2 inches (5.5 centimeters) will generally require surgical repair.

A thoracic aortic aneurysm occurs in the stretch of the aorta that lies within the chest cavity. The critical size for surgical intervention of a thoracic aortic aneurysm is 2.3 inches (6 centimeters). As with all surgeries in such close proximity to the heart, the risk-to-benefit ratio must be carefully weighed.

Treatment Options

If the AAA is small and slow-growing, a watch-and-wait approach is often taken. An abdominal ultrasound, computed tomography (CT), and MRI will aid in the determination of the most appropriate treatment. Surgical repair involves removing the damaged portion of the aorta and replacing it with a graft. Another minimally-invasive technique involves reinforcing the weakened area with metal mesh.

Brain

Bulging or ballooning in a blood vessel within the brain is the second most common site for an aneurysm. Another common site for aneurysms is where the internal carotid artery (ICA) enters the cranium; it branches into a system of arteries that provide blood flow to the brain, known as the *circle of Willis*. Most small brain aneurysms do not rupture and are found during various tests. An aneurysm may press on brain tissue and present with ocular pain or symptoms. However, a rupture is a medical emergency that can lead to stroke or hemorrhage. The most common symptom described by patients is "the *worst* headache of my life." A sudden, severe headache, stiff neck, blurred or double vision, photophobia, seizure, loss of consciousness, and confusion may also be reported.

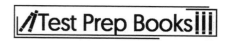
Here's a graphic of the circle of Willis, which are interconnecting arteries at the base of the brain:

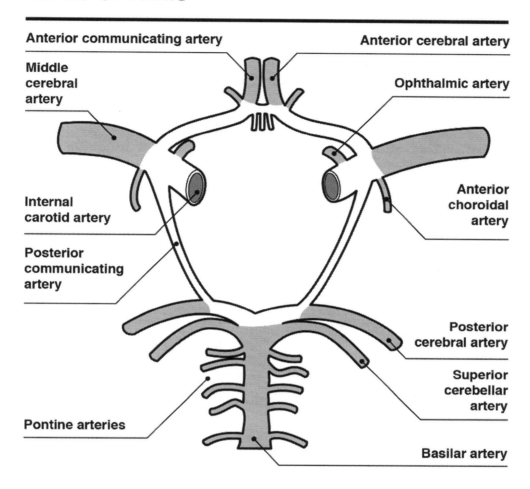

Circle of Willis

Anterior communicating artery

Anterior cerebral artery

Middle cerebral artery

Ophthalmic artery

Internal carotid artery

Anterior choroidal artery

Posterior communicating artery

Posterior cerebral artery

Superior cerebellar artery

Pontine arteries

Basilar artery

Risk Factors

A family history of aneurysm and certain other aneurysm risk factors are genetic. Other predisposing factors are an arteriovenous malformation (AVM) at the circle of Willis, polycystic kidney disease (PKD), and Marfan syndrome. Poor lifestyle choices, such as smoking and cocaine use, greatly increase the risk for aneurysm formation. There is a higher risk for individuals over the age of forty, women, patients who have experienced a traumatic head injury, and patients with hypertension.

Treatment Options

Depending on a brain aneurysm's cause, size, and symptoms and the patient's general health, there are several treatment options. The most common surgical treatment is clipping. The bulge is clipped at the base to prevent blood from entering. The clip remains in place for life. Eventually, the bulge will shrink.

If the artery has been damaged by the aneurysm, an occlusion and bypass surgical procedure may be performed. The affected artery is closed off, and a new route that allows circulation to bypass the damage is created. The artificial development of an embolism, known as **endovascular embolization**, is another treatment option. A variety

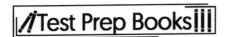
of substances such as plastic particles, glue, metal, foam, or balloons are coiled and inserted into the aneurysm to block blood flow.

A liquid embolic surgical glue is a new option to the standard coiling procedure: Onyx HD 500 is a vinyl alcohol copolymer that solidifies on contact with the blood in the aneurysm, sealing it. In the case of smaller aneurysms, a watch-and-wait approach may be taken. Bleeding, vasospasm, seizures, and hydrocephalus are the main complications related to a brain aneurysm.

Spleen

The **spleen** plays an important role in the regulation of red blood cells. The filtration action of the spleen removes worn-out or damaged red blood cells and microbes. It is also an important organ in the immune system, producing the white blood cells that fight infection and synthesize antibodies.

Although very rare, the spleen is the third most common site of an aneurysm. The exact cause of a splenic arterial aneurysm is unknown. However, the aneurysm represents a damaged splenic artery. Portal hypertension and multiple pregnancies produce an increase in intra-abdominal pressure that is thought to damage the splenic artery, leading to the formation of an aneurysm. Trauma and autoimmune disease are also known causes.

A splenic aneurysm is generally asymptomatic and found incidentally on diagnostic studies. An aneurysm of the splenic artery is treated by clipping.

Dissection

Dissection is a condition in which the layers of the arterial wall become separated and blood leaks in between the layers of the vessel. A dissection represents damage through at least the first layer of an artery. It is a more serious form of aneurysm because all the layers are compromised.

A dissection is different from a rupture. With a dissection, blood leaks in and through the layers of an artery, but the artery remains structurally intact, albeit weakened. Blood is still contained within the vessel. When a rupture occurs, it is similar to the popping of a balloon. The integrity of the artery is disrupted, and blood leaks out of the artery. Dissections increase the risk of rupture. Medical management with beta-blockers is the treatment of choice for stable aortic dissections.

Summary

Symptoms of an aneurysm/dissection may be absent, vague, or difficult to identify. The consequences of a rupture are life-threatening. The expert clinician will ascertain a thorough patient and family history, including social factors and lifestyle choices. Autoimmune disorders, age, gender, a sedentary lifestyle, smoking, and drug or alcohol abuse are contributing factors to the development of an aneurysm. Rapid assessment, diagnosis, and treatment are essential. Vital signs, neurological status, and loss of consciousness should be closely monitored.

Dysrhythmias

Dysrhythmia, also known as **arrhythmia**, is abnormal electrical activity of the heart. The abnormal heartbeat may be irregular, too fast, or too slow.

Normally, the electrical conduction system of the heart begins with an impulse known as the **action potential** at the pacemaker sinoatrial (SA) node. The impulse travels across the right and left atria before activating the atrioventricular (AV) node.

Cardiac Conduction Cycle

A.

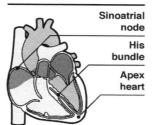

Sinoatrial node

His bundle

Apex heart

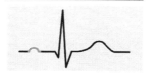

An electrical impulse travels from the sinoatrial node to the walls of the atria, causing them to contract.

B.

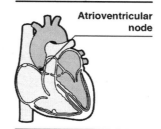

Atrioventricular node

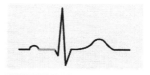

The impulse reaches the atrioventricular node, which delays it by about 0.1 second.

C.

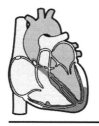

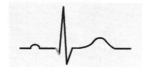

Bundle branches carry signals from the atrioventricular node to the heart apex.

D.

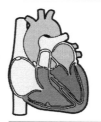

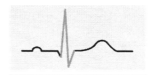

The signal spreads through the ventricular walls, causing them to contract.

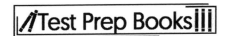
The pathway from the SA to the AV node is visualized on the ECG as the P wave. From the AV node, the impulse continues down the septum along cardiac fibers. These fibers are known as the **bundle of His**. The impulse then spreads out and across the ventricles via the Purkinje fibers. This is represented on the ECG as the QRS complex. The T wave represents the repolarization or recovery of the ventricles.

Electrical Events of the Cardiac Cycle

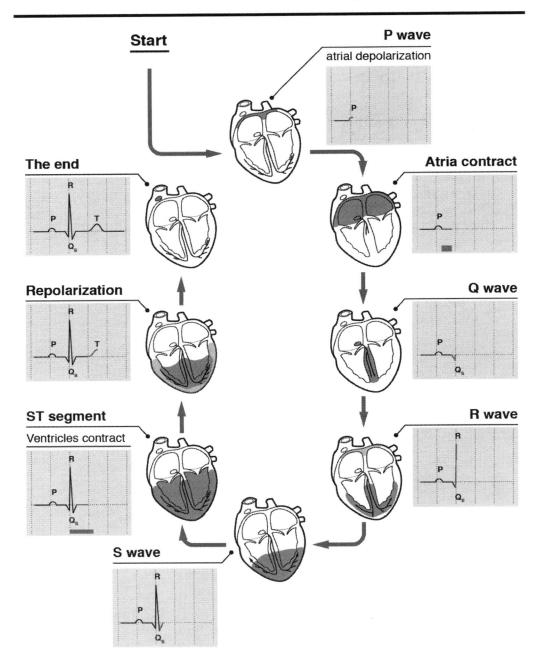

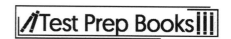

Properties of Cardiac Cells

Cardiac cells have four important properties: excitability, conductivity, contractility, and automaticity. **Excitability** allows the heart to respond to stimuli and maintain homeostasis. **Conductivity** is the ability to transfer the electrical impulse initiated at the SA node across cardiac cells. **Contractility** is the cardiac cells' ability to transform an action potential into the mechanical action of contraction and relaxation. **Automaticity** is the ability of cardiac cells to contract without direct nerve stimulation. In other words, the heart initiates its own impulse. If the SA node fails to initiate the impulse, the AV node will fire the impulse at a slower rate. If neither the SA nor the AV node fires the impulse, the cells within the bundle of His and the Purkinje fibers will fire to start the impulse at an even slower rate.

Action Potential

The **action potential** is a representation of the changes in voltage of a single cardiac cell. Action potentials are formed as a result of ion fluxes through cellular membrane channels, most importantly, the sodium (Na+), potassium (K+), and calcium (Ca+) channels. Electrical activity requires an action potential. Contraction of the cardiac muscle fibers immediately follows electrical activity.

Phases of an Action Potential

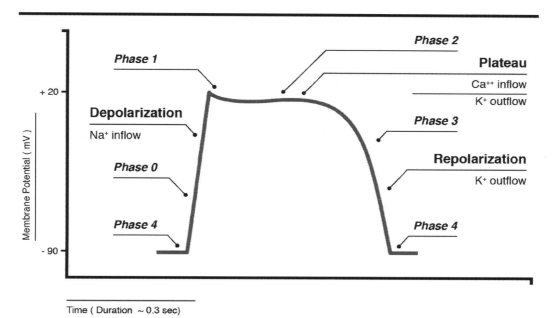

Phase 0: Depolarization

- Rapid Na+ channels are stimulated to open.

- The cardiac cell is flooded with Na+ ions, which change the transmembrane potential.

- The shift in potential is reflected by the initial spike of the action potential.

- Depolarization of one cell triggers the Na+ channels in surrounding cells to open, which causes the depolarization wave to propagate cell by cell throughout the heart.

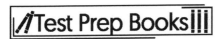

Phases 1–3: Repolarization phases

During these phases, represented as the plateau, Ca+ and some K+ channels open.

Ca+ flows into the cells, and K+ flows out.

The cell remains polarized, and the increased Ca+ within the cell trigger contraction of the cardiac muscle.

Phase 4: Completion of repolarization

- Ca+ channels close.
- K+ outflow continues.
- The cardiac cell returns to its normal state.

The cardiac cycle of **atrial depolarization-ventricular depolarization-repolarization** is represented on the ECG by the P wave, QRS complex, and T wave. A dysrhythmia can occur anywhere along the conduction system. It can be caused when an impulse from between the nodes or fibers is delayed or blocked. Arrhythmias also occur when an ectopic focus initiates an impulse, thereby disrupting the normal conduction cycle. Additional sources of damage to the conduction system include MIs, hypertension, coronary artery disease (CAD), and congenital heart defects.

Overview of Dysrhythmias

Abnormalities in the electrical conduction system of the heart may occur at the SA node, the AV node, or the His-Purkinje system of the ventricles. Careful evaluation of the ECG will aid in determining the location and subsequent cause of the dysrhythmia.

Dysrhythmias that occur above the ventricles in either the atria or the SA/AV nodes are known as **supraventricular dysrhythmias**. Common arrhythmias in this category are sinus bradycardia, sinus tachycardia, atrial fibrillation, atrial flutter, junctional rhythm, and sustained supraventricular tachycardia (SVT). **Atrioventricular** (AV) **blocks**, known as **heart blocks**, occur when the impulse is delayed or blocked at the AV node. The three types of heart block are first degree, second degree, and third degree, with first degree being the least severe and third degree being the most severe.

Ventricular dysrhythmias can be life-threatening because they severely impact the heart's ability to pump and maintain adequate cardiac output (CO). A bundle branch block (BBB), premature ventricular complexes (PVCs), sustained ventricular tachycardia (V-tach), ventricular fibrillation (V-fib), Torsades de pointes, and digoxin-induced ventricular dysrhythmias are the most common ventricular arrhythmias.

Supraventricular Dysrhythmias

Sinus Bradycardia

Sinus bradycardia occurs when the SA node creates an impulse at a slower-than-normal rate—less than 60 beats per minute (bpm). Causes include metabolic conditions, calcium channel blockers (CCB) and beta-blocker medications, MIs, and increased intracranial pressure. If symptomatic, treatment involves transcutaneous pacing and atropine.

Sinus Tachycardia

Sinus tachycardia occurs when the SA node creates an impulse at a faster-than-normal rate, also characterized as a rate greater than 100 bpm. Causes include physiological stress such as shock, volume loss, and heart failure as well as medications and illicit drugs. Sinus tachycardia is typically treated by treating the underlying cause.

Atrial Fibrillation

Atrial fibrillation is the most common sustained dysrhythmia. It is caused when multiple foci in the atria fire randomly, thereby stimulating various parts of the atria simultaneously. The result is a highly irregular atrial rhythm. Ventricular rate may be rapid or normal. Fatigue, lightheadedness, chest pain, dyspnea, and hypotension may be

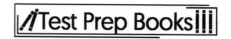
present. Treatment goals are to improve ventricular pumping and prevent stroke. Beta-blockers and CCBs impede conduction through the AV node, thereby controlling ventricular rates, so they are the medications of choice. Cardioversion and ablation are also treatment options.

Atrial Fibrillation and Flutter ECG Tracings

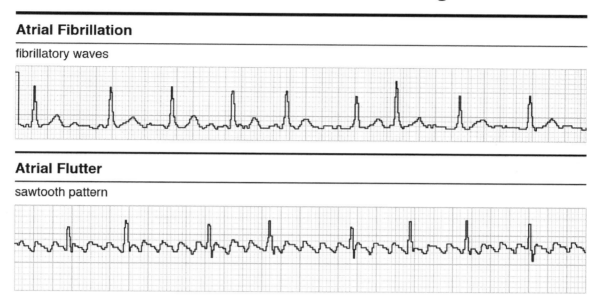

Atrial Flutter

Atrial flutter is caused by an ectopic atrial focus that fires between 250 and 350 times a minute. The AV node is unable to transmit impulses at that speed, so typically only one out of every two impulses reach the ventricles. Cardioversion is the treatment of choice to convert atrial flutter back to a sinus rhythm. CCBs and beta-blockers are used to manage ventricular rates.

Junctional Dysrhythmias

If either the SA node slows or its impulse is not properly conducted, the AV node will become the pacemaker. The heart rate for an impulse initiated at the AV junction will be between 40 and 60 bmp. The P wave will be absent on an EKG. Suggested treatment is similar to that of sinus bradycardia: transcutaneous pacing, atropine, and epinephrine.

Supraventricular Tachycardia

Sustained **supraventricular tachycardia** (SVT) is usually caused by an AV nodal reentry circuit. Heart rate can increase to 150 to 250 bpm. Interventions that increase vagal tone such as the Valsalva maneuver or carotid massage may slow the heart rate. Beta-blockers and CCBs may be given intravenously for immediate treatment or may be taken orally to prevent reoccurrence.

Heart Block

In **first-degree heart block**, the impulse from the SA node is slowed as it moves across the atria. On an ECG, the P and R waves will be longer and flatter. First-degree block is often asymptomatic.

Second-degree heart block is divided into two categories known as Mobitz type I and Mobitz type II. In Mobitz type I, the impulse from the SA node is increasingly delayed with each heartbeat until eventually a beat is skipped

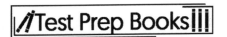

entirely. On an ECG, this is visible as a delay in the PR interval. The normal PR interval is 0.12–0.20. The PR interval will get longer until the QRS wave does not follow the P wave. Patients may experience mild symptoms with this dysrhythmia.

When some of the impulses from the SA node fail to reach the ventricles, the arrhythmia is a Mobitz type II heart block. Some impulses move across the atria and reach the ventricles normally, and others do not. On an ECG, the QRS follows the P wave at normal speed, but some QRS complexes are missing because the signal is blocked. Patients experiencing this dysrhythmia usually need a pacemaker.

A **third-degree heart block** is also known as complete heart block, or complete AV block. The SA node may continue to initiate the impulses between 80 and 100 bpm, but none of the impulses reach the ventricles. The automaticity of cardiac cells in the Purkinje fibers will prompt the ventricles to initiate an impulse; however, beats initiated in this area are between 20 and 40 bpm. The slower impulses initiated from the ventricles are not coordinated with the impulses from the SA node. Therefore, third-degree heart block is a medical emergency that requires a temporary to permanent pacemaker.

Bundle Branch Block

A **bundle branch block** (BBB) occurs when there is a delay or defect in the conduction system within the ventricles; a BBB may be designated as "left" or "right" to specify the ventricle at fault or as "complete" or "partial." The QRS complex will be widened or prolonged. Treating the underlying cause is the goal.

Premature Ventricular Complex

A **premature ventricular complex** (PVC) occurs when a ventricular impulse is conducted through the ventricle before the next sinus impulse. This may be caused by cardiac ischemia, heart failure, hypoxia, or hypokalemia. Treatment is to correct the cause, and long-term treatment is not indicated unless the patient is symptomatic.

Ventricular Tachycardia

Ventricular tachycardia (V-tach) occurs from a single, rapidly firing ectopic ventricular focus that is typically at the border of an old infarct (MI). This dysrhythmia is usually associated with CAD. Ventricular rates can be 150 to 250 bpm. However, the heart cannot pump effectively at those increased rates. Immediate cardioversion is the treatment of choice. Antidysrhythmic medications such as amiodarone, lidocaine, or procainamide may be given. An implantable cardioverter defibrillator (ICD) may be necessary.

Ventricular Tachycardia and Fibrillation ECG Tracings

VT - Ventricular Tachycardia

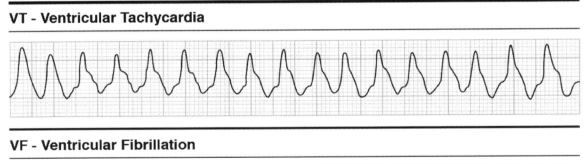

VF - Ventricular Fibrillation

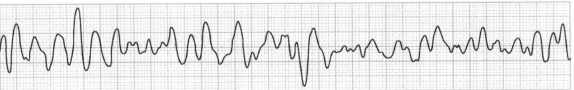

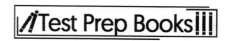
Ventricular Fibrillation

Ventricular fibrillation (V-fib) is a life-threatening emergency that requires immediate treatment. It is caused by multiple ventricular ectopic foci firing simultaneously, which forces the ventricles to contract asynchronously. Coordinated ventricular contraction is impossible in this scenario. The result is reduced cardiac output, and defibrillation is required. Lidocaine, amiodarone, and procainamide may be used.

Torsade de Pointes

Torsade de pointes is an atypical rapid undulating ventricular tachydysrhythmia. This rhythm has a prolonged QT interval. A variety of drugs cause QT-interval prolongation. The treatment is intravenous magnesium and cardioversion for sustained V-tach.

Torsade de Pointes ECG Tracing

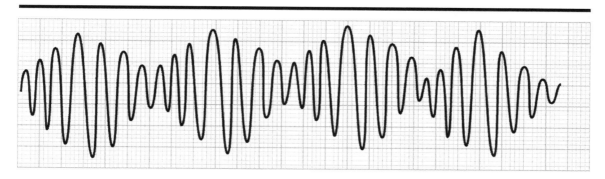

Digoxin-Induced Ventricular Dysrhythmias

Digoxin is a cardiac glycoside medication that increases the strength and regularity of the cardiac rhythm. It has a very narrow therapeutic range. Toxicity occurs when therapeutic levels are exceeded. Digoxin toxicity can mimic all types of dysrhythmias. Digoxin acts by increasing automaticity in the atria, ventricles, and the His-Purkinje system. It also decreases conduction through the AV node. Therefore, an AV block is the most common form of presenting dysrhythmia in the general population. Among the elderly, chronic toxicity is common as well, as it can be easily caused by drug-to-drug interactions and declining renal function.

Summary

Dysrhythmias range from asymptomatic to life-threatening. They can be divided into three major groups: supraventricular dysrhythmias, heart block, and ventricular dysrhythmias. Treatment is necessary when ventricular pumping and cardiac output are impacted. There are two phases of treatment. The first is to terminate the dysrhythmia using medications, defibrillation, or both. The second is long-term suppression with medications.

A complete medical history with an emphasis on current medications, comorbidities, and family history is paramount. Immediate nursing priorities include establishing IV access, monitoring vital signs, and administering oxygen as needed. Evaluation of the ECG, chest x-ray, and both laboratory and diagnostic values is required. Defibrillation, cardioversion, and transcutaneous pacing are other possibilities.

Endocarditis

By definition, endocarditis is the inflammation of the endocardium, or innermost lining of the heart chambers and valves. It is also called **infective endocarditis** or **bacterial endocarditis**.

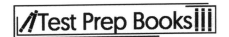
To review, there are three layers of tissue that comprise the heart. A double-layer serous membrane, known as the **pericardium**, is the outermost layer. The pericardium forms the pericardial sac that surrounds the heart. The middle and largest layer is the **myocardium**. Since an MI occurs when the heart muscle is deprived of oxygen, the myocardial layer of the heart is where the damage due to lack of oxygen occurs. The innermost layer that lines the heart chambers and also the heart valves is called the **endocardium**. Endocarditis occurs when the endocardial layer and heart valves become infected and inflamed.

The most common cause of endocarditis is a bloodstream invasion of bacteria. **Staphylococci** and **Streptococci** account for the majority of infective endocarditis occurrences. During medical or dental procedures—such as a colonoscopy, cystoscopy, or professional teeth cleaning—bacteria may enter the bloodstream and travel to the heart. Inflammatory bowel disease and sexually transmitted diseases also foster bacterial transmission to the bloodstream and, ultimately, the heart.

Risk factors for the development of endocarditis include valve and septal defects of the heart, an artificial heart valve, a history of endocarditis, an indwelling long-term dialysis catheter, parenteral nutrition or central lines in the right atrium, IV drug use, and body piercings. Patients taking steroids or immunosuppressive medications are susceptible to fungal endocarditis. Regardless of the source, the bacteria infect the inside of the heart chambers and valves. Clumps of infective bacteria, or vegetation, develop within the heart at the site of infection. The heart valves are a common infection site, which often results in incomplete closure of the valves.

The classic symptoms of endocarditis are fever, cardiac murmur, petechial lesions of the skin, conjunctiva, and oral mucosa. However, symptoms can range in severity. Flu-like symptoms, weight loss, and back pain may be present. Dyspnea and swelling of the feet and ankles may be evident. Endocarditis caused by Staphylococcus has a rapid onset, whereas Streptococcus occurs more slowly with a prolonged course.

Layers of the Heart Wall

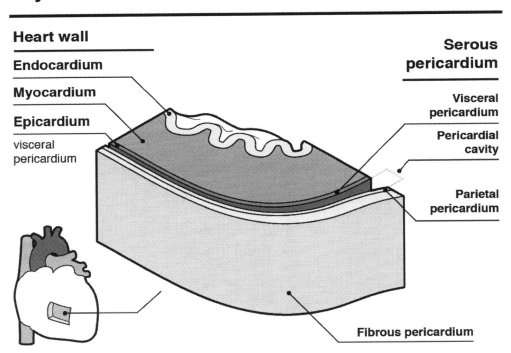

Antimicrobial treatment for four to six weeks is the standard of care. In some cases, two antimicrobials are used to treat the infection and prevent drug resistance. The objective of treatment is to eradicate the infection and treat

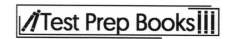
complications. Surgery may be required for persistent recurring infections or one or more embolic occurrences or if heart failure develops.

Left untreated, endocarditis can result in stroke or organ damage, as the vegetation breaks off and travels through the bloodstream and blocks circulation. The spread of infection and subsequent formation of abscesses throughout the body may also occur. Heart failure may develop when the infection hampers the heart's ability to pump effectively or with perforation of a valve.

A complete history and physical that includes inquiry about medications, recent surgeries, screening, and diagnostic testing may provide the crucial piece of information that identifies endocarditis in the face of otherwise vague symptom presentation. The nurse should anticipate the order for blood cultures, an erythrocyte sedimentation rate (ESR), a CBC, an ECG, a chest x-ray, and a transthoracic or transesophageal echocardiogram to identify the location of the infected area.

An in-depth patient interview and assessment by the nurse are essential. Diagnostic and laboratory results coupled with data from the patient interview will aid in early recognition and treatment of endocarditis. Because an incident of endocarditis places one at a higher risk for future infections, patient teaching should include informing all providers and dentists prior to treatment. Antibiotic prophylaxis may be indicated.

Heart Failure
Mechanism
Defined as the failure of the heart to meet the metabolic demands of the body, **heart failure** (HF) is a general term that refers to the failure of the heart as a pump. HF is a syndrome with diverse clinical features and various etiologies. The syndrome is progressive and often fatal. It may involve either or both sides of the heart. Based on ejection fraction (EF), it can be further categorized as diastolic or systolic HF.

Left-sided HF is also referred to as congestive heart failure (CHF) because the congestion occurs in the pulmonary capillary beds. As mentioned previously, oxygenated blood flows from the pulmonary artery into the left atrium, then the LV, and into the aorta for distribution through the systemic circulation.

Once the oxygenated blood has been delivered to end-point tissues and organs, it arrives at the capillary bed. The now-deoxygenated blood begins the return journey back to the heart by passing from the capillary beds into small veins that feed into progressively larger veins and, ultimately, into the superior and inferior vena cava. The vena cava empties into the right atrium. From the right atrium, blood flows into the right ventricle and then into the pulmonary system for oxygenation.

When the right ventricle is impaired, it cannot effectively pump blood forward into the pulmonary system. The ineffective forward movement of blood causes an increase of venous pressure. When venous pressure rises, the blood backs up and leaks into the tissues and the liver. The end result is edema in the extremities and congestion within the liver.

When the LV is impaired, it cannot effectively pump blood forward into the aorta for systemic circulation. The ineffective forward movement of blood causes an increase in the pulmonary venous blood volume, which forces fluids from the capillaries to back up and leak into the pulmonary tissues. This results in pulmonary edema and impaired oxygenation.

Ejection fraction (EF) is the percentage of blood volume pumped out by the ventricles with each contraction. The normal EF is 50 to 70 percent. An EF of 60 percent means that 60 percent of the available blood volume was pumped out of the LV during contraction. It is an important measurement for diagnosing and tracking the progression of HF. The EF also differentiates between diastolic and systolic HF.

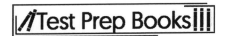

Diastolic HF is currently referred to as HF with normal ejection fraction (HFNEF). The heart muscle contracts normally, but the ventricles do not adequately relax during ventricular filling. In systolic HF, or heart failure with reduced ejection fraction (HFrEF), the heart muscle does not contract effectively, so less blood is pumped out to the body.

Variables

There are several variables that both impact and are impacted by HF. A review of these variables will provide the backdrop for a closer look at the classification, sequelae, symptoms, and treatment of HF.

Cardiac output (CO, or Q) is the volume of blood being pumped by the heart in one minute. It is the product of heart rate multiplied by stroke volume. **Stroke volume** (SV) is the amount of blood pumped out of the ventricles per beat; $CO = HR \times SV$. Normal CO is between four and eight liters per minute. Both CO and SV are reduced in HF.

Systemic vascular resistance (SVR) is related to the diameter and elasticity of blood vessels and the viscosity of blood. For example, narrow and stiff vessels and/or thicker blood will cause an increase in SVR. An increase in SVR causes the LV to work harder to overcome the pressure at the aortic valve. Conversely, larger and more elastic vessels and/or thin blood will decrease SVR and reduce cardiac workload.

Pulmonary vascular resistance (PVR) is the vascular resistance of the pulmonary circulation. It is the difference between the mean pulmonary arterial pressure and the left atrial filling pressure. Resistance and blood viscosity impact both SVR and PVR. However, pulmonary blood flow, lung volume, and hypoxic vasoconstriction are unique to the pulmonary vasculature.

Preload is defined as the amount of ventricular stretch at the end of diastole, or when the chambers are filling. In other words, preload is the amount of pressure from the blood that is being exerted against the inside of the LV. It is also known as left ventricular end-diastolic pressure (LVEDP) and reflects the amount of stretch of cardiac muscle sarcomeres. **Afterload** is the amount of resistance the heart must overcome to open the aortic valve and push the blood volume into the systemic circulation.

Classification

HF is closely associated with chronic hypertension, CAD, and diabetes mellitus. The New York Heart Association (NYHA) classification tool is most frequently used to categorize the stages and symptom progression of HF as it relates to heart disease:

- Stage I: Cardiac disease; no symptoms during physical activity
- Stage II: Cardiac disease; slight limitations on physical activity
- Stage III: Cardiac disease; marked limitations during physical activity
- Stage IV: Cardiac disease; unable to perform physical activity; symptoms at rest

Sequelae

HF may have an acute or chronic onset, but it is progressive. When CO is diminished, tissues are not adequately perfused, and organs ultimately fail. When the LV works harder because of increased preload or afterload, its muscular walls become thick and enlarged, resulting in ventricular hypertrophy. Ventricular hypertrophy causes ventricular remodeling (cardiac remodeling), which is a change to the heart's size, shape, structure, and physiological functioning.

The sympathetic nervous system responds to a diminished CO by increasing the heart rate, constricting arteries, and activating the renin-angiotensin-aldosterone system (RAAS). Elevated angiotensin levels raise BP and afterload, thereby prompting the heart to work harder. The reduced CO caused by HF can diminish blood flow to the kidneys. The kidneys respond to the decreased perfusion by secreting renin and activating the RAAS. As a result, the increase in aldosterone signals the body to retain Na+ and water. Retained Na+ and water leads to volume overload,

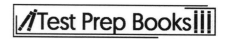
pulmonary congestion, and hypertension. The body's response to reduced CO caused by HF can perpetuate a downward spiral. However, there are naturally-occurring natriuretic peptides that are secreted in response to elevated pressures within the heart. These peptides counteract fluid retention and vasoconstriction.

Atrial natriuretic peptide (ANP) is secreted by the atria. **B-type natriuretic peptide** (BNP) is secreted by the ventricles. Both ANP and BNP cause diuresis, vasodilation, and decreased aldosterone secretion, thereby balancing the effects of sympathetic nervous system response and RAAS activation. Elevated levels of BNP are a diagnostic indication of HF.

Symptoms of Heart Failure

Either an MI or a dysrhythmia can precipitate HF. The clinical presentation reflects congestion in the pulmonary and/or systemic vasculature. Treatment depends on the clinical stage of the disease. Common symptoms include the following:

- Dyspnea on exertion
- Fatigue
- Pulmonary congestion, which causes a cough and difficulty breathing when lying down
- Feelings of suffocation and anxiety that are worse at night
- Peripheral edema

The most common cause of HF exacerbation is fluid overload due to nonadherence to sodium and water restrictions. Patient education is extremely critical to avoiding and managing exacerbations. Congestive heart failure is a core measure, tied to patient satisfaction, patient education, subsequent readmissions in a defined period of time, and ultimately, to reimbursements.

Treatment

Therapy for HF focuses on three primary goals: reduction of preload, reduction of afterload (SVR), and inhibition of the RAAS and vasoconstrictive mechanisms of the sympathetic nervous system. Pharmacotherapy includes ACE inhibitors, angiotensin II receptor blockers (ARBs), diuretics, beta-blockers, vasodilators, and a cardiac glycoside.

The ACE inhibitors and ARBs interfere with the RAAS by preventing the body's normal mechanism to retain fluids and constrict blood vessels. Diuretics decrease fluid volume and relieve both pulmonary and systemic congestion. Beta-blockers and cardiac glycosides slow the HR and strengthen the myocardium to improve contractility. Vasodilators decrease SVR. In addition to a thorough physical exam and complete medical history, a clinical work-up will include a chest x-ray, a BNP and other laboratory values, an ECG, and perhaps an echocardiogram or MUGA scan to measure EF.

Summary

HF is a common debilitating syndrome characterized by high mortality, frequent hospitalizations, multiple comorbidities, and poor quality of life. A partnership between providers, nurses, and patients is paramount to managing and slowing disease progression. Patient education should include a discussion of the disease process, prescribed medications, diet restrictions, and weight management. Patients should know which symptoms require immediate medical care. Self-care can be the most important aspect of HF management. The nurse as educator performs an essential role in this and all disease management.

Hypertension

Hypertension (HTN) is an abnormally high BP (140/90 mmHg or higher). The diagnosis is based on two or more accurate readings that are elevated. HTN is known as "the silent killer" because it is asymptomatic. Several variables impact BP and understanding them is essential.

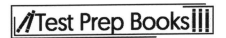
Variables

BP is the product of CO multiplied by SVR; *BP = CO × SVR*. CO is the volume of blood being pumped by the heart in one minute. It is the product of HR multiplied by SV; *HR × SV = CO*. SV is the amount of blood pumped out of the ventricles per beat.

SVR is related to the diameter of blood vessels and the viscosity of blood. The narrower the vessels or the thicker the blood, the higher the SVR. Conversely, larger-diameter vessels and thinner blood decrease SVR.

Mechanism

For HTN to develop, there must be a change in one or more factors affecting SVR or CO and a problem with the control system responsible for regulating BP. The body normally maintains and adjusts BP by either increasing the HR or the strength of myocardial contraction or by dilating or constricting the veins and arterioles.

When veins are dilated, less blood returns to the heart, and subsequently, less blood is pumped out of the heart. The result is a decrease in CO. Conversely, when veins are constricted, more blood is returned to the heart, and CO is increased. The arterioles also dilate or constrict. An expanded arteriole reduces resistance, and a constricted arteriole increases resistance. The veins and arterioles impact both CO and SVR. The kidneys contribute to the maintenance and adjustment of BP by controlling Na+, chloride, and water excretion and through the RAAS. Management of HTN will focus on one or more of the factors that regulate BP. Those regulatory factors are SVR, fluid volume, and the strength and rate of myocardial contraction.

Classification

HTN is classified as primary or secondary depending on the etiology. In **primary HTN**, the cause is unknown, but the primary factors include problems related to the natriuretic hormones or RAAS or electrolyte disturbances. Primary HTN is also known as essential or idiopathic HTN.

In **secondary HTN**, there is an identifiable cause. Associated disease states include kidney disease, adrenal gland tumors, thyroid disease, congenital blood vessel disorders, alcohol abuse, and obstructive sleep apnea. Products associated with secondary HTN are nonsteroidal anti-inflammatory drugs (NSAIDs), birth control pills, decongestants, cocaine, amphetamines, and corticosteroids.

HTN normally increases with age, and it is more prominent among African Americans. BP is classified according to treatment guidelines as normal, pre-HTN, Stage 1 HTN, and Stage 2 HTN. **Pre-HTN** is defined as systolic pressures ranging from 120 to 139 mmHg and diastolic pressures ranging from 80 to 89 mmHg. **Stage 1 HTN** ranges from 140 to 159 mmHg systolic and 90 to 99 mmHg diastolic pressures. In the more severe **Stage 2 HTN**, systolic pressures are 160 mmHg or higher, and diastolic pressures are 100 mmHg or higher.

Sequelae

Systolic pressure is the amount of pressure exerted on arterial walls immediately after ventricular contraction and emptying. This represents the highest level of pressure during the cardiac cycle. Diastolic pressure is the amount of pressure exerted on arterials walls when the heart is filling. This represents the lowest pressure during the cardiac cycle. In general, hypertension increases the risk of cardiovascular disease; diastolic HTN poses a greater risk.

Prolonged HTN damages the delicate endothelial layer of vessels. The damaged endothelium initiates the inflammatory response and clotting cascade. As mentioned, the diameter of veins, arterioles, and arteries changes SVR. When SVR is increased, the heart must work harder to pump against the increased pressure. In other words, the pressure in the LV must be higher than the pressure being exerted on the opposite side of the aortic valve by systemic vascular pressure. The ventricular pressure must overcome the aortic pressure for contraction and ventricular emptying to occur. When the myocardium works against an elevated systemic pressure for a prolonged period of time, the LV will enlarge, and HF may ensue.

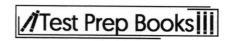
Risk Factors

There are both modifiable and nonmodifiable risk factors associated with the development of HTN. Modifiable risk factors include obesity, a sedentary lifestyle, tobacco use, a diet high in sodium, dyslipidemia, excessive alcohol consumption, stress, sleep apnea, and diabetes. Age, race, and family history are nonmodifiable risk factors.

Treatment

First-line treatments include lifestyle changes and pharmacologic therapy.

Initial therapy includes diuretics, CCBs, ACE inhibitors, and ARBs. Diuretics decrease fluid volume. CCBs decrease myocardial contractility. Both ACE inhibitors and ARBs interfere with the RAAS by preventing the normal mechanism that retains fluids and narrows blood vessels. The result is decreased volume and SVR.

Hypertensive Crisis/Emergency

A **hypertensive crisis** is defined as a BP higher than 180/120 mmHg. BP must be lowered quickly to prevent end organ damage. Pregnancy, an acute MI, a dissecting aortic aneurysm, and an intracranial hemorrhage are associated with a hypertensive crisis. The therapeutic goal is to reduce the BP by 25 percent within the first hour of treatment with a continual reduction over the following 2 to 6 hours and an ongoing reduction to the target goal over a period of days. Short-acting antihypertensive medications administered intravenously is the primary treatment.

Summary

The astute nurse will conduct an in-depth patient interview to identify prescribed and illicit drug use, alcohol and tobacco use, family history, sleep patterns, and dietary habits. Patient education should include information about the Dietary Approach to Stop Hypertension (DASH) diet and alcohol in moderation with a limit of one to two drinks per day. Aerobic exercise and resistance training three to four times weekly for an average of 40 minutes is recommended. Information about prescribed hypertensive medications should also be reviewed with the patient.

Pericardial Tamponade

Cardiac tamponade, or **pericardial tamponade**, is a syndrome caused by the excessive accumulation of blood or fluid in the pericardial sac, resulting in the compression of the myocardium and reduced ventricular filling. It is a medical emergency with complications of pulmonary edema, shock, and death, if left untreated.

The pericardium, or outer layer of the heart wall, is a two-layer membrane that forms the pericardial sac, which envelops the heart. The parietal (outer) layer of the pericardium is made of tough, thickened fibrous tissue. This layer is attached to the mid-diaphragm and to the back of the sternum. These attachments keep the heart in place during acceleration or deceleration. The fibrous nature of the parietal layer prevents cardiac distention into the mediastinal region of the chest.

The visceral (inner) layer of the pericardium is a double-layered membrane. One layer is affixed to the heart. The second layer lines the inside of the parietal (outer) layer. The small space between the parietal and visceral layers is the pericardial space. The space normally contains between 15 and 50 milliliters of pericardial fluid. The pericardial fluid lubricates the membranes and allows the two layers to slide over one another as the heart beats.

A pericardial effusion develops when excess blood or fluid accumulates in the pericardial sac. If the effusion progresses, a pericardial tamponade will ensue. Because the fibrous parietal layer prevents cardiac distention, the pressure from the excessive blood or fluid is exerted inward, compressing the myocardium and reducing space for blood to fill the chambers. The normally low-pressure right ventricle and atrium are the first structures to be impacted by tamponade. Therefore, signs of right-sided HF such as jugular vein distention, edema, and hepatomegaly may be present.

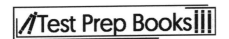
Symptoms of a pericardial tamponade are dyspnea, chest tightness, dizziness, tachycardia, muffled heart sounds, and restlessness. Pulsus paradoxus is an important clinical finding in tamponade; it represents an abnormal BP variation during the respiration cycle and is evidenced by a decrease of 10 mmHg or more in systolic BP during inspiration. Pulsus paradoxus represents decreased diastolic ventricular filling and reduced volume in all four chambers of the heart. The clinical signs associated with tamponade are distended neck veins, muffled heart sounds, and hypotension. These clustered symptoms are known as **Beck's triad**.

Removal of the pericardial fluid via pericardiocentesis is the definitive therapy. A pericardiectomy or pericardial window may be performed to remove part of the pericardium. Fluid removed during the procedure is analyzed to determine the cause of the effusion. Malignancies, metastatic disease, and trauma are major causes of the development of pericardial effusions.

Identification and treatment of a tamponade requires emergent medical intervention. A rapid focused assessment of heart sounds and BP, including assessing for pulsus paradoxus, is a critical first step. An in-depth medical and surgical history can aid in identifying the etiology.

Pericarditis

Pericarditis is inflammation of the pericardium, which forms the pericardial sac that surrounds the heart.

Layers of the Heart Wall

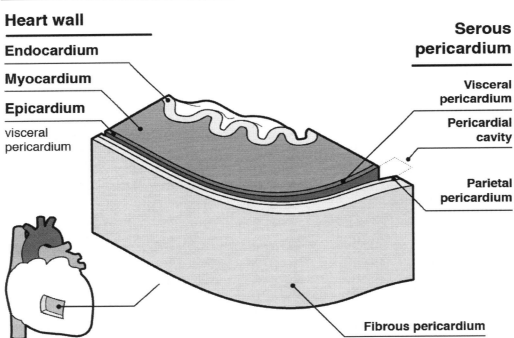

The pericardial sac consists of two layers. The pericardium, or outer layer of the heart wall, is a two-layer membrane that forms the pericardial sac, which envelops the heart.

The visceral (inner) layer of the pericardium is a double-layered membrane. One layer is affixed to the heart. The second layer lines the inside of the parietal layer (outer layer). The small space between the parietal and visceral

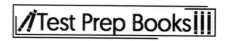

layers is the pericardial space. The space normally contains between 15 and 50 milliliters of pericardial fluid. The pericardial fluid lubricates the membranes and allows the two layers to slide over one another as the heart beats.

The parietal (outer) layer of the pericardium is made of tough, thickened fibrous tissue. This layer is attached to the mid-diaphragm and to the back of the sternum.

These attachments keep the heart in place during acceleration or deceleration. The fibrous nature of the parietal layer prevents cardiac distention into the mediastinal region of the chest. It separates the heart from the surrounding structures, and it protects the heart against infection and inflammation from the lungs. The pericardium contains pain receptors and mechanoreceptors, both of which prompt reflex changes in the BP and HR.

Pericarditis can be either acute or chronic in presentation. Causes are varied and include an acute MI; bacterial, fungal, and viral infections; certain medications; chest trauma; connective tissue disorders such as lupus or rheumatic fever; metastatic lesions from lung or breast tumors; and a history of radiation therapy of the chest and upper torso. Frequent or prolonged episodes of pericarditis can lead to thickening and scarring of the pericardium and loss of elasticity. These conditions limit the heart's ability to fill with blood and, therefore, limit the amount of blood being pumped out to the body. The result is a decrease in CO. Pericarditis can also cause fluid to accumulate in the pericardial cavity, known as **pericardial effusion**.

A characteristic symptom of pericarditis is chest pain. The pain is persistent, sharp, pleuritic, felt in the mid-chest, and aggravated by deep inhalation. Pericarditis may also cause ST elevation, thereby mimicking an acute MI, or it may be asymptomatic.

A pericardial friction rub is diagnostic of pericarditis. It is a creaky or scratchy sound heard at the end of exhalation. The rub is best heard when the patient is sitting and leaning forward. Stethoscope placement should be at the left lower sternal border in the fourth intercostal space. The rub is audible on auscultation and synchronous to the heartbeat. A pericardial friction rub is differentiated from a pleural friction rub by having patients hold their breath. The pericardial friction rub will remain constant with the heartbeat. Other presenting symptoms include a mild fever, cough, and dyspnea. Common laboratory findings are elevated white blood cell (WBC), ESR, or CRP levels.

The diagnosis of pericarditis is based on history, signs, and symptoms. Treatment goals are to determine the cause, administer therapy for treatment and symptom relief, and detect signs of complications. A thorough medical and surgical history will identify patients at risk for developing pericarditis. The physical assessment should evaluate the reported pain level during position changes, inspiration, expiration, coughing, swallowing, and breath holding. In addition, flexion, extension, and rotation of the neck and spine should be assessed for their influence on reported pain.

Peripheral Vascular Disease

Peripheral vascular disease (PVD) refers to diseases of the blood vessels that are outside the heart and brain. The term PVD is used interchangeably with **peripheral arterial disease** (PAD). It is the narrowing of peripheral vessels caused by atherosclerosis. The narrowing can be compounded by emboli or thrombi. Limb ischemia due to reduced blood flow can result in loss of limb or life. The primary factor for the development of PVD is atherosclerosis.

PVD encompasses several conditions: atherosclerosis, Buerger's disease, chronic venous insufficiency, deep vein thrombosis (DVT), Raynaud's phenomenon, thrombophlebitis, and varicose veins.

Risk Factors

CAD, atrial fibrillation, cerebrovascular disease (stroke), and renal disease are common comorbidities. Risk factors include smoking, phlebitis, injury, surgery, and hyperviscosity of the blood. Autoimmune disorders and

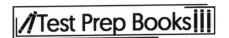

hyperlipidemia are also common factors. The two major complications of PVD are limb complications or loss and the risk for stroke or heart attack.

Symptoms

Intermittent claudication (cramping pain in the leg during exercise) may be the sole manifestation of early symptomatic PVD. It occurs with exercise and stops with rest. Physical findings during examination may include the classic five Ps: pulselessness, paralysis, paresthesia, pain, and pallor of the extremity.

The most critical symptom of PVD is critical limb ischemia (CLI), which is pain that occurs in the affected limb during rest. Manifestations of PVD may include the following symptoms:

- Feet that are cool or cold to the touch
- Aching or burning in the legs that is relieved by sitting
- Pale color when legs are elevated
- Redness when legs are in a hanging-down (dependent) position
- Brittle, thin, or shiny skin on the legs and feet
- Loss of hair on feet
- Nonhealing wounds or ulcers over pressure points
- Loss of muscle or fatty tissue
- Numbness, weakness, or heaviness in muscles
- Reddish-blue discoloration of the extremities
- Restricted mobility
- Thickened, opaque toenails

Diagnostics

The ankle-brachial index (ABI) should be measured. The ABI is the systolic pressure at the ankle, divided by the systolic pressure at the arm. It is a specific and sensitive indicator of peripheral artery disease (PAD). The Allen test looks for an occlusion of either the radial or ulnar arteries. A Doppler ultrasonography flow study can determine the patency of peripheral arteries.

The patient should be assessed for heart murmurs, and all peripheral pulses should be evaluated for quality and bruit. An ECG may reveal an arrhythmia. Because the presence of atherosclerosis initiates an inflammatory response, inflammatory markers such as the D-dimer, CRP, interleukin 6, and homocysteine may be present. Blood urea nitrogen (BUN) and creatinine levels may provide indications of decreased organ perfusion. A lipid profile may reveal the risk for atherosclerosis. A stress test or angiogram may be necessary.

Treatment

The two main goals for treatment of PVD are to control the symptoms and halt the progression to lower the risk of heart attack and stroke. Specific treatment modalities depend on the extent and severity of the disease, the patient's age, overall medical history, clinical signs, and their preferences. Lifestyle modifications include smoking cessation, improved nutrition, and regular exercise. Aggressive treatment of comorbidities can also aid in stopping the progression. Pharmacotherapy may include anticoagulants and vasodilators.

Summary

The primary factor in PVD is atherosclerosis. Prevention should begin early and be centered on balanced nutrition and exercise, alcohol in moderation, and smoking cessation. Once diagnosed, management of PVD will include preventive measures and the incorporation of pharmacotherapeutics. Providing patient education about proper diet and exercise should occur during every patient encounter. The conscientious nurse will take advantage of an encounter to improve patient outcomes through education and referral.

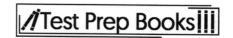

Thromboembolic Disease

In the simplest terms, a **thrombus** is a blood clot that forms in a vein. Clots can be caused by either a fat globule, gas bubble, amniotic fluid, or any foreign material that gets into the bloodstream. A DVT usually forms in the leg. A thrombus becomes an **embolus** when a fragment dislodges and travels through the circulatory system. The embolus will remain in the circulatory system until it reaches a vessel too narrow for its passage. An **embolism** occurs when the embolus lodges and prevents blood flow. In the cardiac cycle, veins begin at the capillary bed and get progressively larger as they return deoxygenated blood to the right side of the heart. From the right side of the heart, blood flows to the lungs.

A **pulmonary embolism** (PE) occurs when the embolus, or a fragment of the embolus, becomes lodged in the pulmonary circulation. A DVT frequently results in a PE. A **fat embolism** may form when fat globules pass into the small vessels and damage the endothelial lining. As the fat breaks down to free fatty acids, it causes toxic damage. When the damage occurs in the lungs, acute respiratory failure ensues.

Mechanism

A strong clinical link exists between clot formation and atherosclerosis, PAD, diabetes, and other factors contributing to heart disease. Anything that damages a vein's endothelial lining may cause a DVT to form. Damage to vessel lining can occur from smoking, cancer, chemotherapy, injury, or surgery. In addition to a damaged endothelial layer, increased age, dehydration, and viscous or slow-flowing blood increase the risk of DVT formation. Factors that slow blood flow are prolonged bed rest, sitting for extended periods, smoking, obesity, and HF. In the presence of atrial fibrillation, the atria do not empty adequately. Blood pools in the upper chambers, increasing the risk for clots to form.

Closed long-bone fractures carry a high risk for a fat embolism to develop because when the bone marrow is exposed as a result of a fracture, its particles can enter the bloodstream. Orthopedic procedures, a bone marrow biopsy, massive soft tissue injury, and severe burns are also associated with the development of an embolus. In addition, there are nontraumatic conditions associated with a fat embolism, such as prolonged corticosteroid therapy, pancreatitis, liposuction, fatty liver, and osteomyelitis.

Women who are pregnant or taking oral contraceptives are at risk for the development of an embolus. Estrogen increases plasma fibrinogen, some coagulation factors, and platelet formation, which lead to the hypercoagulability of the blood. During pregnancy, the expanding uterus can slow blood flow in the veins. The combined effects of hypercoagulability and slowed blood flow exacerbate the risk. During delivery, an embolus can form from the amniotic fluid and travel through maternal circulation. Therefore, during pregnancy and the subsequent postpartum period, women are at increased risk for DVT formation.

Symptoms

Swelling of the leg below the knee is a common symptom of a DVT. There may also be redness, tenderness, or pain over the area around the clot, but a DVT may be asymptomatic. When a DVT becomes a PE, the patient may experience difficulty breathing and a rapid HR. Reported symptoms may include chest pain, coughing up blood, fainting, and low BP. There is a 24- to 72-hour latent period from injury to onset in the development of a fat embolism.

Diagnosis and Treatment

The clinician will consider presenting signs and symptoms, the patient's and family's medical history, and an ultrasound to evaluate blood flow to identify a DVT. The differential diagnoses are pneumonia and a thrombus. A vena cava filter may be placed in the inferior vena cava to capture a clot or fragments. In life-threatening situations such as a PE, an IV thrombolytic may be used to break up the clot. Indications for thrombolytic therapy are chest pain lasting longer than 20 minutes, ST elevation in two leads, and less than 6 hours from the pain's onset. However,

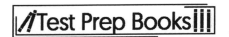

thrombolytic medications are absolutely contraindicated in a patient with active bleeding. Prior to the administration of a thrombolytic, the international normalized ration (INR) must be calculated to determine clotting time. In healthy people, an INR of 1.1 or below is considered normal. An INR range of 2.0 to 3.0 is an effective acceptable therapeutic range for people taking warfarin.

For long-term management, patient education should include anticoagulant medication therapy, the use of compression stockings, and avoidance of tight clothing. Patients should be instructed to regularly elevate their feet, avoid prolonged periods of sitting, and increase their exercise to counteract slowed blood flow.

Trauma

The causes of trauma can be categorized into three types, according to their potential degree of injury: penetrating injuries, blunt nonpenetrating injuries, and medical injuries that occur during an invasive procedure. **Penetrating injuries** are associated with knife and gunshot wounds. **Blunt nonpenetrating** injuries are most commonly due to automobile accidents. **Medical injuries** may occur during the implantation of a medical device, an endomyocardial biopsy, the placement of a Swan-Ganz catheter, and cardiopulmonary resuscitation (CPR).

Trauma is evaluated according to a prioritized systematic assessment approach that starts with the primary survey and proceeds to the secondary survey. The findings gathered during the surveys in conjunction with the type of injury identified will direct the treatment approach.

Types of Injuries

A penetrating injury is categorized by the mechanism of injury as low, medium, or high velocity. A knife wound is low velocity, disrupting just the surface penetrated. A handgun wound, or medium-velocity injury, damages more than the penetrated surface, but less than a high-velocity injury. A high-velocity injury is related to rifles and military weapons.

Penetrating chest trauma comprises a broad spectrum of injury and severity. Any structure within the thoracic cavity may be impacted, such as the heart and great vessels, the tracheobronchial tree, the esophagus, the diaphragm, and surrounding bony structures.

The following conditions may result from penetrating chest trauma: hemothorax, pneumothorax, or pneumomediastinum. These conditions compromise oxygenation and ventilation. A diaphragmatic rupture, pulmonary contusion, rib or sternal fractures, and esophageal or thoracic tears may be present.

A blunt nonpenetrating injury can also affect any of the components of the thoracic cavity. The major damage from both penetrating and nonpenetrating injuries involves derangement in the flow of air, blood, or both. If esophageal perforations are present, alimentary contents may leak into the bloodstream, causing sepsis. Blunt injuries can be further categorized according to the area of impact:

- Chest wall fractures, dislocations, or diaphragmatic injuries
- The pleural lining, the lungs, and upper digestive tract
- The heart, great arteries, veins, and lymphatics

Trauma Survey

The **primary survey** begins with the ABCDE resuscitation system: airway, breathing, circulation, disability or neurological status, and exposure. Adjuncts to the primary survey are x-rays, an EKG, laboratory testing, and the focused assessment with sonography in trauma (FAST) examinations.

Trauma patients may not be able to provide a historical account or verbalize symptoms. Injuries within the thoracic cavity can quickly become life-threatening. Hypoxia and hypoventilation are the major causes of death in chest trauma. Therefore, the FAST examinations can provide a timely diagnosis when compared to older methods of

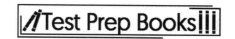

assessment. Blood and fluid tend to pool in dependent areas within the body. The primary FAST examination includes the hepatorenal recess (Morison's pouch), the perisplenic view, the subxiphoid pericardial window, and the suprapubic window (pouch of Douglas). The extended version (E-FAST) incorporates additional views of the thoracic cavity to assess for hemothorax and pneumothorax. These specific views can rapidly identify injuries and bleeding in the pericardial, pleural, and peritoneal areas. The ease and noninvasiveness of the FAST approach allows for serial examinations to observe changes and monitor progression.

The **secondary survey** incorporates the physical assessment beginning with the ample history acronym. Allergies; medication; past illnesses; last meal; and events, environment, or mechanism of injury are assessed. The head-to-toe physical assessment should be done using inspection, auscultation, percussion, and palpation, as appropriate.

The head, face, and neck are first assessed for injury. The presence of Battle's sign or raccoon eyes may indicate intracranial bleeding. Central nervous system function is evaluated using the Glasgow Coma Scale (GCS). Motor, verbal, and eye responses are graded from total paralysis (3) to normal strength (15). Next, the chest, abdomen, pelvis, perineal, rectal, and genital areas are assessed for injury. Finally, the neurovascular status of the musculoskeletal system is evaluated.

In addition to sonographic and physical assessments, trauma scoring systems are used by clinicians to identify the severity of the trauma and to guide treatment, ensure continuous quality improvement, and direct future research.

Severity Scoring

Scoring the level of injury in a trauma patient has several applications, and there are a variety of tools available for use. **Field trauma** scoring can guide prehospital triage decisions, reduce time of transfer and treatment, and maximize resources. It also serves as a quality assurance measure between facilities and during transfer.

Trauma scoring tools are categorized according to the data points they evaluate as either physiologic, anatomical, or combined.

Physiologic Scoring Tools

The **Revised Trauma Score** (RTS) is the most common physiologic scoring tool in use. The RTS combines three parameters: the GCS, systolic blood pressure (SBP), and respiratory rate (RR). The best motor or eye-opening response can be substituted for the GCS in the presence of central nervous system influences such as drugs or alcohol.

Revised Trauma Score			
Coded Value	**GCS**	**Systolic Blood Pressure (mmHg)**	**Respiratory Rate (breaths per minute)**
0	3	0	0
1	4-5	< 50	< 5
2	6-8	50-75	5-9
3	9-12	76-90	> 30
4	13-15	> 90	10-30

The **Acute Physiology and Chronic Health Evaluation** (APACHE II) scoring tool incorporates the chronic health evaluation and comorbid conditions with the Acute Physiology Score (APS).

The **Emergency Trauma Score** (EMTRAS) uses patient data that is quickly available, and it does not require knowledge of anatomic injuries. EMTRAS comprises patient age, GCS, base excess, and prothrombin time (PT) to accurately predict mortality.

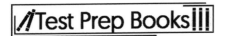
Anatomic and Combined Scoring Tools

The **Injury Severity Score** (ISS) tool is based on the Abbreviated Injury Scale (AIS). The ISS uses an anatomical scoring system to give an overall score for patients who have sustained multiple injuries, each of which is assigned an AIS score. Only the highest AIS score for each of six different body regions (head, face, chest, abdomen, extremities and pelvis, and external) is used. The ISS tool grades the severity of injury from minor injury (1) to lethal injury (6); the three most severely injured body regions have their score squared and added together to produce the ISS score. The Trauma and Injury Severity Scoring (TRISS) tool combines ISS, RTS, and the age of the patient to grade severity and predict mortality.

Summary

Regardless of the cause or degree of injury, the astute clinician begins the assessment with the primary survey. The secondary survey focusing on the head-to-toe physical assessment also includes evaluation of the FAST examination, x-rays, laboratory testing, and severity scoring tools. Although there is no universally accepted tool for scoring the severity of trauma, there are many valid tools. Coupled with clinician judgment, the assessment findings and severity scoring tools can improve and predict mortality.

Shock
Cardiogenic Shock

The clinical definition of **cardiogenic shock** is decreased CO and evidence of tissue hypoxia in the presence of adequate intravascular volume. It is a medical emergency and the most severe expression of LV failure. It is the leading cause of death following an MI with mortality rates between 70 and 90 percent without aggressive treatment. When a large area of the myocardium becomes ischemic, the heart cannot pump effectively. Therefore, SV, CO, and BP drastically decline. The result is end-point hypoperfusion and organ failure. Characteristics of cardiogenic shock include ashen, cyanotic, or mottled extremities; distant heart sounds; and rapid and faint peripheral pulses. Additional signs of hypoperfusion such as altered mental status and decreased urine output may be present.

Work-Up/Treatment

The key to survival in cardiogenic shock is rapid diagnosis, supportive therapy, and coronary artery revascularization. Diagnosis is based on clinical presentation, cardiac and metabolic laboratory studies, chest x-ray, ECG, echocardiogram, and invasive hemodynamic monitoring. Treatment is the restoration of coronary blood flow and correction of electrolyte and acid-base abnormalities.

Obstructive Shock

Obstructive shock occurs when the heart or the great vessels are mechanically obstructed. A cardiac tamponade or massive PE is a frequent cause of obstructive shock. Systemic circulatory collapse occurs because blood flow in or out of the heart is blocked. Generalized treatment goals for shock are to identify and correct the underlying cause. In the case of obstructive shock, the goal is to remove the obstruction.

Treatment begins simultaneously with evaluation. Stabilization of the airway, breathing, and circulation are primary, followed by fluid resuscitation to increase BP. Vital signs, urine flow, and mental status using the GCS should be monitored. Shock patients should be kept warm. Serial measurements of renal and hepatic function, electrolyte levels, and ABGs should be monitored.

Summary

Shock is characterized by organ blood flow that is inadequate to meet the oxygen demands of the tissue. The management goal for shock is to restore oxygen delivery to the tissues and reverse the perfusion deficit. This is accomplished through fluid resuscitation, increasing CO with inotropes, and raising the SVR with vasopressors.

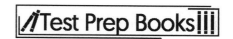

Endocrine and Immunological

Endocrine Conditions

The endocrine system is responsible for hormone production and messaging. These hormones are produced by glands through the brain and body. They regulate a vast number of mental, emotional, and physiological functions, such as mood, growth, metabolism, sleep, sexual function, and reproduction. Consequently, some pathological conditions can have system-wide repercussions.

Adrenal Conditions

Located on top of each kidney, the adrenal glands are responsible for producing a number of hormones. These include sex hormones, such as DHEA and androstenedione; corticosteroids, such as cortisol; and mineralocorticoids, such as aldosterone. These hormones influence sexual function, metabolism, electrolyte balance, blood volume, blood pressure, immunity, and stress management. Dysfunctional conditions of the adrenal glands include the following:

- Cushing's syndrome: This disease results from an excess of glucocorticoid, which is responsible for producing steroids that manage inflammation and other stresses in the body. One example of a glucocorticoid is cortisol. Symptoms of Cushing's syndrome include excessive weight gain that cannot be managed, excessive growth of body hair, high blood pressure, and decreased elasticity in the skin. This disease is typically treated with medication that controls hormone production. In severe cases, adrenal surgery may be required.

- Addison's disease: This disease may be referred to as adrenal insufficiency. It results when the adrenal glands produce insufficient amounts of glucocorticoids and mineralocorticoids. Mineralocorticoids are another group of steroids influencing electrolyte and fluid balance. This can be the result of an underlying autoimmune disorder or systemic infection. Symptoms include fatigue and skin discoloration. Addison's disease is usually treated with steroid injections but may become a medical crisis if the patient goes into shock, a stupor, or a coma. This can occur if the patient does not realize he or she has the disease, as some of the primary symptoms can be quite generic.

- Conn's syndrome: This disease is characterized by excess aldosterone production. Symptoms include hypertension, muscle cramping, weakness, dehydration, and excessive thirst. It is usually treated by surgically removing any tumors on the adrenal glands, and the patient may be asked to minimize table salt consumption. If Conn's syndrome goes untreated, it can result in serious cardiovascular and kidney disease.

- Adrenal tumors: The presence of malignant or benign tumors on the adrenal glands may affect hormone production, which can cause one of the above disorders to develop.

Glucose-Related Conditions

The endocrine system handles processes related to the metabolism of glucose. Disorders relating to glucose include the following:

- Diabetes mellitus: This is a condition that affects how the body responds to the presence of glucose. Glucose is needed for cell functioning, and all consumable calories eventually are converted to glucose in the body. A hormone produced by the pancreas, called **insulin**, is needed to break down food and drink into glucose molecules. In patients with type 1 diabetes, the pancreas fails to produce insulin, leading to high levels of glucose in the bloodstream. This can lead to organ damage, organ failure, or nerve damage. Patients with type 1 diabetes receive daily insulin injections or have a pump that

81

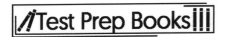
continuously monitors their blood insulin levels and releases insulin as needed. These patients need to be careful to not administer excess insulin, as this will cause their blood sugar to become too low. Low blood sugar can lead to fainting and exhaustion and may require hospitalization.

- In patients with type 2 diabetes, the pancreas produces insulin, but the body is unable to use it effectively. Patients with type 2 diabetes typically need to manage their condition through lifestyle changes, such as losing weight and eating fewer carbohydrate-rich and sugary foods. There are also some medications that help the body use the insulin that is present in the bloodstream. Gestational diabetes is a form of diabetes that some women develop during the second to third trimester of pregnancy, when their systems temporarily become resistant to insulin. High blood sugar in a pregnant woman can affect fetal growth and influence the baby's risk of becoming obese. Pregnant women with gestational diabetes are encouraged to exercise daily, avoid excessive weight gain, and carefully monitor their diet. Gestational diabetes is similar to type 2 diabetes in the way symptoms present and in treatment options.

- Diabetic Ketoacidosis: This is an acute complication that primarily occurs in patients with type 1 diabetes who lack adequate insulin. When the body does not have enough insulin in the blood to break down macronutrients into glucose, it defaults to breaking down fatty acids into ketones for energy. This typically does not cause major issues in a person who does not have diabetes, as eventual insulin production and uptake will balance the level of ketones in the blood. In a patient with diabetes who cannot produce enough insulin, the body will continue to release fatty acids into the bloodstream. Eventually, this will result in too many ketones in the blood and will shift the body's pH level to an excessively acidic one. This is a crisis situation, and the patient may eventually go into a coma if left untreated. Symptoms include dehydration, nausea, sweet-smelling breath, confusion, and fatigue. Treatment includes oral or IV electrolyte and insulin administration. Diabetic ketoacidosis can occur with type 2 diabetes but occurs more frequently with type 1 diabetes. Often, a ketoacidosis event is the first indicator that a person may have diabetes.

- Glycogenoses: **Glycogenoses** refer to a number of hereditary disorders in which the body is unable to convert stored glycogen to glucose when glucose is needed by the body. This inability is the result of the absence of an enzyme, although the specific enzyme that is missing can vary from patient to patient. Symptoms include growth and development issues, kidney stones, confusion, and general weakness. More severe cases can result in chronic gout, seizures, coma, intestinal sores, and kidney failure. These disorders are usually treated by timing carbohydrate consumption so that blood sugar levels remain stable throughout the day.

- Metabolic Syndrome/Syndrome X: **Metabolic syndrome**, or **Syndrome X**, refers to the presence of comorbid cardiovascular and insulin-related conditions. Patients diagnosed with metabolic syndrome must have three or more of the following conditions: hypertension, elevated fasting blood glucose levels, low HDL cholesterol, high triglycerides, and excess belly fat. This syndrome is believed to result from insulin resistance, causing high blood glucose, insulin, and lipid levels. Patients with metabolic syndrome tend to be overweight or obese and at an increased risk of organ failure, heart attacks, and strokes. They often suffer from another underlying condition, such as diabetes or polycystic ovary syndrome, that leads to metabolic syndrome. Metabolic syndrome is often treated with prescription medications that lower cholesterol and blood pressure, but diet and exercise changes are strongly recommended. Weight loss is a key component in managing metabolic syndrome.

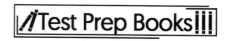
Diabetic Situations

Diabetes is a common diagnosis among patients in the United States. It is a disease in which the body's natural insulin response to blood glucose is compromised, causing hyperglycemia. **Hyperglycemia** is a dangerously high blood sugar that can damage the organs and tissues of the body.

The nurse will become accustomed to taking care of patients with diabetes. These patients may have a special diabetic diet that restricts or counts carbohydrates; may need blood sugar levels taken before meals, upon rising, and before going to bed, depending on their specific orders; and will need special care in case their blood sugar becomes dangerously low or high.

Insulin is a hormone secreted by the pancreas in the body. No other organ secretes insulin. The **pancreas** is positioned behind the stomach in the body, making it conveniently situated to assist with the absorption and distribution of glucose that enters the body. Glucose enters the body through the food that one eats, is a type of sugar, and is necessary for metabolic functioning in the body. Insulin works in the blood stream to allow glucose to be absorbed into the cells of the body.

When the insulin response is compromised, as is the case in diabetes, it is no longer effective in moving glucose from the bloodstream into the cells of the body. The glucose then accumulates in the blood stream with nowhere to go, and the resulting state is called **hyperglycemia.** The cells of the body need glucose to survive and are unable to function if they are unable to obtain glucose from the bloodstream.

There are two main types of diabetic emergencies: **hypoglycemia**, in which the blood sugar is too low; and **hyperglycemia**, in which the blood sugar is too high.

Hypoglycemia is when the blood sugar of a patient drops below 70 milligrams per deciliter (mg/dL). Patients may develop this if they have had too much insulin or have not ingested enough dietary glucose. This can sometimes occur in a hospital or facility if a patient misses meals due to scheduled tests or procedures. The nurse should be vigilant about the patient getting regular meals or adjusting insulin dosages.

Symptoms of hypoglycemia include decreased level of consciousness, tremors, fatigue, excessive sweating, dizziness, and syncope (fainting). The patient may also become anxious, report blurred vision and/or a headache, or have slurred speech.

If the medical-surgical nurse sees signs of hypoglycemia, they should expect to collect a blood glucose reading and a set of vital signs. The nurse will likely administer prescribed oral glucose, IV dextrose, or perhaps parenteral glucagon to correct the blood sugar.

Hyperglycemia is a blood sugar level greater than 200 milligrams per deciliter. Normal blood sugar recommendations are usually between 70 and 130 milligrams per deciliter, but symptoms of hyperglycemia may not manifest until the blood sugar level is greater than 200 milligrams per deciliter. Hyperglycemia may go unnoticed since the patient may not have symptoms of high blood sugar. It is therefore important to obtain blood sugar levels as necessary, even if the patient is not showing symptoms.

Hyperglycemia can be caused by the patient not having adequate insulin and/or anti-diabetic medication management, ingesting more glucose than normal, illness that changes normal routine, or a personal crisis that has occurred causing emotional stress in the body.

The medical-surgical nurse should recognize the most common symptoms of hyperglycemia: an increased need to urinate, called **polyuria**, and excessive thirst, called **polydipsia**. If hyperglycemia has caused complications such as **diabetic ketoacidosis** (an acidotic metabolic state in the body), a patient may display these two symptoms, as well as nausea, abdominal pain, fruity-scented breath, and/or confusion.

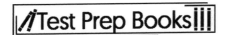

Diabetic ketoacidosis is a metabolic imbalance that can cause a condition called **diabetic coma**, when the blood sugar becomes so high that the patient loses consciousness. If diabetic coma is not treated, the patient may not survive.

If signs and symptoms of either hypoglycemia or hyperglycemia are present in the patient, the medical-surgical nurse must stabilize the patient's blood glucose.

Thyroid Conditions

Located at the front of the throat, the thyroid is one of the most influential glands in the endocrine system. The hormones it produces are involved in a multitude of functions throughout the body, including an assortment of metabolic, muscle, and digestive functions. Thyroid hormones also play a key role in neurological processes. When thyroid conditions develop, they can cause systemic effects. Testing for thyroid conditions goes beyond simply testing thyroid hormone levels. It can also include a physical exam, blood tests to determine how much thyroid-stimulating hormone (TSH) is being produced by the pituitary gland, tests to determine blood antibody levels, ultrasounds to check for tumors, and uptake tests to determine the rate at which the thyroid uses iodine.

Hyperthyroidism

When patients are diagnosed with **hyperthyroidism**, they may also be referred to as having an **overactive thyroid**, which results in the overproduction of T4 and/or T3 hormones. Symptoms include feelings of anxiety, trouble focusing, feeling overheated, gastrointestinal problems such as diarrhea, insomnia, elevated heart rate, and unexplained weight loss. Hyperthyroidism is commonly caused by Grave's disease, an autoimmune disorder. The extent to which symptoms of Grave's disease manifest can be broad, depending on the severity of the disease. Family history, stress, smoking, and pregnancy can increase the risk of developing Grave's disease. Women under the age of forty are most likely to be diagnosed. Medical treatment options can include methimazole and propylthiouracil, two common antithyroid medications. Prescription corticosteroids may also be used. In nonpregnant patients, radioactive iodine may be used. This is a long-term, repeat-dose solution that can sometimes result in hypothyroidism, which can be easier to treat. In serious cases, some or all of the thyroid may be removed, although this also usually results in hypothyroidism. It is also recommended that most patients with Grave's disease modify their lifestyle to limit stress, eat a healthy diet, and exercise regularly.

Hypothyroidism

When patients are diagnosed with **hypothyroidism**, they may also be referred to as having an underactive thyroid, which results in the underproduction of T4 and/or T3 hormones. Symptoms include depression, excessive fatigue, chills, dry skin, lowered heart rate, gastrointestinal problems such as constipation, and unexplained weight gain. Hypothyroidism is commonly caused by Hashimoto's disease, another autoimmune disease that affects thyroid functioning. This disease is usually treated with synthetic thyroid hormone replacement therapy, which involves taking a daily dose of the T4 hormone. T3 supplementation is rare, as it is derived from T4. Hypothyroidism can also be caused by the presence of too much iodine. The thyroid uses iodine to make T4 and T3 hormones. If there is too much iodine in the blood, the pituitary gland releases less TSH. The low levels of TSH can later result in the thyroid not producing enough T4 and/or T3 hormones. In some cases of hypothyroidism, surgery is required.

Goiter

A **goiter** refers to any enlargement in the thyroid gland. Goiters can occur in healthy thyroids or in thyroids producing abnormal levels of hormones. Their presence can indicate a lack of iodine, an autoimmune disease, an injury, or cancer.

Thyroid Cancer

Thyroid cancer is rare but can result in goiters and thyroid dysfunction. Thyroid cancer is more common in people who have nodes or goiters already present on the thyroid, which later turn malignant. The disease is also more prevalent in people who have been exposed to radiation. Thyroid cancer is usually treated through surgery, and thyroid hormone replacement therapy is a part of follow-up treatment.

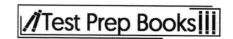
Immunocompromised Patients

An **immunocompromised** person refers to any individual who has a less than optimally functioning immune system. This could be the result of a genetic disorder, a viral or cancerous disease, medication, injury, surgery, age, or nutrition. An immunocompromised person is more susceptible to infection and illness than someone whose immune system is functioning optimally.

HIV/AIDS

The human immunodeficiency virus (HIV) is a sphere-shaped virus that is a fraction of the size of a red blood cell. There are primarily two types of HIV: HIV-1 and HIV-2. HIV-2 is not highly transmissible and is poorly understood. It has mainly affected people in West Africa. HIV-1 is more severe and more highly transmissible. It is the dominant strain among global HIV cases, and when literature and media refer to HIV, this is usually the type that is being referred to.

HIV is highly contagious. It is found in human bodily fluids and can be transmitted through infected breast milk, blood, mucus, and sexual fluids. The most common forms of transmission are through anal or vaginal sex, but transmission can also occur through contaminated syringe use, blood transfusions, or any other method where membranes are compromised. Once in the body, HIV attacks and destroys CD4/T cells. These cells are responsible for attacking foreign bodies (e.g., bacteria, infections, other viruses). As the body's CD4/T-cell count diminishes, the patient is left immunocompromised.

The HIV-1 type can be broken further into four groups: M, N, O, and P. M is the most commonly seen group globally. Within group M, there are nine different subtypes of HIV. These are noted as A, B, C, D, E, F, G, H, J, and K. Subtype B is prevalent in the Western world, and most research has been conducted on this subtype. This research has led to the manufacturing of antiretroviral (ARV) drugs. Antiretroviral therapy (ART) has been a major breakthrough in the management of HIV and in the quality of life for patients with HIV. In conjunction with medical care, many patients with HIV are able to have completely normal, healthy, active lives. It is important to treat HIV as early as possible. The better a patient's HIV is managed, the lower their viral load. Viral load refers to how much HIV is present in a patient's blood; when a viral load is low, transmission of the disease is far less likely to occur. With ART, many patients with HIV are viral-suppressed, and some even have an undetectable viral load. Viral load in other transmitting fluids, such as semen, cannot be detected but the virus is still present. Therefore, transmission is still possible, and all precautions should be taken.

Globally, most HIV patients have subtype C, but subtypes are mixing as travel and migration become more widespread. Most subtypes can be treated with ART, though these drugs were researched and manufactured to treat subtype B. However, ART is not always physically available or financially accessible in countries that need it most.

Without early intervention or adequate managed care of HIV, the virus can deteriorate the host body's immune system to a point where it cannot be rehabilitated. This stage is marked by extremely low levels of CD4/T cells (less than two hundred cells per cubic millimeter of blood) and is referred to as **acquired immunodeficiency syndrome (AIDS)**. When a patient's HIV diagnosis progresses to AIDS, he or she often succumbs to serious chronic diseases, such as cancer. Mild illnesses, such as a cold or flu, can also be fatal to someone with AIDS. Not everyone who is diagnosed with HIV will also be diagnosed with AIDS. Once diagnosed with AIDS, the patient has approximately one to three years to live unless he or she receives adequate treatment.

Patients Receiving Chemotherapy

Chemotherapy is a broad term referring to the use of drugs in cancer treatment. This type of therapy is intended to target and treat the entire body, especially in advanced stages of cancer where malignant cells may be widespread. However, it may also be used in earlier stages of cancer to eliminate many of the cancerous cells. This is done with the intention that the patient will go into remission and potentially not experience cancer again in the future. If this

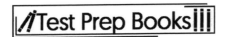

does not seem like a viable prognosis, chemotherapy can be used to control early stages of cancer from advancing. In advanced stages of cancer, chemotherapy can be used to manage pain and suffering from cancerous tumors, even if the patient's prognosis is poor.

The aggressiveness of chemotherapy (such as which drugs are used, dosing amount, and frequency) is contingent on many factors, such as the type and stage of cancer. Chemotherapy treatment plans also consider the patient's personal and medical history. Since this form of treatment is so aggressive, it is often effective in reducing or eliminating cancer cells. However, chemotherapy can also kill healthy cells in the process. The intensity of this side effect varies by person, but almost all patients experience some degree of immunocompromise. This is because chemotherapy almost always inadvertently targets bone marrow, where white blood cells are made.

White blood cells, especially neutrophils, play an important role in fighting infection. When there are not enough white blood cells present in the patient's blood, he or she can become seriously ill from sickness or infection that would be mild in a healthy person. Medical personnel usually monitor neutrophil counts during and between chemotherapy cycles to make sure these levels do not fall too low. Chemotherapy cycles can last up to six months, and patients are considered to have a compromised immune system for the entire time they are undergoing chemotherapy. Once a full cycle of chemotherapy ends, it takes approximately one month for the immune system to return to its normal state.

Patients undergoing chemotherapy should be especially mindful of personal hygiene habits such as handwashing and showering, as well as avoiding cuts, scrapes, insect bites, or other instances where the skin may break. They may also need help taking care of a pet and handling pet waste or other trash. Additionally, it is important to practice extra caution when handling foods, such as cooking meats well, avoiding unpasteurized foods, washing produce with produce cleaner, cooking many foods that typically could be eaten raw, and avoiding certain moldy cheeses. They also need to be more careful of their surroundings in public places; since these areas tend to be dirtier and more populated, there is an increased risk of contracting infections. Medical personnel and those visiting the patient should be aware of these practices as well.

Urological/Renal

Genitourinary

Foreign Bodies

The emergency care of the male patient who presents with purulent or mucopurulent penile discharge, dysuria, hematuria, or painful intercourse is focused on identifying the cause. Prompt treatment is necessary to prevent renal damage and systemic complications. In addition to obtaining routine lab studies and cultures, the provider will inquire if the patient has a recent history of catheterization of the urethra due to medical intervention or self-induced. Anecdotal reports indicate that insertion of foreign bodies into the urethra for autoerotic purposes is a rare occurrence, and in most cases, is associated with preexisting psychiatric disease.

Depending on the dimensions of the object, a local reaction may not be apparent immediately, which means that any infection may be advanced by the time the patient seeks treatment. The diagnosis is most often identified by the physical examination and patient report. Diagnostic imaging studies and laboratory data are collected to assess the extent of infection and inflammation and to determine the optimal method for retrieval of the foreign body. Common methods of retrieval include endoscopy, surgical removal by suprapubic cystotomy, and urethrotomy. Treatment for localized effects of the existence of the foreign body will include antimicrobial therapy appropriate to results of the cultures and referral for psychiatric care. If the condition has progressed beyond the urethra and bladder, aggressive management is necessary to prevent sepsis.

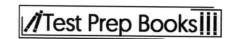

Infection

Infections of the male genitourinary (GU) tract are considered to be complicated infections because the infective process has overcome the naturally robust defenses of the male urinary tract. Common conditions resulting in infection include the inflammation of the prostate gland, epididymis, testes, kidney, bladder, and urethra; unprotected sexual intercourse; and the use of urinary catheters. Additional contributing factors to the incidence of infection include a history of previous urinary tract infections (UTIs), enlargement of the prostate gland, changes in voiding habits such as the onset of nocturia, comorbid diabetes or HIV infection, immunosuppressive therapy, and previous surgical intervention of the urinary tract. Painful urination, defined as *dysuria*, is the most common presenting manifestation, and complaints of coexisting dysuria, urinary frequency, and urgency are considered to be 75 percent predictive for UTI. Additional manifestations are dependent on the cause but may include fever, tachycardia, flank pain, suprapubic pain, penile discharge, scrotal masses and tenderness, and enlargement of the inguinal lymph nodes.

The diagnosis depends on the patient's history; presenting manifestations and physical examination; cultures of the urine, penile discharge, and blood; and assessment of kidney function. If obstruction of any portion of the urinary tract is suspected, additional diagnostic studies may include ultrasound, CT scans, and IV pyelogram (IVP). The infection will be treated with third-generation antimicrobial therapy, fluid resuscitation, antipyretics, analgesics, and urinary analgesics. The successful treatment of sexually transmitted infections requires adherence to the agent-specific medication regimen and the protocol for the treatment of all sexual partners and follow-up care. Emergency care of the patient with a UTI is focused on prompt identification of any obstructive pathology, treatment of infection and pain, preservation of kidney function, and prevention of systemic disease.

Priapism

Priapism is a urological emergency manifested by the enlargement of the penis that is unrelated to sexual stimulation and is unrelieved by ejaculation. Low-flow priapism is the most common form and is not associated with evidence of trauma but is due to dysfunction of the detumescence mechanism that is responsible for the relaxation of the erect penis. High-flow priapism results from abnormal arterial blood to the penis as a result of trauma to the GU system. The cause of low-flow priapism is most often idiopathic; however, the most common cause of the condition in children is sickle cell disease. Additional conditions that may cause this form of priapism include dialysis, vasculitis, spinal cord stenosis, bladder and renal cancer, and some medications, including heparin, cocaine, and omeprazole. High-flow priapism is due to straddle injuries or, most commonly, injury to the arteries of the penis by the injection of medications into the vasculature of the penis.

Prompt treatment of low-flow priapism within 12 hours of the onset of symptoms is necessary to prevent long-term alterations in erectile function. The primary cause is identified and treated if possible, followed by aspiration of fluid from the corpora cavernosa at the base of the penis, with or without saline irrigation, which is an effective treatment in 30 percent of cases. If aspiration and irrigation are unsuccessful, a vasoconstrictive agent such as phenylephrine can be instilled at 5-minute intervals until the erection is entirely resolved. If these interventions fail to eradicate the priapism, temporary or permanent surgical placement of a shunt between the corpus cavernosum and the glans penis or corpus spongiosum is necessary to restore venous drainage. Treatment of high-flow priapism involves cauterization and/or evacuation of areas of bleeding. Emergency treatment is focused on identification of the specific condition and prompt resolution of the erection.

Renal Calculi

Nephrolithiasis is defined as the process of stone or calculi formation in the pelvis of the kidney. The pain associated with this condition is referred to as **renal colic** and most often reflects the stretching and distention of the ureter when the stone leaves the kidney. The most common cause is insufficient fluid intake that concentrates stone-forming substances in the kidney. In order of occurrence, calculi are composed of calcium (75 percent) due to increased absorption of calcium by the GI tract, struvite (15 percent) as a result of repeated UTIs, uric acid (6

87

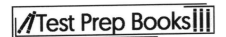

percent) due to increased purine intact, and cysteine (1 percent) due to an intrinsic metabolic defect in susceptible individuals. In addition, AIDS medications, some antacids, and sulfa drugs are also associated with stone formation. Renal calculi are more common in men than women, are associated with obesity and insulin resistance, and have a familial tendency.

Diagnosis is based on the patient's history and physical examination. Common lab studies include CBC, coagulation studies, kidney function tests, and C-reactive protein. Imaging studies may include ultrasonography, KUB films, and CT scans. Treatment options are based on the likelihood that the stone will be expelled spontaneously from the urinary system, given the size and location of the stone. Common interventions include aggressive fluid management, antimicrobial therapy, and pain management. If necessary, to prevent mechanical damage to the organs or the progression of the condition to urosepsis, the stone may be surgically removed, or the patient may undergo extracorporeal shock wave lithotripsy. The emergency care is focused on preventing damage to the urinary tract, restoring fluid volume, managing pain, and preventing progression of the illness to systemic urosepsis. Patient education regarding the essential follow-up care is critical to the prevention of recurrent calculi formation.

Torsion

Torsion refers to the abnormal twisting of the structures of the spermatic cord, which results in ischemia in the ipsilateral testicle that causes irreversible damage to fertility if not relieved within 6 hours. The condition is most common in infants, due to the mobility of the undescended testicles, and in adolescents, due to the abnormal attachment of fascia and muscles to the spermatic cord. The Testicular Workup for Ischemia and Suspected Torsion (TWIST) is the scoring system used to quantify the risk associated with the condition. The TWIST is used by emergency providers and then validated by the physician, most commonly a urologist, and the score is based on swelling of the testicle, hardened texture of the testicle, absence of the cremasteric reflex, nausea and vomiting, and placement of the testicles at a higher than normal position in the scrotum. The resulting risk factor may be low, intermediate, or high. A low TWIST score may indicate an alternative cause for the patient's manifestations. An intermediate risk requires the use of ultrasound to confirm the diagnosis, while the patient with a high-risk TWIST score requires immediate surgical intervention to prevent long-term dysfunction.

Nonoperative treatments include manual manipulation of the testicle guided by Doppler imaging. If the procedure is successful, surgical stabilization of the spermatic cord structures is required. Immediate surgical repair is required if the procedure is unsuccessful. If the affected testicle is nonviable and is removed, a testicular prosthesis will be inserted after wound healing is complete. Analgesics and antianxiety medications will be included in the treatment plan. Caregivers must be aware that the condition can reoccur. Emergency care of the patient requires immediate intervention based on the calculation of the TWIST score to prevent necrosis of the affected testicle.

Trauma

Organs of the GU tract include the bladder, urethra, and external genitalia, all of which are subject to varied sources of trauma. The bladder is commonly injured by blunt trauma that results from pelvic fractures and is also affected less commonly by penetrating trauma. The different segments of the male urethra can be injured as a result of pelvic fractures, straddle-type injuries, or from penetrating injuries that may be self-inflicted. The penis and scrotum are subject to blunt trauma, often due to sports injuries and other varied injuries that may be self-inflicted.

The diagnosis depends on the history of the precipitating event and the physical examination. Trauma to the GU tract may not be life-threatening; however, the GU injuries are often secondary to other injuries affecting the pelvis, spine, kidney, and abdomen, which warrant immediate attention. Common lab studies include CBC, prothrombin time, type and cross match, and urinalysis. Ultrasonography and CT scans are used in addition to studies specific to the bladder and testes, which include retrograde urethrogram, retrograde cystogram, and nuclear med studies. Established prehospital trauma care is required. Emergency treatment is aimed at identifying and correcting the underlying injury and preserving the function of the GU tract and includes fluid replacement, antimicrobial therapy,

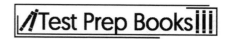
and pain management. Referrals to urologists, orthopedists, and other specialists must be made as necessary. In the event of self-inflicted injuries, psychiatric referrals are also appropriate.

Urinary Retention

Urinary retention may be acute or chronic and is defined as cessation of urination or incomplete emptying of the bladder. It occurs more often in older men, and common causes include prostate gland enlargement, neurogenic bladder due to diabetes or other chronic diseases, urethral strictures and other anatomic abnormalities, and the use of anticholinergic medications. Urinary retention in younger men is most commonly due to pelvic or spinal cord trauma. Unrelieved urinary retention can result in urinary tract infections due to stasis of the urine or renal failure due to the retrograde pressure of the accumulated urine. Common manifestations include suprapubic distension, pain, a history of contributing neurological diseases, and possible systemic signs such as fever and tachycardia. The condition also may be asymptomatic or characterized by urinary frequency or overflow incontinence, with loss of small amounts of urine accompanied by sensations of bladder fullness.

Diagnosis depends on the patient's history, including the presence of causative conditions and physical examination. Common lab studies include CBC, BUN, creatinine, electrolytes, urinalysis, ultrasound, urodynamic testing, and cystoscopy. The emergency treatment of acute urinary retention is aimed at draining the accumulated urine, protecting kidney function, addressing the underlying issue, and preventing systemic effects and recurrence. Urethral or suprapubic catheterization or a percutaneous nephrostomy may be done to drain the urine from the bladder, while urethral catheterization can also be used to obtain urodynamic measurements and to evaluate postvoid volumes after treatment. Clean technique self-catheterization is done by patients with chronic urinary retention due to neurogenic causes. If surgical removal of a portion or all of the bladder is required to repair traumatic damage or to remove malignant tumors, a urinary diversion will be created to maintain kidney function.

Urinary Incontinence

The inability of the body to control voluntary sphincters is known as **incontinence**. One form of incontinence is the inability to control urine excretion, or **urinary incontinence**. An acute form of incontinence is known as **transient incontinence**, which lasts 6 months or less. Intra-abdominal pressure causes another form of urinary incontinence known as **stress incontinence**. **Overflow incontinence** occurs when the bladder is filled and can no longer hold urine. **Functional incontinence** is the lack of proper toileting. **Reflex incontinence** occurs when the body cannot feel the release of urine. **Total incontinence** happens when the urine loss is continuous and the patient does not have the ability to stop its flow.

Mixed incontinence occurs when a patient experiences one or more types of incontinence. Many factors can contribute to urinary incontinence. Some are medically induced, others are due to illness or an acute change in health status, and some are psychologically driven. Patients who are dehydrated may require intravenous fluids that increase fluid volume in the body. Diuretic medications that treat HTN are used to excrete excess fluid from the systemic circulation. This increases urine volume in the bladder. Activities that produce pressure in the intra-abdominal cavity, such as sneezing or coughing, can lead to stress incontinence. Obesity and pregnancy increase the weight that is pressed onto the bladder and can also lead to stress incontinence. The bladder empties when the stretch receptors along the bladder wall are activated by urine. The stretch receptors are controlled by the nervous system.

Patients who have spinal cord injuries or nerve damage do not have an intact nervous system, leading to overflow, or reflex incontinence. Patients who have conditions affecting orientation can have functional incontinence. Dementia, Alzheimer's, acute psychotic episodes, or confusion may lead to decreased toileting. Patients may not utilize the restroom appropriately and suffer incontinence in inappropriate places. Patients who suffer trauma or develop cancers in the pelvic area may have a urostomy. Artificial openings do not have sphincters. A urostomy does not provide control over urine excretion and is a form of total incontinence.

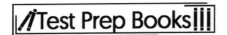

Musculoskeletal/Neurological/Integumentary

Dementia/Alzheimer's Disease

Dementia

Dementia is a general term used to describe a state of general cognitive decline. Although Alzheimer's disease accounts for up to 80 percent of all cases of dementia in the United States, the remaining two million cases may result from any one of several additional causes. The destruction of cortical tissue resulting from a stroke, or more commonly from multiple small strokes, often results in altered cognitive and physical function, while repetitive head injuries over an extended period also potentially result in permanent damage, limiting normal brain activity. Less common causes of dementia include infection of the brain by prions (abnormal protein fragments), as in Creutzfeldt-Jakob disease or the human immunodeficiency virus (HIV); deposition of Lewy bodies in the cerebral cortex as in Parkinson's disease; and reversible conditions such as vitamin B-12 deficiency and altered function of the thyroid gland. The onset and progression of the disease relate to the underlying cause and associated patient comorbidities.

Alzheimer's Disease

Alzheimer's disease is a chronic progressive form of dementia with an insidious onset that is caused by the abnormal accumulation of amyloid-β plaque in the brain. The accumulation of this plaque eventually interferes with neural functioning, which is responsible for the progressive manifestations of the disease. Although the exact etiology is unknown, environmental toxins, vascular alterations due to hemorrhagic or embolic events, infections, and genetic factors have all been proposed as the triggering mechanism for the plaque formation. The progression of the disease and the associated manifestations are specific to the individual; however, in all individuals, there is measurable decline over time in cognitive functioning, including short-term and long-term memory, behavior and mood, and the ability to perform activities of daily living (ADLs).

The diagnosis is based on the patient's presenting history and manifestations, imaging studies of the brain, protein analysis of the cerebrospinal fluid (CSF), and cognitive assessment with measures such as the Mini-Mental State Exam. Current treatments are only supportive, although cholinesterase inhibitors and N Methyl D aspartate receptor antagonists may slow the progression of the manifestations for a limited period if administered early in the course of the disease. All patients will suffer an eventual decline in all aspects of cognitive functioning, with the average survival rate dependent on the presence of comorbidities and the level of care and support available to the patient.

Experiencing a fall with or without a resulting fracture, somatic illnesses, and caregiver strain are the most common reasons for emergency department visits in this population. The nursing care of the patient with Alzheimer's disease must focus on patient safety because the environment of the hospital or facility can be disorienting to the confused patient. Safeguards against increased confusion and wandering, which is a common behavior in this patient population, should be implemented. In addition, the entire family unit should be assessed by the interdisciplinary health team to identify any alterations of family process or additional resources that are required for adequate patient care after discharge.

Chronic Neurological Disorders

Multiple Sclerosis

Multiple sclerosis (MS) is a chronic disease manifested by progressive destruction of the myelin sheath and resulting plaque formation in the central nervous system (CNS). The precipitating event of this autoimmune disease is the migration of activated T cells to the CNS, which disrupts the blood-brain barrier. Exposure to environmental toxins is considered to be the likely trigger for this immune response. These alterations facilitate the antigen-antibody reactions that result in the demyelination of the axons. The onset of this disease is insidious, with symptoms occurring intermittently over a period of months or years. Sensory manifestations may include numbness

90

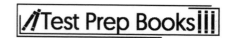

and tingling of the extremities, blurred vision, vertigo, tinnitus, impaired hearing, and chronic neuropathic pain. Motor manifestations may include weakness or paralysis of limbs, trunk, and head; diplopia; scanning speech; and muscle spasticity. Cerebellar manifestations include nystagmus, ataxia, dysarthria, dysphagia, and fatigue.

The progress of the disease and presenting clinical manifestations vary greatly from one individual to another; however, there are common forms of the disease that relate to the expression of the clinical manifestations or disability and the disease activity over time. An initial episode of neurological manifestations due to demyelination that lasts for at least 24 hours is identified as a clinically isolated episode of MS. The potential for progression of the disease to the relapsing-remitting form of MS is predicted by magnetic resonance imaging (MRI) studies indicating the presence or absence of plaque formation. The remaining forms of MS are all associated with increasing disability related to the disease over time. The relapsing-remitting form is common to 85 percent of all patients diagnosed with MS and presents a variable pattern of active and inactive disease. The manifestations may resolve, decrease in severity, or become permanent after a relapse. In the primary-progressive form of MS that affects 10 percent of patients diagnosed with MS, the disease is constantly active without periods of remission. The secondary-progressive form of MS is identified as the progression of the relapsing-remitting form to a state of permanently active disease without remission.

Acute exacerbations of MS are treated with interferon or another of the seven disease-modifying drugs (DMDs), which are used to decrease the frequency of relapses and slow the progression of the disease. Research indicates that the medications are most effective when therapy is begun as soon as the diagnosis is confirmed. Other treatments are symptomatic and may treat conditions such as bladder infections, gastrointestinal (GI) disorders, and muscle spasticity.

Patients with MS most commonly access care in the emergency department for non-neurological conditions, including GI disorders, falls, and bladder infections, and management of the manifestations associated with acute relapses.

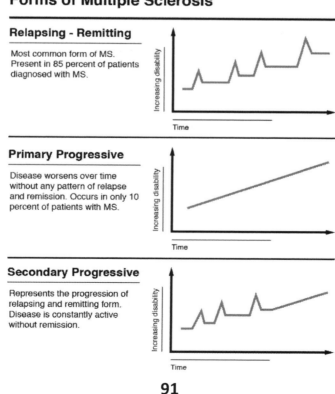

Forms of Multiple Sclerosis

Relapsing - Remitting

Most common form of MS. Present in 85 percent of patients diagnosed with MS.

Primary Progressive

Disease worsens over time without any pattern of relapse and remission. Occurs in only 10 percent of patients with MS.

Secondary Progressive

Represents the progression of relapsing and remitting form. Disease is constantly active without remission.

91

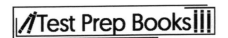

Myasthenia Gravis

Myasthenia gravis is also an autoimmune disease of the CNS that is manifested by severe muscle weakness resulting from altered transmission of acetylcholine at the neuromuscular junction due to antibody formation. Relapses and remissions are common, and these relapses may be triggered by infection, increases in body temperature due to immersion in hot water, stress, and pregnancy. Subjective manifestations include weakness, diplopia, dysphagia, fatigue on exertion, and bowel and bladder dysfunction. Objective manifestations include unilateral or bilateral ptosis of the eye, impaired respiratory function, impaired swallowing, and decreased muscle strength. Tensilon testing and electromyography, which measures muscle activity over time, are used to diagnose this disorder, while anticholinesterase agents and immunosuppressant agents are the mainstays of treatment. Additional treatments include plasmapheresis to decrease circulating antibodies and removal of the thymus gland to slow T-cell production.

Patients in myasthenic crisis due to a lack of cholinesterase may present with hypertension and severe muscle weakness that requires mechanical ventilation. Tensilon therapy may temporarily reduce the symptoms. Patients in cholinergic crisis due to an excess of cholinesterase exhibit hypotension, hypersecretion, and severe muscle twitching, which eventually results in respiratory muscle fatigue requiring ventilatory support. Atropine is used to control manifestations of this complication.

Guillain-Barré Syndrome

The most common form of **Guillain-Barré syndrome** (GBS) is acute immune-mediated demyelinating polyneuropathy. This rare syndrome may develop two to four weeks after a bacterial or viral infection of the respiratory or GI systems or following surgery. The most common causative organisms are *C. jejuni* and cytomegalovirus that may produce a subclinical infection that occurs unnoticed by the patient prior to the development of the acute onset of GBS. Other causative agents that are associated with GBS include the Epstein-Barr virus, *Mycoplasma pneumoniae*, and varicella-zoster virus. There is also an association between GBS and HIV. Current research is focused on investigating any association between the Zika virus and GBS; however, to date, there is little evidence of that relationship because there are few laboratories in the United States with the technology needed to identify the virus. The incidence of GBS has also been associated with vaccine administration; however, accumulated data does not support these claims.

The manifestations present as an acute onset of progressive, bilateral muscle weakness of the limbs that begins distally and continues proximally. The syndrome is the result of segmental demyelination of the nerves with edema, resulting from the inflammatory process. Additional presenting manifestations include pain, paresthesia, and abnormal sensations in the fingers. The progressive muscle weakness peaks at four weeks and potentially involves the arms, the muscles of the core, the cranial nerves, and the respiratory muscles. Involvement of the cranial nerves may result in facial drooping, diplopia, dysphagia, weakness or paralysis of the eye muscles, and pupillary alterations. Alterations in the autonomic nervous system also may result in orthostatic hypotension, paroxysmal hypertension, heart block, bradycardia, tachycardia, and asystole. Respiratory manifestations include dyspnea, shortness of breath, and dysphagia. In addition, as many as 30 percent of patients will progress to respiratory failure requiring ventilatory support due to the demyelination of the nerves that innervate the respiratory muscles.

The syndrome is diagnosed by the patient's history and laboratory studies to include electrolytes, liver function analysis, erythrocyte sedimentation rate (ESR), pulmonary function studies, and the assessment of CSF for the presence of excess protein content. In addition, electromyography and nerve conduction studies are used to identify the signs of demyelination, which confirms the diagnosis.

The emergency care of the patient with Guillain-Barré syndrome follows the Airway, Breathing, Circulation (ABC) protocol. Intubation with assisted ventilation is indicated in the event of hypoxia or decreasing respiratory muscle function as evidenced by an ineffective cough or aspiration. Cardiac manifestations vary according to the progression of the disease and are treated symptomatically. Placement of a temporary cardiac pacemaker may be

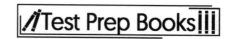

necessary to treat second- or third-degree heart block. Treatment with plasmapheresis to remove the antibodies and intravenous (IV) immunoglobulin (Ig) to interfere with the antigen expression must be initiated within two to four weeks of the onset of symptoms to induce progression to the recovery phase of the syndrome. Care of the patient in the recovery phase must also address the common complications of immobility. The healthcare team must be alert for the presenting manifestations that can progress rapidly to respiratory failure.

Headaches and Head Conditions

Temporal Arteritis

Temporal arteritis, also known as **giant cell arteritis**, is an inflammatory disorder of unknown origin that manifests as inflammatory changes in the intima, media, and adventitia layers of the artery as well as scattered accumulations of lymphocytes and macrophages that result in ischemic changes distal to the damaged areas. The condition is more common in women over fifty years of age, and current research indicates that infection and genetics also may be related to the development of the disease. The onset may be acute or insidious, and common signs and symptoms include head pain, neck pain, jaw claudication (jaw pain caused by ischemia of the maxillary artery), visual disturbances, shoulder and pelvic girdle pain, and general malaise and fever. The condition is diagnosed by a patient history of the onset of the headaches or the change in the characteristics of the headache in patients with chronic headaches, elevated ESR, and temporal artery biopsy that confirms the diagnosis. The condition is immediately treated with steroids if possible, or alternatively with cyclosporine, azathioprine, or methotrexate.

The onset of ophthalmic alterations requires emergency care because any loss of vision before treatment is initiated will be irreversible. In addition, if treatment is delayed beyond two weeks after the onset of the initial vision loss, vision in the unaffected eye will be lost as well. Additional complications are related to steroid therapy and include stroke, myocardial infarction, small-bowel infarction, vertebral body fractures, and steroid psychoses. Even with successful treatment that prevents irreversible vision alterations, the patient with temporal arteritis has a lifelong risk of inflammatory disease of the large vessels.

Migraine

Migraine headaches are often preceded by an aura, which may be visual or sensory. The pulsatile pain associated with migraine headaches is described as throbbing and constant and most often localizes to one side of the head. Other manifestations include photophobia, sound sensitivity, nausea and vomiting, and anorexia. The pain increases over a period of one to two hours and then may last from 4 to 72 hours. The exact cause of the migraine headache syndrome is not well understood; however, there is strong evidence of a genetic link and some support for the role of alterations in neurovascular function and neurotransmitter regulation. Risk factors include elevated C-reactive protein and homocysteine levels, increased levels of TNF-alpha and adhesion molecules (systemic inflammation markers), increased body weight, hypertension, impaired insulin sensitivity, and coronary artery disease. The diagnosis is determined by the patient's history, laboratory testing for inflammatory markers, and imaging studies and lumbar puncture, as indicated by the severity of the patient's condition.

The treatment for migraine headaches may be preventive, therapeutic, and/or symptomatic. Medications used to prevent migraine headaches are used for those patients with chronic disease who have fourteen or more headaches per month. Antiemetics are used to lessen nausea and vomiting, while opioids may be prescribed even though their use in migraine management is not recommended. The emergency care of the patient with a migraine headache is focused on establishing the differential diagnosis and correcting fluid volume alterations that may result from vomiting. Although most patients who seek care are diagnosed with migraine headaches, the importance of early intervention for temporal arteritis, stroke, or brain tumor requires a prompt diagnosis.

Increased Intracranial Pressure

Under normal circumstances, there is a dynamic equilibrium among the bony structure of the cranium, brain tissue, and extracellular fluid that comprise approximately 85 percent of the intracranial volume; the blood volume that

93

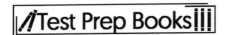

comprises 10 percent of the volume; and the CSF that occupies the remaining 5 percent of the volume of the cranium. If any one of these volumes increases, there must be a compensatory decrease in one or more of the remaining volumes to maintain normal intracranial pressure (ICP) and optimal cerebral perfusion pressure (CPP).

The CPP represents the pressure gradient for cerebral perfusion and is equal to the difference between the mean arterial pressure (MAP) and the ICP ($MAP - ICP = CPP$). The process of autoregulation maintains optimal CPP by dilation and constriction of the cerebral arterioles; however, if the MAP falls below 65 millimeters of mercury or rises above 150 millimeters of mercury, autoregulation is ineffective, and cerebral blood flow is dependent on blood pressure (BP). Once this mechanism fails, any increase in volume potentially will cause an increase in the ICP. For instance, normal ICP may be maintained in the presence of a slow-growing tumor; however, a sudden small accumulation of blood will cause a sharp increase in the ICP. Eventually, all autoregulatory mechanisms will be exhausted in either circumstance, and the ICP will be increased. In an adult in the supine position, the normal ICP is 7 to 15 millimeters of mercury, while an ICP greater than 15 millimeters of mercury is considered abnormal, and pressures greater than 20 millimeters of mercury require intervention.

Conditions associated with increased ICP include space-occupying lesions such as tumors and hematomas; obstruction of CSF or hydrocephalus; increased production of CSF due to tumor formation; cerebral edema resulting from head injuries, strokes, infection, or surgery; hyponatremia; hepatic encephalopathy; and idiopathic intracranial hypertension. Early manifestations of increased ICP include blurred vision with gradual dilation of the pupil and slowed pupillary response, restlessness, and confusion with progressive disorientation as to time, then to place, and finally to person.

Later signs include initially ipsilateral pupillary dilation and fixation, which progresses to bilateral dilation and fixation; decorticate or decerebrate posturing; and Cushing's triad of manifestations that include bradycardia, widening pulse pressure, and Cheyne-Stokes respirations. ICP monitoring will be used to assess all patients requiring emergency care for any condition that is potentially associated with increased ICP. Depending on the underlying pathology, common interventions for increased ICP include sedation and paralysis, intubation and hyperventilation to decrease the $PaCO_2$, infusion of mannitol, an osmotic diuretic, and hypertonic saline IV solutions. Healthcare providers understand that sustained elevations of ICP are associated with a poor prognosis, and therefore, the underlying cause and manifestations must be treated aggressively.

Meningitis

Meningitis is defined as the infection and resulting inflammation of the three layers of the meninges, the membranous covering of the brain and spinal cord. The causative agent may be bacterial, viral, parasitic, or fungal, which commonly occurs in patients who are HIV positive. The most common bacterial agent is *S. pneumoniae*, while meningococcal meningitis is common in crowded living spaces. However, the development and use of the meningococcal vaccine (MCV 4) has reduced the incidence in college students and military personnel. The *Haemophilus influenzae* type B (Hib) vaccine has decreased the incidence and morbidity of the HI meningitis in infants, and the pneumococcal polysaccharide vaccine (PPSV) is being used to prevent meningitis in at-risk populations, such as immunocompromised adults, smokers, residents in long-term care facilities, and adults with chronic disease.

General risk factors for bacterial infection of the meninges include loss of, or decreased function of, the spleen; chronic glucocorticoid use; deficiency of the complement system; diabetes; renal insufficiency; alcoholism; chronic liver disease; otitis media; and trauma associated with leakage of the CSF. Bacterial meningitis is infectious, and early diagnosis and treatment are essential for survival and recovery. Healthcare providers understand that even with adequate treatment, 50 percent of patients with bacterial meningitis will develop complications within two to three weeks of the acute infection, and long-term deficits are common in 30 percent of the surviving patients. The complications are specific to the causative organism, but may include hearing loss, blindness, paralysis, seizure disorder, muscular deficiencies, ataxia, hydrocephalus, and subdural effusions. In contrast, the incidence of viral meningitis is often associated with other viral conditions such as mumps, measles, herpes, and infections due to

94

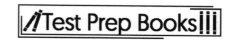

arboviruses such as the West Nile virus. The treatment is supportive, and the majority of patients recover without long-term complications; however, the outcome is less certain for patients who are immunocompromised, less than two years old, or more than sixty years old.

The classic manifestations of bacterial meningitis include fever, nuchal rigidity, and headache. Additional findings may include nausea and vomiting, photophobia, confusion, and a decreased level of consciousness. Patients with viral meningitis may report the incidence of fatigue, muscle aches, and decreased appetite prior to the illness.

The diagnosis of meningitis is determined by lumbar puncture; CSF analysis; cultures of the blood, nose, and respiratory secretions and any skin lesions that are present; complete blood count (CBC); electrolytes; coagulation studies; serum glucose to compare with CSF glucose; and procalcitonin to differentiate bacterial meningitis from aseptic meningitis in children. There is a small risk of herniation of the brain when the CSF is removed during the lumbar puncture, and while a computerized tomography (CT) scan may be done to assess the risk, healthcare providers understand that effective antibiotic treatment must be initiated as quickly as possible to prevent the morbidity associated with bacterial meningitis. The results of the Gram stain of the CSF and blood will dictate the initial antibiotic therapy, which will be modified when the specific agent is identified. Additional interventions include seizure precautions, cardiac monitoring, and ongoing assessment of respiratory and neurological function. Patients with bacterial meningitis may require long-term rehabilitation.

Seizure Disorders

A **seizure** is defined as a chaotic period of uncoordinated electrical activity in the brain, which results in one of several characteristic behaviors. Although the exact cause is unknown, several possible triggers have been proposed as noted below. The recently revised classification system categorizes seizure activity according to the area of the brain where the seizure initiates, the patient's level of awareness during the seizure, and other descriptive features such as the presence of an aura. The unclassified category includes seizure patterns that do not conform to the primary categories. Seizures that originate in a single area of the brain are designated as **focal seizures**, while seizures that originate in two or more different networks are designated as **generalized seizures**. The remaining seizures in the onset category include seizures without an identified point of onset and seizures that progress from focal seizures to generalized seizures.

Risk factors associated with seizures include genetic predisposition, illnesses with severe temperature elevation, head trauma, cerebral edema, inappropriate use or discontinuance of antiepileptic drugs (AEDs), intracerebral infection, excess or deficiency of sodium and glucose, toxin exposure, hypoxia, and acute drug or alcohol withdrawal. Patients are encouraged to identify any conditions that may be triggers for their seizure activity. Although the triggers vary greatly from one patient to another, commonly identified events include increased physical activity, excessive stress, hyperventilation, fatigue, acute ETOH (ethyl alcohol) ingestion, exposure to flashing lights, and inhaled chemicals, including cocaine.

The tonic phase presents as stiffening of the limbs for a brief period, while the clonic phase is evidenced by jerking motions of the limbs. These manifestations may be accompanied by a decreased level of consciousness, respiratory alterations and cyanosis, incontinence, and biting of the tongue. Absence seizures are manifested by a decreased level of awareness without abnormal muscular activity. The manifestations of the postictal phase include alterations in consciousness and awareness and increased oral secretions. Seizure disorders are diagnosed by serum lab studies to assess AED levels and to identify excess alcohol and recreational drugs, metabolic alterations, and kidney and liver function. Electroencephalography (EEG) and the enhanced magnetoencephalography are used to identify the origin of the altered electrical activity in the brain, and MRI, skull films, and CSF analysis are used to rule out possible sources of the seizure disorder such as tumor formation.

Seizure disorders are treated with AEDs that stabilize the neuron cell membrane by facilitating the inhibitory mechanisms or opposing the excitatory mechanisms. Patients with a chronic seizure disorder, or epilepsy, usually

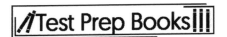

require a combination of medications to minimize seizure activity. Elderly patients respond differently to the AEDs and may require frequent assessment and revision of the care plan. The emergency care of the patient with seizures is focused on patient safety during and after the seizure and the cessation and prevention of the seizure activity. Prolonged seizure activity is defined as *status epilepticus*, which is the occurrence of multiple seizures, each lasting more than 5 minutes over a 30-minute period. This life-threatening condition is commonly the result of incorrect usage of AEDs or the use of recreational drugs. Emergency care of this condition includes the immediate administration of phenytoin and benzodiazepines, in addition to possible general anesthesia if the medication therapy is not effective.

Shunt Dysfunctions

Increased production or decreased absorption and drainage of CSF results in hydrocephalus. This condition develops in infants, due to premature birth, intracranial hemorrhage, and genetic defects such as spina bifida, while in older children and adults, CSF accumulations due to hemorrhagic disease and tumor formation result in a significant increase in ICP due to the presence of a rigid cranium. In any event, emergency care of hydrocephalus is necessary to prevent physical and intellectual deficits.

If tumor formation is responsible for the development of hydrocephalus, removal of the tumor commonly results in an 88 percent reduction in the ICP. Research indicates that medical interventions are only minimally effective, and while surgical interventions have greater efficacy in select patients, 75 percent of patients with hydrocephalus will require the placement of a shunt for long-term drainage of the CSF. A CSF shunt facilitates the flow of excess CSF from the ventricle to a distant anatomical site such as the peritoneum (the most common site), the atria, and the pleural space. The catheter has a one-way flow pressure valve that limits the rate of flow of the CSF from the cerebral ventricle to the distant absorption site and a reservoir that provides percutaneous access to the shunt. The catheter is positioned in the ventricle and then tunneled subcutaneously to the collection site, allowing the excess CSF to flow from the ventricle to be reabsorbed, thereby decreasing the ICP.

Infections of the shunt manifest with similar signs of increased ICP in addition to possible purulent drainage, skin erosion and erythema, abdominal pain, and signs of peritonitis. Fever may or may not be present and is not necessary to confirm the diagnosis. Noninfectious complications related to the catheter include mechanical failure, migration of the distal catheter due to the patient's growth, and initial mispositioning of the catheter. Obstruction of the catheter accounts for 50 to 80 percent of all shunt failures, with the proximal catheter and shunt valve identified as the most common sites of obstruction due to choroid ingrowth or deposition of blood and cellular debris. Obstruction of the distal catheter, which occurs most often at the abdominal entry site, is less common and may be due to twisting of the catheter or from obstruction by inflammatory cellular debris or pseudocyst formation.

The medical-surgical nurse understands the expected signs of increased ICP, such as headache, vomiting without nausea, changes in the level of consciousness, irritability, bradycardia, seizures, and visual alterations. Patients and care providers must be alert for these changes to access appropriate emergency care. Previous shunt revision or infection are associated with an increased risk of shunt failure, which typically occurs two to four months after insertion of the catheter. MRI scans, shunt series radiographs and nuclear medicine studies, and ultrasounds are used to assess the integrity and position of the catheter. Emergency management includes initiating a neurosurgical consultation, close observation of all vital signs for the advancement of the increased ICP, identification of the cause of the malfunction, treatment of any infection, and drainage of the excess CSF through the reservoir.

Spinal Cord Injuries

Injuries to the spinal cord are associated with severe and often irreversible neurological deficits and disabilities. **Spinal cord injuries** (SCIs) may be due to one or a combination of the following types of injury: direct traumatic injuries of the spinal cord, compression of the spinal cord by bone fragments or hematoma formation, or ischemia resulting from damage to the spinal arteries. The anatomical location of the SCI predicts the degree of sensory and motor function that will be lost. In addition, the injury will be labeled as **paraplegia** if the lesion is at the T1 to the T5

96

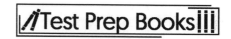

level, affecting only the lower extremities, or **tetraplegia** if the lesion is at the C1 to the C7 level, affecting both the upper and lower extremities in addition to respiratory function. SCIs may be categorized as complete or incomplete depending on the degree of impairment.

While complete SCIs are associated with complete loss of sensory-motor function, incomplete lesions are determined by the actual portion of the spinal cord that is affected. Central spinal cord syndrome is an incomplete SCI that involves upper extremity weakness or paralysis with little or no deficit noted in the lower extremities. Anterior spinal cord syndrome is also an incomplete SCI that is associated with loss of motor function, pain, and sensation below the injury; however, the sensations of light touch, proprioception, and vibration remain intact. In addition, Brown-Sequard syndrome is an incomplete lesion of one-half of the spinal cord, which results in paralysis on the side of the injury and loss of pain and temperature sensation on the opposite side of the injury.

Healthcare providers understand that the injury to the spinal cord is an evolving process, which means that the level of the injury can rise one to two spinal levels within 48 to 72 hours after the initial insult. An incomplete injury may progress to a complete injury during this time due to the effects of altered blood flow and resulting edema and the presence of abnormal free radicals. Essential interventions aimed at minimizing or preventing this progression include establishing and maintaining normal oxygenation, arterial blood gas (ABG) values, and perfusion of the spinal cord.

SCIs are also associated with three shock syndromes, including hemorrhagic shock, spinal shock, and neurogenic shock. Hemorrhagic shock from an acute or occult source must be suspected in all SCIs below the T6 level that present with hypotension. Spinal shock refers to the loss of sensory-motor function that may be temporary or permanent depending on the specific injury. At the same time, the patient must be monitored for signs of neurogenic shock, which presents with a triad of symptoms that include hypotension, bradycardia, and peripheral vasodilation. This complication is due to alterations in autonomic nervous system function, which causes loss of vagal tone. Most often, it occurs with an injury above the T6 level, resulting in decreased vascular resistance and vasodilation. Neurogenic shock may also be associated with hypothermia due to vasodilation; rapid, shallow respirations; difficulty breathing; cold, clammy, pale skin; nausea; vomiting; and dizziness. Emergency treatment of neurogenic shock includes IV fluids and inotropic medications to support the BP and IV atropine and/or pacemaker insertion, as needed, to treat the bradycardia. If a patient presents with neurological deficits eight or more hours after sustaining an SCI, high-dose prednisone may be administered to reverse the manifestations of neurogenic shock.

Emergency management of SCIs is focused on preventing extension of the injury and long-term deficits with immobilization and interventions based on the Airway, Breathing, and Circulation protocol. Cervical SCIs result in an 80 to 95 percent decrease in vital capacity, and mechanical ventilation is often required for lesions at this level. Support of circulation is addressed in the treatment of neurogenic shock. Other supportive treatment interventions are aimed at minimizing the effects of immobility. Healthcare providers are aware that patients with complete SCIs have less than a 5 percent chance of recovery; however, more than 90 percent of all patients with SCIs eventually return home and regain some measure of independence.

Stroke

A **stroke** is defined as the death of brain tissue due to ischemic or hemorrhagic injury. Ischemic strokes are more common than hemorrhagic strokes; however, the differential diagnosis of these conditions requires careful attention to the patient's history and physical examination. In general, an acute onset of neurological symptoms and seizures is more common with hemorrhagic stroke, while ischemic stroke is more frequently associated with a history of some form of trauma. The National Institutes of Health (NIH) Stroke Scale represents an international effort to standardize the assessment and treatment protocols for stroke. The scale includes detailed criteria and the protocol for assessment of the neurological system. The stroke scale items are to be administered in the official order listed and there are directions that denote how to score each item.

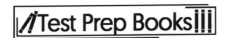
Ischemic Stroke

Ischemic strokes result from occlusion of the cerebral vasculature as a result of a thrombotic or embolic event. At the cellular level, the ischemia leads to hypoxia that rapidly depletes the ATP stores. As a result, the cellular membrane pressure gradient is lost, and there is an influx of sodium, calcium, and water into the cell, which leads to cytotoxic edema. This process creates scattered regions of ischemia in the affected area, containing cells that are dead within minutes of the precipitating event. This core of ischemic tissue is surrounded by an area with minimally-adequate perfusion that may remain viable for several hours after the event. These necrotic areas are eventually liquefied and acted upon by macrophages, resulting in the loss of brain parenchyma. These affected sites, if sufficiently large, may be prone to hemorrhage, due to the formation of collateral vascular supply with or without the use of medications such as recombinant tissue plasminogen activator (rtPA). The ischemic process also compromises the blood-brain barrier, which leads to the movement of water and protein into the extracellular space within 4 to 6 hours after the onset of the stroke, resulting in vasogenic edema.

Nonmodifiable risk factors for ischemic stroke include age, gender, ethnicity, history of migraine headaches with aura, and a family history of stroke or transient ischemic attacks (TIAs). Modifiable risk factors include hypertension, diabetes, hypercholesterolemia, cardiac disease including atrial fibrillation, valvular disease and heart failure, elevated homocysteine levels, obesity, illicit drug use, alcohol abuse, smoking, and sedentary lifestyle. The research related to the occurrence of stroke in women indicates the need to treat hypertension aggressively prior to and during pregnancy and prior to the use of contraceptives to prevent irreversible damage to the microvasculature. In addition, it is recommended that to reduce their risk of stroke, women with a history of migraine headaches preceded by an aura should ameliorate all modifiable risk factors, and all women over seventy-five years old should be routinely assessed for the onset of atrial fibrillation.

Heredity is associated with identified gene mutations and the process of atherosclerosis and cholesterol metabolism. Hypercholesterolemia and the progression of atherosclerosis in genetically-susceptible individuals are now regarded as active inflammatory processes that contribute to endothelial damage of the cerebral vasculature, thereby increasing the risk for strokes. There are also early indications that infection also contributes to the development and advancement of atherosclerosis.

The presenting manifestations of ischemic stroke must be differentiated from other common diseases, including brain tumor formation, hyponatremia, hypoglycemia, seizure disorders, and systemic infection. The sudden onset of hemisensory losses, visual alterations, hemiparesis, ataxia, nystagmus, and aphasia are commonly, although not exclusively, associated with ischemic strokes. The availability of reperfusion therapies dictates the emergent use of diagnostic imaging studies, including CT and MRI scans, carotid duplex scans, and digital subtraction angiography to confirm the data obtained from the patient's history and physical examination. Laboratory studies include CBC, coagulation studies, chemistry panels, cardiac biomarkers, toxicology assays, and pregnancy testing as appropriate.

The emergency care of the patient who presents with an ischemic stroke is focused on the stabilization of the patient's ABCs, completion of the physical examination and appropriate diagnostic studies, and initiation of reperfusion therapy as appropriate, within 60 minutes of arrival in the emergency department. Reperfusion therapies include the use of alteplase (the only fibrinolytic agent that is approved for the treatment of ischemic stroke), antiplatelet agents, and mechanical thrombectomy. Healthcare providers must also be alert for hyperthermia, hypoxia, hypertension or hypotension, and signs of cardiac ischemia or cardiac arrhythmias.

Hemorrhagic Stroke

Hemorrhagic strokes are less common than ischemic strokes; however, a hemorrhagic stroke is more likely to be fatal than an ischemic stroke. A hemorrhagic stroke is the result of bleeding into the parenchymal tissue of the brain due to leakage of blood from damaged intracerebral arteries. These hemorrhagic events occur more often in specific areas of the brain, including the thalamus, cerebellum, and brain stem. The tissue surrounding the hemorrhagic area is also subject to injury due to the mass effect of the accumulated blood volume. In the event of subarachnoid hemorrhage, ICP becomes elevated with resulting dysfunction of the autoregulation response, which

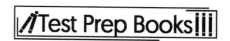

leads to abnormal vasoconstriction, platelet aggregation, and decreased perfusion and blood flow, resulting in cerebral ischemia.

Risk factors for hemorrhagic stroke include older age; a history of hypertension, which is present in 60 percent of patients; personal history of stroke; alcohol abuse; and illicit drug use. Common conditions associated with hemorrhagic stroke include hypertension, cerebral amyloidosis, coagulopathies, vascular alterations including arteriovenous malformation, vasculitis, intracranial neoplasm, and a history of anticoagulant or antithrombotic therapy.

Although the presenting manifestations for hemorrhagic stroke differ in some respect from the those associated with ischemic stroke, none of these manifestations is an absolute predictor of one or the other. In general, patients with hemorrhagic stroke present with a headache that may be severe, significant alterations in the level of consciousness and neurological function, hypertension, seizures, and nausea and vomiting. The specific neurological defects depend on the anatomical site of the hemorrhage and may include hemisensory loss, hemiparesis, aphasia, and visual alterations.

Diagnostic studies include CBC, chemistry panel, coagulation studies, and blood glucose. Non-contrast CT scan or MRI are the preferred imaging studies. CT or magnetic resonance angiography may also be used to obtain images of the cerebral vasculature. Close observation of the patient's vital signs, neurological vital signs, and ICP is necessary.

The emergency management of the patient with hemorrhagic stroke is focused on the ABC protocol, in addition to the control of bleeding, seizure activity, and increased ICP. There is no single medication used to treat hemorrhagic stroke; however, recent data suggests that aggressive emergency management of hypertension initiated early and aimed at reducing the systolic BP to less than 140 millimeters of mercury may be effective in reducing the growth of the hematoma at the site, which decreases the mass effect. Beta-blockers and ACE inhibitors are recommended to facilitate this reduction. Endotracheal intubation for ventilatory support may be necessary; however, hyperventilation is not recommended due to the resulting suppression of cerebral blood flow. While seizure activity will be treated with AEDs, there is controversy related to the prophylactic use of these medicines. Increased ICP requires osmotic diuretic therapy, elevation of the head of the bed to 30 degrees, sedation and analgesics as appropriate, and antacids. Steroid therapy is not effective and is not recommended.

Patients who present with manifestations of hemorrhagic stroke with a history of anticoagulation therapy present a special therapeutic challenge due to the extension of the hematoma formation. More than 50 percent of patients taking warfarin who suffer a hemorrhagic stroke will die within thirty days. This statistic is consistent in patients with international normalized ratio (INR) levels within the therapeutic range, with increased mortality noted in patients with INRs that exceed the therapeutic level. Emergency treatment includes fresh frozen plasma, IV vitamin K, prothrombin complex concentrates, and recombinant factor VIIa (rFVIIa). There are administration concerns with each of these therapies that must be addressed to prevent any delays in the reversal of the effects of the warfarin.

Transient Ischemic Attack

A **transient ischemic attack** (TIA) is defined as a short-term episode of altered neurological function that lasts for less than one hour; it may be imperceptible to the patient. The deficit may be related to speech, movement, behavior, or memory and may be caused by an ischemic event in the brain, spinal cord, or retina. The patient's history and neurological assessment according to the NIH Stroke Scale establish the diagnosis. Additional diagnostic studies include CBC, glucose, sedimentation rate, electrolytes, lipid profile, toxicology screen, 12-lead ECG, and CSF analysis. Imaging studies include non-contrast MRI or CT, carotid Doppler exam, and angiography.

Care of the patient with a TIA is focused on the assessment of any neurological deficits and the identification of comorbid conditions that may be related to the attack. Hospital admission is required in the event of an attack that lasts more than one hour, if the patient has experienced more than a single attack in a one-week period or if the

99

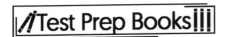

attack is related to a cardiac source such as atrial fibrillation or a myocardial infarction. The ABCD^2 stroke risk score calculates the patient's risk for experiencing a true stroke within two days after the TIA based on five factors (see the table below). Interventions aimed at stroke prevention in relation to the risk stratification as calculated by the ABCD^2 score are specific to underlying comorbidities; however, treatment with ASA and clopidogrel is commonly prescribed.

ABCD^2 Stroke Risk Score		
	1 Point	**2 Points**
Age	≥ 60 years	
Blood Pressure	SBP ≥ 140 mmHg DBP ≥ 90 mmHg	
Clinical Features	Speech impairment but no focal weakness	Focal weakness
Duration of Symptoms	≤ 59 minutes	≥ 60 minutes
Diabetes	Diagnosed	
Total Score (denotes risk for stroke [CVA] within 2 days after TIA)	0-3 points = 1% risk 4-5 points = 4.1% risk 6-7 points = 8.1% risk	

Sudden Onset of Confusion or Agitation

Patients who have entered a facility or hospital may experience periods of confusion or agitation. This may be an acute situation for the individual or part of an ongoing diagnosis of dementia or Alzheimer's disease. A severe and acute situation that involves confusion and agitation is called **delirium**. The medical-surgical nurse should be aware of these different situations, their causes, and what can be done to assist the patient back to normal functioning.

Confusion and agitation are symptoms of an underlying condition or disease. Patients who once were oriented to who they were, where they were, what circumstances brought them to the facility, and the time may become confused on one or all of these points. They will suddenly not understand and become uncertain about the facts of their situation.

A patient who is agitated may display an acute anxiety about seemingly small details of their stay at the hospital or facility, perhaps even becoming verbally or physically abusive toward staff. In either of these situations, if the confusion and agitation are new, they should be reported to the nurse immediately for further investigation. Usually if the cause can be found, the situation can be corrected.

Delirium is a mental disturbance involving confusion, decreased awareness of surroundings, and sometimes agitation that causes a patient to lose focus and attention. This condition is usually transient in nature, not lasting for long if appropriate interventions are applied. Delirium usually occurs in the presence of an illness, as a sign of drug toxicity, and in situations of dehydration, where the body's fluids and electrolytes are out of balance. A patient who is older, has Parkinson's disease, dementia, or a history of stroke may be at a greater risk to develop delirium.

Patients with dementia or Alzheimer's disease may be prone to periods of heightened agitation or confusion. A person with these conditions is also more prone to acute periods of delirium. **Dementia** is a chronic, long-term condition that involves decreased cognitive ability over time, while delirium happens quickly and usually does not last long.

The medical-surgical nurse should work with the rest of the health care team to create an environment around the confused patient that is conducive to calm, collected behavior. This includes making the environment around the patient as stable as possible, without bright lights, loud and/or sudden noises, and unexpected interruptions to the patient's expected routine.

100

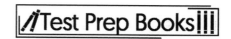

Including items in a patient's room such as family photographs and other familiar objects can be visual reminders to the patient about their circumstances.

If the patient has sensory deficits such as visual or hearing loss, the medical-surgical nurse should ensure that these are addressed. The patient's hearing aid batteries should be kept refreshed, glasses and dentures in a place where they can be easily accessed, and assistive walking devices such as canes or walkers at hand if appropriate. Granting the patient as much freedom and familiarity as possible will assist the patient in functioning while in the facility.

The medical-surgical nurse can help patients with confusion and agitation by listening to their needs, maintaining a calm, collected, and professional attitude, talking about what the daily tasks and expectations are, and reorienting the patient whenever necessary. The nurse must work with patients based on their cognitive abilities to assure that they can work with the health care team effectively without becoming overwhelmed and confused.

Family members and/or friends of the patient are valuable resources when dealing with confusion, especially if it is a long-standing issue. The patient's loved ones may have developed some tips and tricks for helping the patient regain orientation that can be used by the health care team.

Patient Safety Protocols

Ensuring patient safety is one of the most important jobs for nurses. Nurses are the professionals who have the most patient contact and can best assess and prevent safety issues, such as bed sores, falls, and suicidal patients. Because nurses have the most interaction with a patient, they are able to implement measures to ensure safety and prevent common injuries from happening. Patient safety is a major area of quality improvement, which reinforces its systemic importance and the vital role nurses play in implementing it.

Rounding
Rounding is the timely process of checking on a patient's well-being, assessing their needs, and addressing any issues. Common timeframes for rounding are hourly or every two hours. While rounding, the nurse inspects the patient's room and environment looking for any potential sources of injury, such as wires that can be tripped on. They assess the patient for such aspects of care as IV lines being intact, the patient being alert or resting comfortably, and any changes in patient disposition. A systematic rounding policy reduces fall rates, call bell rings, and interruptions for the nurse. It also increases patient satisfaction because it ensures they are getting their needs met and interacting with a member of their healthcare team regularly.

As part of customer satisfaction, patients expect their call bell to be answered promptly. In many cases this is difficult for nurses, as they may be either charting or attending to another patient. Frequent rounding helps address patient needs earlier on, preventing numerous call bells later. This proactive approach addresses patient's needs faster, leading to increased satisfaction and in the long run, better healing.

A common mnemonic to remember what to address during rounding is the Three P's, which stand for pain, potty, and position. During each rounding, the nurse should assess pain by asking the patient to rate their pain from zero to ten. If necessary, the nurse can then administer medication following provider orders and document medications given. Reassuring the patient that their pain will be rounded on and addressed at frequent time intervals is comforting to patients and families. For potty, the nurse should ask if the patient needs assistance to the restroom and provide education on not getting out of bed without assistance. Lastly, ask the patient if their position is comfortable. Remember to turn patients every two hours to prevent bed sores and skin breakdown.

Skin Integrity
Skin integrity refers to the health of a patient's skin. Skin with high integrity is free of open wounds, moisture, and infection. This is an important factor in patient health as the skin is the largest barrier between external harmful

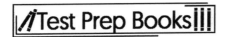

agents and internal organs, bones, and tissues. When skin integrity is low, patients become more susceptible to infection, therefore reducing recovery time and quality of care while increasing poor health outcomes (including death). When providing care to patients, nurses should ensure that surgical and recovery positioning do not compromise the skin (i.e., leaving patients in a way that would make them prone to pressure ulcers). If patients already have compromised areas, medical staff should ensure that all precautions are made to keep the wound clean, bandaged, and free of pressure or friction.

Elderly Patients

Elderly patients have an increased risk for skin injuries due to the fragility of their skin, decreased circulation, poor nutrition, decreased sensation, mental changes, and altered mobility. As the body ages, the skin becomes thinner due to decreased adipose tissue and has less elasticity. The **epidermis**, which is the outer layer of the skin, is only 0.1 millimeters thick and becomes thinner with time. Loss of collagen as the skin ages decreases the skin's elasticity, making it more vulnerable to friction and force. **Dry skin** is caused by loss of sweat and oil, and also due to a decrease in blood flow to the skin. All of these factors contribute to skin that is fragile and prone to tears. If any skin injuries are observed on a patient, the injuries must be assessed, documented, treated, and monitored for changes. Patients who require total care have the greatest risk of developing a skin tear or a pressure ulcer.

Risks for developing a skin tear or pressure ulcer include the following:

- Bedridden patient
- Wheelchair dependent
- Limited mobility
- Spinal-cord injury
- Poor nutrition
- Poor circulation to the skin, commonly due to a heart condition or diabetes
- Dependence on others for care
- Weakened immune system
- Elderly population
- Excessive pressure on the skin or on bony areas

Braden Scale

The **Braden Scale** is used to assess the risk of patients developing pressure ulcers (commonly known as bedsores). A pressure ulcer refers to internal and/or external damage that can occur in areas of the body where areas of bone are poorly cushioned by soft or adipose tissue (such as the tailbone). This is normally the result of low mobility in a patient, resulting in constant pressure placed on the bony area and therefore resulting in bruising of or breakage in the corresponding soft tissue, blood vessels, or skin.

The Braden Scale takes into account patients' sensory perception (whether they can feel areas of pressure), moisture (how damp an area is), activity (how much patients are able to generally move on their own or with assistance), mobility (how well patients are able to generally move on their own or with assistance), nutrition (patient intake of macronutrients, vitamins, and minerals that support bodily functions), and friction (if any areas are exposed to repeated rubbing or chafing). Based on this scale, patients will be categorized as at risk, moderate risk, high risk, or very high risk of developing a pressure ulcer. Nurse monitoring and patient care should be tailored to the patient's risk category.

Bruising

Bruises or **ecchymosis** are caused by blunt force or clotting abnormalities that cause capillaries under the skin to leak blood into the tissue, causing a discolored area. Bruises can range in color from blue, brown, or purple to even green and yellow depending on the stage of healing. Bruising can occur in patients as a result of bumping into objects, multiple or failed intravenous-access attempts, medication side effects, or falling. Significant bruising that

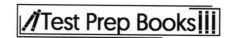

occurs without a known cause could indicate an underlying medical condition, such as a blood-clotting disorder. Bruising can also be a result of physical abuse. If suspicious bruises are noticed, it is important to ask the patient questions about the bruising. Family members should also ask staff about bruises they notice on their loved one.

Risks for bruising include the following:

- Elderly population
- Frail, thin skin
- Blood-thinner medications that cause slower blood clotting times, resulting in quicker and easier bruising
- Altered mental status or disorientation (may cause a person to be unsteady or to be unaware of their surroundings)
- Environmental hazards in the patient's room, such as corners of tables, furniture, or cords that could cause tripping and bumping
- Visual or other sensory impairment (may cause falling or bumping into objects)

Restraints

Restraints can be defined as anything that is used, done, or said to intentionally limits a person's ability to move freely. Restraints, when applied properly, cannot be easily removed or controlled by the person. In addition to physical form, restraints can also be emotional, chemical, or environmental. Use of restraints is very controversial due to the ethical issue of personal freedom. These are a temporary solution to a problem and must always be used as a last resort. Restraints are used to limit a patient's movement to prevent injury to themselves or others, and they always require a physician's order.

Types of restraints include the following:

- Physical: vests, wrist restraints, straps, or anything that confines the body
- Emotional: verbal cues or emotions used to coerce the patient to act a certain way
- Environmental: side rails, locked doors, closed windows, locked beds
- Chemical: any medication used to change a patient's behavior

The medical doctor or practitioner is responsible for ordering the use of restraints. Nurses are responsible for applying restraints safely and for the management of a patient with a restraint. After an order is given, the physician must visit the patient within twenty-four hours of placing the order to assess its further necessity.

The following are circumstances under which restraints are used:

- Signs of patient aggression toward self, staff, or other patients
- Interference with important medical devices, such as an IV or a catheter
- Patient movements that are potentially harmful to their health or may cause further injury
- Potential for a patient to interfere with a procedure

When applying restraints:

- always follow the facility's restraint policy.
- obtain an order from a physician or medical practitioner, unless it is an emergency situation.
- obtain consent from the patient or from next of kin if the patient is not capable of understanding.
- explain to the patient what is going to happen, even if the patient is unable to understand due to confusion or dementia.

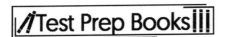
- always monitor the patient per facility policy—check the positioning of the restraint every thirty minutes and remove every two hours for range of motion. Remember to reposition the patient and offer toileting every two hours.
- explain the need for restraints and how long the restraints will be used.

Vests have holes for the arms and the opening crosses in the back. The straps will be secured on either side of the bed or chair, depending on the patient's location. Tie it in a quick-release knot to a lower part of the bed that does not move. Make sure that two fingers fit underneath the vest on the patient's chest so that it is not too tight.

Wrist or **ankle restraints** are cloths that wrap around each wrist or ankle. They have a strap that is tied to a lower, immovable part of the bed or chair. Tie it in a quick-release knot. Ensure the restraints aren't too tight and that the patient's arms or legs aren't in an awkward position. Usually, a pillow will be placed under the arms and/or the knees and heels.

Possible injuries from restraints can include the following:

- Broken bones
- Bruises
- Falls
- Skin tears or pressure sores
- Depression or fear due to lack of freedom
- Death from strangulation

Fall Prevention

Risk for falls is a serious consideration for all patients entering into a facility or hospital. A fall can cause injuries that worsen the patient's condition and may even lead to death. The medical-surgical nurse should be able to identify patients at risk for falls and implement the proper fall precautions to ensure the patient's safety.

Risk factors for falls include the following:

- Muscle weakness
- Balance and gait problems
- Dizziness related to low blood pressure, heart conditions, or medication side effects
- Slower reflexes
- Confusion or memory loss
- Foot problems and/or unsafe shoes
- Vision problems
- History of falls (Patients who have fallen before are two to three times more likely to fall again.)

A fall may occur for a number of reasons. Older adults are at risk for falls more so than younger people due to weakening muscles and bones. This weakness in the musculoskeletal system leads to an unsteady gait and poor balance. People with a weak musculoskeletal system may not be able to correct themselves as quickly or with as much agility when they lose their balance, nor can they catch themselves as well when they fall, leading to greater injury.

Fluctuations in blood pressure may cause a person to fall, especially if the blood pressure becomes too low. Blood pressure is a reflection of how well the heart is pumping oxygen-rich blood to the tissues of the body, especially the brain. If the brain is not getting enough oxygen from the blood as a result of low blood pressure, among other causes, the person may fall as a result of dizziness and/or fainting. **Orthostatic hypotension** occurs when blood pressure drops suddenly as a result of a change in position, such as from sitting to standing, and does not immediately compensate.

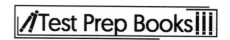

Low blood sugar may cause a decreased level of consciousness in an individual. The brain not only needs oxygen, but it also needs an adequate supply of blood glucose to maintain consciousness and regulate movement and coordination. When blood sugar becomes too low, the resulting altered level of consciousness may cause a person to lose balance and fall to the ground.

Patients in an unfamiliar environment may become confused when in bed or navigating themselves around their room. Confusion is common among hospitalized individuals, resulting from medication side effects and the effects of illness. A patient may suddenly attempt to get out of bed or try and walk to the bathroom, not remembering that they are attached to an intravenous pole, urinary catheter, and/or many other types of equipment, depending on their condition. This brief moment of confusion and unexpected obstacles can lead to a fall and injury.

Patients with sensory deficits may be at risk for a fall, such as those with visual and hearing impairments. Visual impairments may prevent a patient from seeing obstacles in their path. Hearing impairments may prevent a patient from hearing warning sounds or words.

There are certain measures, called **fall precautions**, which can be put in place for a patient who is at risk for a fall. The medical-surgical nurse can create an uncluttered, well-lit environment for the patient. Rooms that are full of clutter, equipment, and obstacles put the patient at risk for a fall. In the same way, if the lighting is not adequate for the patient, they may trip on an unseen object and fall.

Placing the call light in the patient's reach and talking to the patient about using it when needing any sort of assistance can prevent a fall. Some hospitals have a "Call Don't Fall" sign in the patient's room, indicating the patient and family should ask for help using the call light when necessary.

Patients who have displayed confusion and impulsive behavior that may put them at risk for a fall, such as suddenly attempting to get out of bed when they are not physically able or need assistance with equipment, should have special precautions put in place. A **bed alarm** is a device that sets off an alarm when the patient tries to get out of bed unassisted. It is a pad with a sensor that is placed under the patient's buttocks or under the fitted sheet of the bed; the bed itself may be equipped with an alarm device.

Some patients will be put on what is called a **low bed**, a bed that can be lowered close to the floor. This ensures that the patient will not accidentally slide or roll out of bed if they try to get out of bed before the health care staff can assist.

Medical-surgical nurses should encourage patients to use available assistive devices, such as canes, walkers, and wheelchairs. Before leaving a patient's room, make sure any assistive device that the patient can use independently is within their reach.

The use of assistive devices such as **gait belts** (also known as **transfer belts**) benefits both the nurse and the patient. When transferring or walking with a patient who needs assistance, it's advised to use a gait belt to prevent falls. When using a gait belt to assist a patient to walk, fasten the belt around their waist and hold it with both hands while standing to the side and slightly behind the patient. If the patient loses their balance and begins to fall, never attempt to catch them. Instead, continue holding the gait belt, bend at the knees, and slowly lower the patient to the floor.

Safe Transfer Techniques

When transferring a patient, the safety of the patient and the nurse are of the greatest importance. Incorrectly performed transfers can cause injury to both. Be mindful of proper transfer techniques and body mechanics, such as keeping a straight back, bending at the knees, avoiding twisting at the waist, and, most importantly, asking for additional help if needed.

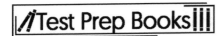

When assisting a patient out of bed, always make sure that the bed is in the lowest position. Then, assist the patient to sit upright on the side of the bed with both feet on the floor. While the patient remains in this seated position, make sure they aren't lightheaded or dizzy from the position change. If the patient needs significant physical assistance other than stabilization, an assistive device should be considered. To assist the patient in standing, the nurse should stand in front of the patient, place their knees in front of the patient's knees, and hug the patient under the arms for lifting. Then instruct the patient to help as much as possible. If transferring the patient to a chair after assisting them to stand, both the nurse and the patient should take small steps, pivoting around to the chair. Make sure the backs of the patient's knees are touching the front of the seat before lowering them into the chair.

When transferring a patient, make sure that all wheels are locked on the bed and/or chair before moving the patient.

Suicide

Patients need to be interviewed regarding their life stressors and coping mechanisms. Life stressors can include losing a job, losing a loved one, divorce, chronic illnesses, and increased family obligations. The goal of risk reduction is keeping the patient safe and helping them avoid self-harm. A **suicide risk assessment** should be performed when patients verbalize suicide ideation or poor coping skills. The patient should be asked if they have a suicide plan and the means to carry it out. The SAD PERSONAS suicide risk assessment can be used to assess a patient's suicide risk. Eleven major areas (sex, age, depression, previous attempt, ethanol abuse, rational thinking loss, social supports lacking, organized plan, no spouse, availability of lethal means, sickness) are assessed and scored. The higher the score, the higher the risk.

Risk Factors

Nurses must acknowledge patient safety risk factors and ensure processes to prevent them. Common types of risk factors that can lead to patient harm include pharmacological (ensuring the five rights of medication administration), environmental (reducing fall and infection rates), equipment (verifying equipment is working properly), and demographic (verifying patient by name and date of birth).

Environmental Risk Factors

Environmental risk factors include anything in the patient's surroundings that can cause harm. This includes the patient's room, infection control, fire safety, and more. Several factors go into ensuring a patient's room is safe and best equipped to prevent falls. One is rooming patients that are more likely to fall, those who are noncompliant, and those with psychiatric conditions or dementia closest to the nurse's station. This allows the nurses to monitor these patients more closely. Another is moving any tripping hazards in the room, including phone chargers and items or spills on the floor. Nurses should also follow policy for setting bed alarms and having patients wear nonslip socks and fall risk bracelets. For infection control, nurses should follow standard precautions including wearing appropriate PPE. No matter the risk to the patient—whether from fall, fire, or infection—the nurse should prevent the risk from occurring, assess the surroundings, then either remove the danger or remove the patient from danger.

Equipment Risk Factors

Common patient safety risk factors that concern equipment include improper decontamination of equipment and equipment that is not labeled properly. Pathogens are present on equipment that is used on multiple patients, such as portable X-ray machines, ultrasound devices, and even stethoscopes. Hospital-acquired infections are harmful to patients and costly to facilities. Nurses should ensure that equipment has been properly sanitized before each use. Another area of concern is untagged equipment, such as IV bags and lines, fire extinguishers, and damaged equipment. When a patient has several IV lines, they should all be properly labeled and include the date the tubing needs to be changed. In an emergency, knowing which line goes to which bag is vital. Damaged equipment should have a label indicating it is damaged and should not be used on patients. This equipment should be stored in a separate location from the functioning equipment.

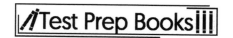

Pharmacological Risk Factors

Pharmacotherapeutic intervention selection is a form of clinical judgment that is based on the findings of the nurse's comprehensive assessment. The selection of pharmacotherapeutic interventions is based on: indications for the therapy; contraindications; cost and compliance; efficacy; adverse effects; dose; duration; and patient directions. The patient's pharmacokinetic response to any drug is related to the patient's inherited metabolic pathways, comorbidities, and the drug characteristics for all prescribed and over the counter (OTC) drugs. The potential for altered drug metabolism can also be the result of the binding of one or more prescribed drugs to liver enzymes, which can decrease (inhibition) or increase (induction) excretion of the drugs through that same enzyme pathway. Inhibition is more common than induction, which potentially results in an adverse drug reaction (ADR) due to increases in the plasma concentration of the drugs. The risk for ADRs also exists when two drugs compete for the same enzyme pathway. These potential sources for ADRs are not always predictable. This means that the medical-surgical nurse will be aware of common ADRs while maintaining close monitoring for patient-specific reactions.

The risk of ADRs resulting from pharmacotherapeutic interventions is greatest for elderly patients. More than 50 percent of patients receiving Medicare take five or more prescribed drugs every day. However, the majority of younger adults report at least occasional use of OTC medications that contain aspirin, acetaminophen, ibuprofen, or naproxen. Many patients underestimate the importance of reporting this use to their care provider, which increases the risk of interactions with prescribed medications. In addition, physician groups have recently requested decreases in the amount of acetaminophen that is contained in OTC combination drugs such as cold and headache preparations. The current levels can potentially result in liver failure even when the patient complies with the recommended dosage schedule. This risk exists for the elderly, patients who consume alcohol, and those patients with undiagnosed susceptibility for this adverse reaction.

The World Health Organization (WHO) and the FDA maintain information related to all reports of drug interaction. The FDA Adverse Events Reporting System (FAERS) also publishes revisions to the black box warnings on all drugs administered in the United States. Identified drug interactions are classified as major, moderate, or minor, according to the documented adverse effects of the interaction. In general, major interactions mean that the combination of drugs should not be used, while the drugs that result in moderate reactions should be used with appropriate caution. Drug interactions are also classified as **pharmacokinetic reactions** (PK reactions) or **pharmacodynamic reactions** (PD reactions). PK reactions refer to drug interactions that occur in one of the four kinetic phases. PD reactions refer to drug interactions that alter the body's response to the drugs.

There are two kinds of contraindication for a pharmacotherapeutic intervention: absolute and relative. An **absolute contraindication** means that the administration of the drug or combination of drugs can result in life-threatening adverse effects that must be avoided. A **relative contraindication** means that the potential for adverse effects should be weighed against the expected therapeutic effect. An absolute contraindication can be related to the reaction of one or more drugs with another drug or with certain patient populations, such as pregnant women, patients with renal failure, and people with other drug allergies. An example of an absolute drug-to-drug contraindication is that warfarin cannot be given with aspirin; one drug potentiates the effect of the other, resulting in an increased risk for bleeding.

Absolute contraindication for pharmacotherapeutic interventions in pregnant women is associated with **teratogenicity**, which is the risk for birth defects due to maternal exposure to the drugs. Patients with renal disease are at risk from the drug interactions because most drugs are excreted by the kidneys, and when there is any degree of altered renal function, the plasma concentration of the drugs, and therefore the risk of adverse effects, will be increased. Patients with identified allergies are at greater risk for hypersensitivity reactions to other drug therapies. Many of the recommended contraindications are contained in condition-specific protocols such as oral contraceptive use, smoking cessation, and obesity therapy. For example, absolute contraindications to oral contraceptive therapy include a known or suspected pregnancy or a history of thrombotic disease. Relative contraindications include the presence of hypertension and current smoking history. In children, there is an

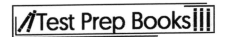

absolute contraindication for the use of aspirin in patients recovering from a viral infection due to the risk of Reye's syndrome, which is rare but often fatal.

Another issue that is associated with the selection of pharmacotherapeutic agents is the use of off-label use of drugs, which means that the drug is being used for a treatment that has not been approved by the FDA. This practice is common in the treatment of cancer when a drug that has been evaluated for the treatment of one form of cancer is used to treat a different form of cancer without being evaluated by the FDA for that specific use. These new therapies can be related to adverse reactions that may be unpredictable. This practice is common in pediatric populations, especially in children with rare diseases because there is insufficient research data to support the providers' clinical decisions.

The **selectivity** of a drug may also be defined as the propensity of a given drug to affect the desired receptor population over others in the body; thus, a highly selective drug reduces the likelihood of possible side effects. **Potency** is a measure of the dosage necessary to produce a standard effect; a more potent drug can be administered in smaller doses than a less potent one. One safety measure of a drug is the **therapeutic index**, which compares the lethal dose of the drug to the therapeutic dose of the drug. Drugs with higher therapeutic indexes are thought to be safer to administer than those with low therapeutic indexes.

This measure is criticized for the use of death as the definition of undesirable adverse effects, and a portion of the supporting data is derived from animal, not human studies. However, it does provide a means of comparing the acceptability of two drugs. The efficacy of a drug is also affected by the **placebo effect**, which is the patient's positive or negative perception of the results of the drug that are not related to the therapeutic outcomes associated with the drug. The availability of generic drugs can also influence the drug selection. Although the inactive ingredients may vary, name brand and generic drugs must contain the active ingredients in the same dosage, potency, and route of administration. The formulation of injectable generic drugs is most often exactly the same as that of the name brand drug.

Genetic Risk Factors

A **genetic risk assessment** estimates an individual's risk for the development of chronic and rare diseases that are genetically linked. This assessment only identifies a statistical probability, not cause and effect, because diseases that result from variants in multiple genes as opposed to a single gene increase the complexity of estimating the risk. There is a wide variation in the degree to which the genetically-linked diseases contribute to the possibility of expression of the disease in the offspring. For instance, the genetic risk associated with the development of melanoma is 21 percent whereas the risk associated with type 1 diabetes is 88 percent. There are two categories of risk: absolute risk and relative risk. **Absolute risk** means that if the patient has a one in ten chance of developing a disease in their lifetime, that person has a 10 percent risk for that disease. **Relative risk** compares the risk for two groups for the same disease. For instance, the risk of breast cancer is higher for descendants of Ashkenazi Jews who emigrated from Eastern Europe than for the average female population in the United States.

There are family patterns that increase the risk for the development of diseases including having multiple first-degree relatives with the same condition, having a relative diagnosed with the condition before the age of 55, having a relative with a disease that is more common in the opposite gender, and having more than one genetically linked disease in the family. The genetic pedigree, which is a visual representation of the patient's family tree, may be used to assess the patient's genetic risk factors. Providers must also support patients and families as they decide whether or not to access formal genetic testing. The Genetic Information Nondiscrimination Act (GINA) and the Health Insurance Portability and Accountability Act (HIPAA) of 1996 provide some protection against discrimination due to the findings of the testing. There also can be ethical questions related to reproductive planning and family dynamics. The patient should be encouraged to seek professional counseling when considering genetic testing. The patient should also understand that direct-to-consumer genetic tests may or may not provide reliable information for the patient's unique circumstances and that none of the commercial products provides counseling.

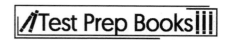
Behavior and Lifestyle Risk Factors

The Centers for Disease Control (CDC) identifies and tracks four lifestyle risk factors: poor exercise habits, inadequate nutrition, smoking, and excessive alcohol intake. Each of these lifestyle behaviors increases the risk of chronic diseases such as HTN, stroke, and respiratory disease. The research clearly implicates smoking as a factor in the development of all of these conditions; yet, adults and young people continue to smoke. The government has enacted age restrictions on the sale of tobacco in addition to imposing a significant tariff that is included in the price of cigarettes, and commercial companies market a wide array of prescription and nonprescription smoking cessation products. There are commercial and medical weight loss programs that provide one-on-one and peer support and twelve-step programs for all forms of addiction. The nurse is responsible for supporting patients' plans to change by providing the necessary information prior to the change in behavior and then to support patients as they initiate and maintain the changed behavior.

The patient should understand that persistent change requires effort continued over time and that even modest reductions in lifestyle risks will have some effect on the progression of chronic diseases. In other words, the patient does not have to run a marathon to gain some benefit from regular, light exercise. Modest dietary improvement and increased activity can lower blood pressure and lipids; however, smoking cessation requires total abstinence to be effective in reducing the development or progression of chronic illness. The nurse will monitor the patient's medication needs as these risk factors are addressed to be sure that medication doses are reduced as necessary. It is not uncommon for patients who eliminate smoking, increase exercise, and improve their nutritional status to be able to discontinue or limit their use of antihypertensive drugs, oral hypoglycemic drugs, or antilipidemic drugs. A patient who has accurate health-promoting information, contacts for needed community resources, and the support of the provider will have the greatest chance for successful change.

Host Risk Factors

Host risk factors, or **host factors**, are terms that refer to a patient's susceptibility to certain diseases. Several factors can affect the probability that someone will develop an acute or chronic illness. Assessing these factors via a health history interview followed by a physical assessment can direct the advanced practice nurse to develop a treatment plan that will prevent possible complications. Microorganisms thrive when they invade the body and overpower the immune response. The first line of defense in the body is the skin. When the skin is broken, it opens up a pathway for microorganisms to enter the body and cause illness. Assessing the patient's skin integrity is an important component of a physical assessment. Patients who have skin integrity issues are more at risk of developing infections. To survive, the body must maintain an acid-base balance. The pH levels vary throughout the body. The stomach is highly acidic, whereas the large intestine is more basic. In females, vaginal pH is moderately acidic. When pH levels in these areas change, microorganisms can grow.

For example, when the vaginal pH turns alkaline, there is an increased risk of developing bacterial vaginosis (BV), which can cause itchiness, discharge, and discomfort. The immune response is activated when a microorganism enters the body. Cell mediators alert the body that there is a potentially harmful organism present. White blood cells (WBCs) help fight off infection in the body. When patients have decreased levels of WBCs, they are more susceptible to infection due to a delayed or weakened immune response. Medications can alter a patient's immune response. Corticosteroids, a class of anti-inflammatory drugs, suppress the immune system. They are helpful in autoimmune illnesses in which the body attacks its own immune system. However, a practitioner should always balance the risks and benefits of suppressing immunity. Age is an important host factor for susceptibility. Older adults go through age-related changes, such as loss of skin elasticity, a decrease in sphincter control of the bladder, and a decreased cough reflex. These changes can increase the risk of skin, urinary tract, and pulmonary infections.

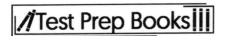
Demographic Risk Factors

It is important for the nurse to know which diseases or conditions ethnic and racial groups are prone to. The white population is more prone to atrial fibrillation than people of other races. The Hispanic population has high rates of obesity and diabetes; in individuals from Puerto Rico, there is an increased incidence of HIV infection and AIDS.

Obesity and type 2 diabetes are common in African Americans, and the death rate from HTN, stroke, HIV infection, and AIDS is higher than the rate in the non-Hispanic white population. Asian Americans have an increased incidence of tuberculosis, and hepatitis B infection occurs more commonly in recent immigrants to the United States. Asian Americans also have an increased rate of chronic obstructive pulmonary disease (COPD), in spite of the fact that smoking rates among Chinese and Japanese Americans are lower than average. Native Americans have a high incidence of alcoholism; recent pharmacologic research indicates that altered metabolic pathways may contribute to this finding. As with the Asian American population, the nurse will be aware of the frequent use of herbal preparations in the Native American population as well.

Patient Safety Culture

A patient safety culture is an environment in which nurses can admit to mistakes without being punished. The goal is to allow nurses to report to strategize prevention measures and teach other nurses ways to avoid the same mistake. Patient safety culture is one of actability, accountability, and learning.

Near-Miss Reporting

Near misses are events during which a medical mistake was almost made but was corrected before any harm was done to the patient. An example would be a nurse almost administering the wrong medication but realizing the error before it was given to the patient. Reporting allows institutions to identify weaknesses and correct them to prevent the near miss from happening again. It is important to learn from near misses to prevent errors that result in harm to patients which are called **adverse events**. The object of reporting is not to be punitive but to improve processes for better patient care.

Just Culture

Just culture is a philosophy that encourages transparency and accountability across many levels of an organizational system. Individuals have responsibility for outcomes in the organization, as do established policies and procedures that guide decision-making and behaviors across the organization. Just culture aims to drive ethical decision-making while acknowledging that a myriad of variables can contribute to poor outcomes. Patient outcomes are affected by the nurse's direct patient care; however, they are also influenced by leadership decisions, hospital-wide policies, federal regulations, and other factors outside of the nurse's control. Instead of blaming people for workplace situations that go wrong, just cultures aim to improve problematic processes.

Just cultures acknowledge that human error is possible with even the best standardized operating procedures in place. When a patient experiences poor outcomes, the situation is sometimes attributed to a mistake made by the nurse. The nurse may be terminated from their role or punished in another way. However, continuously replacing nurses rather than addressing the root cause of errors is a costly and inefficient resolution. Just cultures can be cultivated by establishing the expectation that all individuals within an organization have shared accountability for ensuring patient outcomes and by encouraging open communication from staff members across the organizational hierarchy. For example, entry-level staff members should feel comfortable expressing to senior leadership how system flaws may be contributing to poor patient outcomes.

Frontline workers should feel comfortable reporting when they believe they have made an error on the job, rather than delaying resolution out of fear for their job security or punitive responses. Comparatively, senior leadership should understand frontline roles so that they can best identify gaps and make prompt process changes.

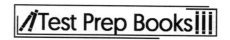
Organizations should regularly review standard operating procedures with input from all staff members to identify gaps and opportunities for process improvement that could lead to better patient outcomes.

Finally, although just culture focuses heavily on improving whole systems rather than solely blaming individuals for healthcare errors, the philosophy encourages personal responsibility where possible. Individual employees should not intentionally work carelessly or with disregard for patient outcomes. Federal regulators now look for just culture practices within hospital safety standards, typically through indicators such as employee reporting standards, risk assessment frameworks, communication standards between healthcare providers and patients, and corrective action and prevention plans that focus on process improvement.

Speak Up

Speak Up is The Joint Commission's patient safety program, which encourages patients and family members to participate in their healthcare. Speak Up is a mnemonic that stands for Speak up, Pay attention, Educate yourself, Advocates can help, Know about your medicine, Use a quality healthcare organization, and Participate in all decisions about your care. Information is available via posters and videos on topics such as vaccinations, new parents, and surgery. The program's goal is to empower patients to become autonomous in their healthcare decision making.

High Accountable Organizations

High Accountable Organizations, also known as Accountable Care Organizations, are groups of providers or hospitals that work together to ensure the best patient care. This includes providing high-quality care, reducing medical costs, and improving health outcomes. These programs originated from the Center for Medicare and Medicaid Services. High Accountable Organizations may focus on a specific geographical location or special population, like people with diabetes. This model allows providers to holistically look at a patient's health history and services that have been provided at other facilities. For the patient, this means less repeat testing and services.

Care Bundles

A **care bundle**, developed by the Institute for Healthcare Improvement, is a succinct set of evidence-based practices to improve patient care for common treatments that pose risks. One example is a central line bundle that has five steps to prevent catheter-related bloodstream infections. Bundles are helpful because they pull together multiple ways of performing a task into one evidence-based process to promote uniformity. The goal of the bundle is to provide the highest possible patient care and outcome.

Bundles have specific formats that are slightly different from checklists and algorithms. Bundles have a stepwise approach in which each step must be completed before moving to the next to achieve the optimum outcome. They are based on Level 1 evidence-based practices, which compare randomized controlled trials to ensure the nurse is using the best data to perform the procedure. Additionally, bundles provide black-and-white, yes-or-no distinctions that leave no gray area up for interpretation. Lastly the bundle must be completed by one healthcare team in one setting. Care bundles are to be repeated as needed until the service is no longer required.

Another example of a bundle is the ventilator bundle, which was created to prevent ventilator-associated pneumonia, a common hospital-acquired infection. Through research, it was found that doing the following four interventions may prevent or delay the onset of this type of pneumonia:

- Administering deep vein thrombosis prophylaxis
- Administering gastric ulceration preventative medications
- Elevating the head or bed to between 30 and 45 degrees
- Assessing whether the patient can breathe on their own daily

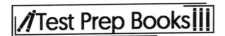

Patient Safety Assessments and Reporting

Nurses are mandated to report certain findings or suspicions, such as child abuse, elder abuse, and human trafficking. Regardless of whether the nurse thinks the patient's claims are true or if there is any proof, they must report. Sometimes patients will divulge this information on their own, but often the nurse must assess for these risks and for social determinants of health.

Abuse and Neglect

Patients can arrive at a clinic or hospital as a result of experiencing abuse or neglect. They may also arrive for some other reason but show signs of having been abused or neglected. Medical-surgical nurses must be able to identify when patients have been experiencing abuse and neglect and know how to provide care while ensuring that the situation is escalated to the necessary authorities. Abuse and neglect most commonly result from domestic violence between partners, violence against children by their parents or caregivers, or against elders by caretakers. Abuse may be physical, emotional, financial, or sexual.

While abuse refers to intentional assaults, neglect refers to inadequate caretaking that endangers someone. This may include not feeding, bathing, or otherwise assisting a person who is unable to take care of themselves. Signs of neglect include poor hygiene, malnourishment, and the presence of bedsores. Neglect may take the form of withholding necessary medications or mobility supports (e.g., a walker) or exposing the person to unsafe situations.

Identifying potential abuse and neglect should be a component of the intake process. Nurses should note any visible signs and ask the patient questions about their care. Nurses should be aware of visible signs of abuse, including bruises, burns, injured limbs, trauma near the patient's private areas, disrespectful treatment by caretakers, and fearfulness shown by the patient near certain visitors. Nurses may consider directly asking the patient about specific instances of abuse. Patients may not feel comfortable answering these questions, and nurses should allow them time and privacy away from their caregivers to complete intake. After intake, a physical examination can also provide clues about patient abuse and neglect.

Physical abuse involves injuries to the body from punching, kicking, etc. If the nurse notes various bruises or cuts in various stages of healing without explanation, it may be a sign of physical abuse. *Sexual abuse* is when sexual contact is made without the consent of one party, including rape, coercion into doing sexual acts, and fondling of genitalia. The nurse should look for unexplained bruising of or bleeding around the perineal area, new difficulty sitting or walking, or increased agitation/aggression as potential signs of sexual abuse. *Emotional* or *mental abuses* are not quite as obvious as physical abuse as the damage inflicted is internal or hidden. Emotional and mental abuses are usually caused by verbal assaults. The abuser may belittle and criticize the victim to the point that the victim feels worthless, insecure, and afraid. If the nurse senses an uncomfortable relationship between an informal caregiver or family member and the patient, this should be monitored, investigated, and reported if abuse is suspected. Financial abuse most commonly affects elders who may have decreased cognitive or physical functioning. In financial abuse situations, relatives, friends, or other caretakers may steal money from the patient, forge the patient's signatures on financial documents, or otherwise give themselves legal authority with unjust cause (e.g., claiming that a patient is not healthy enough to make personal decisions and needs a power of attorney). If the nurse suspects that checks and other financial means meant for the patient are being rerouted and misused by a caregiver, this abuse should be reported right away.

If either abuse or neglect is suspected, evidence should be documented in the patient's medical chart in case an investigation occurs. If the medical-surgical nurse suspects abuse or neglect, they are mandatorily required to report it to the appropriate entity. The charge nurse and/or nurse manager should be notified, so the appropriate action can be taken to right the situation. There are also hotlines that can be called, such as the National Center on Elder Abuse (1-800-677-1116).

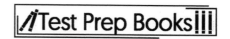
Human Trafficking

Most trafficking victims are women or young men. Many victims are accompanied by their trafficker, which can complicate the processes of identifying and helping them. They generally show signs of physical and mental abuse. A red flag that warrants further attention is when a patient is accompanied by someone who appears overly involved in the case but does not seem to be genuinely concerned about the patient; this is often the trafficker. Their identification may indicate no relation to the patient, but they will insist that they are a friend or romantic partner. They may control all of the patient's personal identification and insist on paying in cash. The trafficker may be highly resistant to letting the patient go anywhere alone with the healthcare provider, yet this is the best way to identify whether someone is a trafficking victim and help them out of the situation. Many victims are seen for medical issues that do not result from trafficked activities but from delays in receiving routine care. For example, a woman who is being trafficked may become pregnant and not receive prenatal care until she is in an emergency situation.

Most healthcare facilities have specific policies and procedures in place to identify and screen trafficking victims. Screening processes should be age appropriate and sensitive in order to help the victim in the most dignified and compassionate manner possible. In most states, adult victims must choose whether they want an intervention. However, all healthcare providers can anonymously and safely report any suspicions of possibly trafficked individuals to the necessary authorities. Intervention can be a traumatic event for the patient and must be handled cautiously, while also ensuring that it is performed quickly and that the trafficker is restrained. Social services, legal services, and law enforcement are often a part of any intervention, making it a highly complex and collaborative initiative.

Social Determinants

Social determinants of health (SDOH) are nonmedical factors that affect a patient's health and well-being. These factors include socioeconomic status, transportation, political climate, and racism, among others. For example, if a patient does not have running water, how can they perform hand hygiene before a dressing change? Screening for these factors helps ensure patient safety and well-being. When screening patients for SDOH, ensure that resources are in place to give to patients or refer them to. For example, if a patient is facing food insecurity, the nurse should have resources to food banks and food assistance programs ready.

Risk Assessment Methods

Root Cause Analysis

Root cause analysis can also be used as a learning exercise for systems theory because this process, which is commonly used to investigate errors, looks at all elements of an institution's relationship with the error. Case studies and reflection are also recommended as useful learning aids for systems thinking. In addition, there are valid assessment instruments that can be used to assess systems thinking skills acquired through these learning activities.

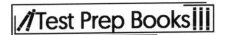
A cause-and-effect diagram can show relationships between factors and can organize potential causes into smaller categories in order to find out why something happened or how it could happen. It is also known as an Ishikawa diagram, named after the man who designed it, Kaoru Ishikawa. Although it was originally developed as a quality control tool, in the healthcare setting the diagram is used to discover the root cause of a problem, uncover bottlenecks in a process or identify where and why a process isn't working. This is called a **root cause analysis** or a **cause-and-effect analysis**.

Example of a Root Cause Analysis

Environment

High noise level

Location of medication room

Communication

Transcription error

Handwritten order illegible

Equipment

Medication dispensing not automated

People

Medication nurse working overtime

Leadership

Equipment needs not met

Budget constraints

Procedures

Pharmacist review not done before dispensing

Order entry not computerized

Medication Error

The root cause analysis (RCA) is used when there is an adverse event, a sentinel event, or close call in the medical setting. It can also be used when there is a concern about a process due to repeated errors, when there is a possibility of serious errors, and when there are high-cost errors. The RCA answers the following critical questions:

- What happened or is still happening?
- How did it happen?
- Why did it happen?
- How can we prevent it from happening again?
- What can we learn from this?

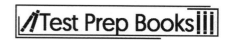

FMEA

Failure mode and effects analysis (FMEA) is a systematic method to discover all the ways something can go wrong in a process and then addressing each of those possibilities. The failure mode is the way something might fail. The effects analysis concerns the consequences of the failure. The overall goal of this system is to identify potential failures and prevent them from happening. FMEA is a team-based tool that includes the following:

- Identifying the steps in the process
- Failure modes (What could go wrong at each step?)
- Failure causes (How could the failures happen?)
- Failure effects (What would the consequences of each failure be?)

Once these have been identified, the next steps are to determine the likelihood of the failure occurring, the likelihood of catching the failure, and the severity of consequences if the failure occurred. Then the potential failures are ranked by risk level so the team knows which to address first.

The FMEA tool can be used at several different junctures, but is best used before a new process is launched to predict potential failure. It can also be used when an existing process needs improvement, when existing processes are being used in a new manner, or when an existing process is being modified.

Let's walk through an example. Say a provider initiates a new drug therapy for a patient. The steps in the process are identified. First, the provider initiates therapy; second, the administration of medication begins; third, the provider monitors the patient's initial response to the new medication; etc. Then potential failures for each step would be identified. So, for the first step (provider initiates therapy), possible failures could include that the order wasn't entered into the electronic health record (EHR) or that the provider did not check the five rights of medication administration. These possible errors would be identified for each step mentioned earlier. Then the team would identify how these mistakes could occur. Maybe the provider got called away to an emergency and could not enter the order, maybe the wrong patient was pulled up on the EHR and the order was entered under the wrong patient's record, or maybe the wrong medication was entered for the correct patient. Next the team would determine the consequences of each failure and rank them in order of severity. If the medication was not ordered, there would be a delay in care. If the medication was urgent, not administering it could have serious consequences. The same applies if the wrong medication or patient was chosen. Along with the severity ranking, the team would evaluate the likelihood of catching these errors before they happen. Lastly, strategies would be developed to prevent these errors from happening. Most EHRs have safety checks built in when prescribing medications. Nurses must scan the patient and the medication before administering. The five rights of medication administration are frequently reviewed on the unit. By breaking up a process into steps and then identifying and preventing potential pitfalls, the workplace and the patients become much safer.

Safety Rounds

In addition to daily rounds from the provider, nursing **safety rounds** are another opportunity to address patient safety. Safety rounds can be performed by the bedside nurse or by a patient safety team. Their frequency depends on the facility. This approach partners the family members with nurses to watch out for patient safety. Since family members are often with the patient for extended periods of time, they are in a great position to notice subtle changes in the patient's disposition that could impact the patient's safety.

Safety Huddles

A **safety huddle** is a short (ten- to fifteen-minute), interdisciplinary debrief of patient safety concerns that were faced yesterday and anticipated ones that may be expected on the current day. This is a way to improve communication between team members and raise awareness around areas of patient concern. It is not a forum to solve safety issues—that responsibility goes to managers or safety committees—but rather to make sure the

115

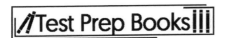
healthcare team is on the same page regarding patients' safety. This opportunity for communication lessens the chances of near misses and patient harm. Huddles foster problem identification and team collaboration, thereby increasing patient safety.

Infection Prevention and Control

Universal Precautions

Universal precautions revolve around blood borne pathogens (BBP) and needle safety. Nurses should treat all blood as if it is infected by a BBP such as HIV or HepB. Protective barriers such as gloves, gowns, masks, surgical caps, shoe or boot covers, and eyewear should be worn when encountering blood. Nurses should never re-cap used needles. All needles should be disposed of in red sharps containers, and all blood-soaked items should be disposed of in red biohazard bins to protect everyone involved in the disposal of waste.

Standard Precautions

Standard precautions are general precautions to be used with all patients in a medical setting. These precautions include personal protection if the patient is suspected to have a contagious disease, environmental cleanliness, disinfection and sterilization of all medical equipment and linens, safe sharps handling, and safe infectious waste disposal techniques. Hand hygiene is one of the most critical precautionary practices. All healthcare providers should wash their hands with soap and water when entering or exiting a patient's room, any time they come into contact with bodily fluids, when removing gloves, before and after touching any medical equipment, before eating, and after using the restroom. In addition to these hand washing guidelines, regular use of alcohol-based hand sanitation throughout the workday is also recommended.

Use standard precautions for the care of all patients

Standard precautions apply to:
- blood
- non-intact skin
- mucous membranes
- all body fluids, secretions, and excretions (except sweat)

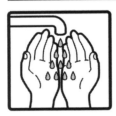	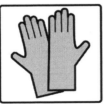	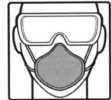	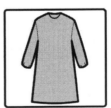	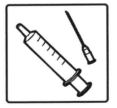
Wash hands	**Wear gloves**	**Wear mask**	**Wear gown**	**Sharps disposal**
Wash hands properly and thoroughly between patient contact and other contact with body fluids or soiled equipment.	Wear gloves when handling blood, body fluids, non-intact skin, or soiled items. Change gloves between patients. Wash hands after removing gloves.	Wear a mask and eye protection or face shield to protect mucous membranes of the eyes, nose, and mouth when likely to be splashed.	Wear a gown to protect skin and prevent soiling of clothing when likely to be splashed or sprayed. Wash hands after removing gown.	Dispose of syringes and other sharps into a designated closed container. **Do not** break or bend needles.

Follow established policies and procedures for patient placement, environmental controls, patient-care equipment, and linen.

116

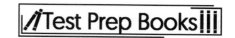

In all healthcare settings, the gold standard in infection prevention is hand hygiene. Hand hygiene includes consistency in hand washing and antisepsis at the correct times and with the proper technique. Although hand hygiene is known to be a simple, effective way to prevent the spread of infectious pathogens (including **multi-drug resistant organisms [MDROs]**), the CDC reports healthcare providers clean their hands less than one half of the times they should.

Healthcare providers use PPE as a way to protect themselves from being exposed to infectious material from the patient and healthcare environment. PPE used in the perioperative setting includes surgical masks, gloves, eye shields, impervious gowns, and shoe covers. PPE is also utilized in patient resuscitation with the use of a bag-valve mask or ambu bag rather than mouth-to-mouth resuscitation. Environmental control is an important aspect of infection prevention because it decreases transmission of pathogens from environmental surfaces to patients and/or healthcare workers. Using approved disinfectants according to manufacturer instructions is an effective environmental control measure in infection control and prevention.

Transmission-Based Precautions

When a patient is colonized or infected with a known MDRO, transmission-based precautions are taken. Transmission-based precautions are used along with standard precautions. These precautions are implemented even while laboratory testing to confirm an infectious agent is conducted. Though this process can take days or weeks, it is necessary in order to control the spread of the infectious agent. Transmission-based precautions encompass contact, droplet, and airborne precaution guidelines. The indication depends on the MDRO.

Contact precautions are used with patients infected or colonized with microorganisms transmitted by direct or indirect contact. These include *Clostridium difficile* (*C. diff*), methicillin resistant *Staphylococcus aureus* (MRSA), and vancomycin resistant *Enterococcus* (VRE).

Droplet precautions are used if a patient has a confirmed or suspected infection transmissible through respiratory droplets. PPE associated with droplet precautions are gloves, gown, and mask. The patient is also placed in a single-patient room. Influenza and respiratory syncytial virus (RSV) are indications for droplet precautions.

Airborne precautions are taken when providing care to a patient with known or suspected infection transmissible via airborne route. The patient's respiratory particles are airborne for prolonged time periods and are carried by normal air currents. The most common airborne-transmissible infections are tuberculosis, measles, and varicella.

Disinfection

Disinfection involves the use of chemical agents that eliminate or kill all pathogenic microorganisms, with the exception of a high number of bacterial spores on inanimate objects. Disinfecting entails using antiseptics and germicides to destroy microorganisms.

The type of disinfectant chosen depends on the action or function that is necessary for the chemical to perform. Also, criteria such as safety, effect on equipment, cost, and impact to the environment should be taken into consideration prior to use.

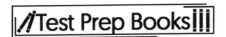

Disinfectants may be split into three categories: high level, intermediate level, and low level. These categories refer to the disinfectant's capabilities.

Level of Disinfectant	Description	Solution
High-Level	High-level disinfectants kill a broad spectrum of microorganisms. However, bacterial spores can survive.	High-level disinfectants receive Food and Drug Administration (FDA) clearance. Example solutions include peracetic acid (PAA), hydrogen peroxides, glutaraldehyde, formaldehyde, and ortho-phthalaldehyde.
Intermediate-Level	Intermediate-level disinfectants kill tubercle bacilli, vegetative bacteria, many viruses, and fungi; however, bacterial spores can survive.	Intermediate-level disinfectants consist of chemical germicides that are registered as tuberculocides by the Environmental Protection Agency (EPA). Solutions consist of alcohols, hypochlorites, iodine, and iodophor disinfectants.
Low-Level	Low-level disinfectants kill vegetative bacteria, some viruses, and fungi.	Chemical germicides are registered as hospital disinfectants by the EPA. Solutions consist of phenolics or quaternary ammonium compounds.

Disinfectants can be irritating to the skin and mucous membranes. Therefore, any use of these chemicals should always take place in an environment with adequate ventilation. Vapor control systems are especially beneficial in protecting staff from irritation.

The Spaulding Classification System

The Spaulding Classification System (named for founder Earle Spaulding) classifies items that require disinfection as being critical, semicritical, or noncritical. These classifications relate to the risk of infection for the patient. Also, the level of disinfection chosen has a direct relationship with the instrument and method of utilization.

Critical Items

Critical items are those devices that enter the sterile tissue or vascular system such as catheters, implants, and ultrasound probes. They have a high risk for infection through microorganism contamination. Institutions purchase these instruments or use steam sterilization. Those instruments that are heat-sensitive receive ethylene oxide or hydrogen peroxide gas plasma.

Semicritical Items

Semicritical items are those instruments or equipment that come in contact with mucous membranes or nonintact skin. Examples of semicritical items include laryngoscope blades, cystoscopes, and anesthesia. Although the lungs and gastrointestinal tract may not be susceptible to bacterial spore infections, they are at risk for infections resulting from bacteria, mycobacteria, and viruses. These items undergo intermediate-level disinfection using chemical disinfectants. Commonly used disinfectants for semicritical items include glutaraldehyde, hydrogen peroxide, ortho-phthalaldehyde, and PAA with hydrogen peroxide.

Endoscopes require flushing with sterile water to prevent any adverse effects that might occur with use of a disinfectant. While tap water or filtered water may also aid in flushing endoscopes and channels, there is a risk for organism contamination, and therefore, sterile water is the preference.

Forced-air drying can assist in the reduction of bacterial contamination, and, therefore, these items should undergo forced-air drying before they are packed and stored away.

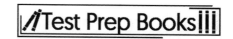
Noncritical Items

Noncritical items are those devices that do not come in contact with mucous membranes but do come in contact with intact skin. Examples of noncritical items include bedpans, blood pressure cuffs, crutches, bedside tables, bed rails, and floors. Low-level disinfectants are appropriate for these items. Decontamination often takes place in the same location of usage. A single-use disposable towel to clean a bedside table surface is an example of surface cleaning in the physical place of use. Transmission of infectious agents to patients from noncritical items is very rare.

Sterilants and Disinfectants

Sterilants, or chemical germicides and **disinfectants**, may fall into a variety of categories. The most common two types include oxidizing agents and alkylating agents.

Oxidizing Agents

Hydrogen peroxide is not only effective in cleaning wounds, but it is also useful as a disinfectant and sterilizing agent for surgical instruments.

Accelerated hydrogen peroxide is effective in fighting against bacteria, viruses, fungi, and spores. Health institutions use it as a disinfectant. Damage to soft metals such as brass, copper, and aluminum is a risk in using accelerated hydrogen peroxide.

Peracetic acid (PAA) is a high-level disinfectant used in aseptic packaging and disinfection. It is a moderately stronger oxidizing agent than hydrogen peroxide. It is effective against bacteria, spores, yeasts, fungi, mycobacteria, and viruses and can reduce microbial populations in wounds that have contamination. PAA is a rapid-acting oxidizer that remains active at low temperatures.

Sodium hypochlorite is one of the most successful disinfecting agents in health care facilities. Low concentrations of this solution can prove to be highly useful as a powerful oxidizing disinfectant as a result of its ability to kill organisms, even with low temperatures. This characteristic makes it especially attractive to health care institutions because it can reduce the transmission of diseases.

Alkylating Agents

One method of sterilization is **gas sterilization**. Instruments undergo exposure to high concentrations of reactive gasses and vapors for a prescribed period within a sealed chamber.

Ethylene oxide sterilization is a low-temperature process in which ethylene oxide gas decreases the number of infectious agents. It is especially beneficial for those instruments that cannot endure the heat of an autoclave sterilization environment. The duration in which the process takes place may vary depending on the type of device that is undergoing sterilization; however, cycles may last between thirty-six and forty-eight hours.

Formaldehyde sterilization is most effective in a highly concentrated gaseous state. It is most useful for those instruments and medical equipment that cannot endure high-temperature sterilization. The staff that uses this method of sterilization may be subject to monitoring if they exceed exposure level limits, as this can lead to injury.

Sterilization

Sterilization is the destruction and removal of microbial life, including spores. Once something is sterile, the probability of microorganism survival is one in one million.

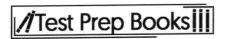

Type of Sterilization	Description
Steam Sterilization	Steam sterilization is the oldest decontamination and sterilization method that uses pressurized steam to kill microorganisms. **Advantages:** • It is a cost-effective form of sterilization. • It works best with devices that are heat and moisture tolerant.
Ethylene Oxide "Gas" Sterilization	This process is used to sterilize those instruments that are not able to withstand high steam sterilization (e.g., plastic packaging, plastic containers, and electronic components). **Advantages:** • Ability to sterilize instruments that are heat sensitive **Disadvantages:** • Cycle time • Cost • Hazards to the patient and staff
Liquid Chemical Sterilization	Liquid chemical sterilization entails the use of a chemical agent to sterilize an instrument. **Advantages:** • Rapid sterilization • Effective for heat-sensitive devices **Disadvantages:** • Cannot fully penetrate barriers such as blood, tissue, and biofilm • Viscosity of some liquids prevents them from reaching pathogens in narrow lumens • Devices may need rinsing after the liquid chemical sterilant, but the water may not be sterile
Ozone Sterilizer	Ozone oxidizes organic matter including bacteria, fungi, and viruses found on instruments. It is able to sterilize equipment at a low temperature and is easy to use. The manufacturer's instructions must be followed closely for proper use. **Advantages:** • Cost-effective • Compatible with aluminum, titanium, ceramic, glass, Teflon, and silicone containers **Disadvantages:** • May be inadequate for killing MERSA
Plasma Sterilization System	The low-temperature hydrogen peroxide gas plasma sterilization can be used with those items that are moisture and heat sensitive. It removes microbial organisms through use of hydrogen peroxide vapor and free radicals that disrupt the microbial cell membranes and enzymes. This system sterilizes instruments within thirty minutes to a little more than an hour using hydrogen peroxide gas. Users must follow the manufacturer's instructions because the system can only be used with certain instruments.

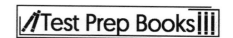

Type of Sterilization	Description
Infrared Radiation	This sterilizer destroys spores. **Advantages:** <ul><li>Short cycle duration</li><li>Alternative for heat-resistant instruments</li></ul> **Not FDA cleared
Gaseous Chlorine Dioxide	The gaseous chlorine dioxide system is a health care sterilization system that has the capacity to sterilize instruments in a short period of time. **Not FDA cleared

Steam Sterilization

Steam sterilization is the oldest decontamination and sterilization method that uses pressurized steam to kill microorganisms. This method of sterilization works best with those items that can withstand heat and moisture.

Steam sterilization requires temperature, time, pressure, and saturated steam to function properly. These things take place in an autoclave or a high-speed prevacuum sterilizer. Autoclaves receive steam at the top or sides of the sterilizing chamber and force the air out of the bottom of the chamber through a drain vent. High-speed prevacuum sterilizers have a vacuum pump that ensures air removal from the sterilizing chamber and loads ahead of steam admission. The prevacuum pump allows for quick steam penetration. The functionality of these machines undergoes the Bowie-Dick test each day to assess for air leaks or poor air removal and includes the use of 100 percent cotton surgical towels that are clean and preconditioned.

Another steam sterilization method is known as the steam flush-pressure pulsing process. This process involves the rapid movement of air through a repeatedly alternating flush of steam and pressure pulse above the atmosphere pressure. Sterilization duration using this method is three to four minutes at 132 to 135 degrees Celsius. The system also undergoes a monitoring process much like the others in which temperature, time, and pressure measurements are reviewed.

The duration in which instruments remain in the system varies by the items requiring sterilization, type of sterilizing system in use, cycle design, bioburden, altitude, package, size, and design. End users must follow the instructions as written by the manufacturer of the sterilizer to achieve the best possible outcome.

While steam sterilization is a commonly utilized method of sterilization, there is some risk that this approach may not be as effective as necessary if it is unable to remove the biofilm adequately. There are some implants and instrument sets that require extended cycles to achieve sterilization.

Dynamic Air Removal and Gravity Displacement

Dynamic air removal and gravity displacement are two methods of steam sterilization that are used to disinfect medical devices. In a dynamic air removal system, instruments that need sterilization are placed in a holding bag which is then placed into a chamber. As steam forcefully enters the chamber, the air that was previously in the chamber is actively removed through a vacuum mechanism. This clears the chamber and allows steam to enter the holding bag and sterilize the instruments. The vacuum mechanism is then used to remove the steam and dry the instruments.

Gravity displacement sterilization uses the force of gravity, rather than an attached vacuum, to remove the air that was previously in the chamber out. As long as the steam is at a hotter temperature than the air in the chamber, the pressure difference will push the air out. The dynamic air removal process allows sterilization to occur in under five

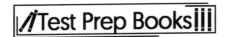

minutes, whereas the gravity displacement process can take about half an hour. When sterilization is complete, the instruments should be left in the chamber until cool and all moisture has evaporated. Touching the instruments before all moisture has evaporated will likely lead to contamination. In gravity displacement systems, complete drying can take two hours or more.

Flash Sterilization

Flash sterilization is another form of sterilization that can prove useful in sterilizing critical medical devices. It is another form of steam sterilization. The item is placed on a tray and undergoes flashing with rapid steaming. This process is done in close proximity to the OR to expedite delivery to the point of service. Flash sterilization is often utilized when there is not enough time to sterilize an item by usual prepackaged methods. It should not be used for "convenience" or instances where there is a risk for infections, nor should it be used with implantable devices.

This method is associated with some adverse episodes such as infections. Also, burns from the instruments have occurred. As a result of these events, policies have been instituted to help avoid preventable burns. Patient burns are avoidable if cooling protocol are followed. Air cooling or immersion in sterile liquid can help with the cooling process.

Heat-Based Sterilization

Heat-based sterilization methods such as a steam autoclave or dry heat oven is a viable option for heat-stable, reusable medical instruments that enter the bloodstream or sterile tissue. Arthroscopic and laparoscopic telescopes should undergo sterilization before use; however, in those instances where this practice is not possible, high-level disinfection is the method of choice. Meanwhile, those components of the endoscopic set such as the trocars and operative instruments can undergo heat-based sterilization methods such as the steam autoclave or dry heat oven.

Safe Handling of Hazardous/Biohazardous Materials

Blood-borne pathogens refer to infectious agents found in human blood that can cause infection and also be easily transmitted upon contact. Most healthcare providers are regularly at risk of exposure to blood-borne pathogens, especially if they regularly work with patients' bodily fluids, in operating rooms, or with sharps. OSHA requires that employers of healthcare providers follow its standards for controlling blood-borne pathogen exposure. These standards include implementing a training program to educate employees about the risks and how to mitigate them, protective clothing and equipment requirements, certain preliminary vaccinations before the employee's first day of work, and using sharps-free medical equipment when possible. The most commonly recognized blood-borne pathogens include the hepatitis viruses and human immunodeficiency virus (HIV).

Safe handling of hazardous and biohazardous materials is a critical function of hospital and clinic staff. Universal-, standard-, and transmission-based precautions each enable staff to adhere to a set of standards that were designed to prevent and protect staff from the transmission of blood-borne infections or diseases.

OSHA requires organizations to develop exposure protocol plans that are shared with staff and undergo a review and revision on an annual basis.

Best practices must be implemented and followed to reduce the risk of employee exposure, which may include a core set of processes and procedures that address:

- Specimen storage and transportation to include warning labels
- Use of personal protective equipment (PPE) and employer provision of those items including gloves, gowns, and masks
- Management of contaminated needles (e.g., not recapping used needles)

- Signage in plain view with biohazard logos

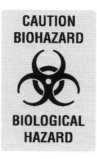

- Housekeeping schedule creation and posting
- Management of contaminated laundry

Antimicrobial Stewardship

Over the years, bacteria have mutated to survive against antibiotics, which make bacterial infections more difficult to treat. **Antimicrobial stewardship** promotes the correct usage of antibiotics to improve patient outcomes, reduce antibiotic resistance, and decrease the spread of antimicrobial resistant infections or "superbugs."

Surgical Scrub

Surgical scrub is the process of washing one's hands and arms in a specific manner prior to entering the operating room. Surgical site infections are one of the leading types of nosocomial infections. Scrubbing before entering the sterile operating room helps prevent pathogens on the nurse's hands and arms from being transmitted to the patient.

Antibiotics

Antibiotics are medications used to kill or stop the growth of bacteria. Antibiotics do not work on viruses and should not be used for viral infections. Many patients believe they should receive an antibiotic for any type of infection they have. Nurses should educate patients on these principles to reduce unnecessary usage of antibiotics, which leads to antimicrobial resistance.

Probiotics

The body, especially the gut, has good bacteria in it that maintains a normal balance for GI health. If antibiotics are taken, they kill good bacteria as well, which disrupts homeostasis and often leads to diarrhea and dehydration. Probiotics can be administered along with or after antibiotic usage to replenish and promote the growth of good bacteria.

Medication Management

Safe Medication Administration Practices

Ongoing assessment and documentation of the effectiveness of the plan of care is an essential function of the medical surgical nurse's professional practice. The initial assessment by the nurse is the foundation for all future assessments and evaluations. With respect to the pharmacotherapeutic plan, patient safety requires a full account of all agents that the patient consumes, including OTC and prescription drugs, herbs, and all other supplements.

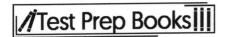

The "seven rights" refer to a set of seven guidelines for healthcare providers to follow when administering medication to patients. These standardize the medication administration process and promote a context of high-quality care. The seven rights are:

- Right medication: Providers check that the medication they are about to administer is the one that was prescribed.
- Right client: Providers check that the patient who is about to receive medication is the correct patient.
- Right dose: Providers check that the dose they are about to administer matches the prescribed dose.
- Right time: Providers check that the medication is given at the pre-determined interval.
- Right route: Providers ensure that medication is delivered in the intended method (e.g., orally).
- Right reason: Providers note that the medication is administered for a specific cause.
- Right documentation: Providers follow institutional protocol to maintain thorough recordkeeping of administered medications.

These rights work to ensure patient safety.

In addition to the rights of the patient, the nurse should ensure that the appropriate physician and pharmacist orders have been given. The nurse will be expected to obtain information about the client's list of prescribed medications, involving the formulary review and consultations with the pharmacist. It is vital that the nurse be able to use critical thinking when expecting certain effects and outcomes of medication administration, including oral, intradermal, subcutaneous, intramuscular, and topical formulations. Over time, the client should be evaluated for their response to their medication regime. This includes a variety of home remedies, their prescription drugs, and any over-the-counter (OTC) drug usage. The response of the client to their medications, whether therapeutic or not, should be evaluated. If adverse reactions or side effects occur, the patient's medications will need to be reevaluated and modified.

The nurse should assess the patient for any allergies. This information can be found in the patient's medical record or chart if they have been previously admitted. The allergy information on the patient should include the specific type of reaction they had, whether it was a mild rash or a severe, anaphylactic reaction.

Most medical facilities have electronic health record systems that, once the client is registered for the first time, will keep track of their medication record. This will need to be modified with each doctor's visit and hospital stay, of course, but is a helpful tool in recording the client's list of medications.

With all medication administration, the nurse should keep their eye on the expected outcome. Identifying the expected outcome, or goal, of the patient's medication regime will assist in keeping the medication list as short and maximally effective as it needs to be. The expected outcome is the overarching goal and principle that will guide the health care team and the patient in their decision-making process. After administration of a drug, observing the rights of the patient, it is important for the nurse to correctly evaluate the treatment and observe if the expected outcome was achieved. This information can be obtained through physical assessment, the taking of the patient's vital signs, lab work, and subjective data from the patient.

The nurse should have access to literature that provides information about drugs, including expected outcomes, mode of action in the body, appropriate dosing, contraindications, and adverse effects. A formulary is an example of this type of literature that gives an official list of medicines that may be prescribed and any related information on the drug. The formulary will give both the generic and the brand name for the drug and is maintained by physicians, nurse practitioners, and pharmacists to ensure it is accurate and up to date. Drugs listed in the formulary have been evaluated for safety and effectiveness by a committee of experts to provide practitioners with those deemed best for patients.

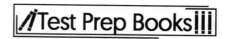
The nurse should use one of the greatest pharmacological references available to them in the health care facility: the pharmacist. Most hospitals have a team of pharmacists on staff whose sole purpose is to oversee the correct dosage, administration, and usage of all the patients' medication needs. Most pharmacists have a doctorate level of education in pharmacy, which the nurse would be wise to make good and often use of. Pharmacists are often found on the floors, overseeing correct antibiotic and other drug dosages and administration, as well as being stationed in the hospital's pharmacy, which is only a phone call away. If the nurse has a question about a medication's use for a patient, they should not hesitate to contact the pharmacist and consult them and their pharmaceutical knowledge. They are a very helpful and valuable member of the health care team.

Prescription drugs are those that may only be prescribed by a qualified health care practitioner. They may be obtained with a prescription from the pharmacy, dispensed by a qualified pharmacist. OTC medications may be obtained without a prescription, at the discretion of the patient. Home remedies include any sort of tonic or home-prepared solution that the patient makes for themselves at home as a cure for an ailment. These are often made with commonly found household or pantry items. Many home remedies are unproven in their effectiveness but rather anecdotally recommended by a friend or family member, often passed down through the generations. An example of a simple home remedy is lemon juice and honey in hot water as a "cure" for a sore throat. These simple ingredients have medicinal properties that may soothe the sore throat and may be preferred by the patient to an OTC or prescription formulation for sore throats. The nurse should obtain information about any home remedies the patient may be using to get a full picture of their health and wellness habits.

Interactions

Drug interaction refers to the alteration in pharmacology (absorption, distribution, metabolism, elimination, efficacy, side effects, etc.) of a medication by various factors including disease conditions, prescription and OTC medications, and foods or nutritional supplements. These interactions may result in either an augmentation or decrease in the efficacy and/or toxicity of the respective medication. Drug interaction should be carefully reviewed in order to avoid serious life-threatening conditions.

Drug interactions are an aspect of pharmacology that the nurse must keep in mind when performing medication administration. A **drug interaction** may occur between many different drugs and substances. These interactions may fall into one of three categories: synergistic, antagonistic, or an interaction in which a whole new action is produced that neither substance could produce on their own.

A **synergistic interaction** is one in which the two concurrently administered substances *enhance* each other's action. Sometimes the prescriber uses the synergistic action of drugs to their advantage when the synergy would be helpful to the patient's condition. In some instances, however, synergy of two drugs is detrimental to the patient. An example of synergistic medications working in the patient's best interest would be the use of multiple antibiotics to treat an infection. Many patients with respiratory infections, such as pneumonia, will be prescribed a combination of different antibiotic therapies for two reasons. One is that the prescriber does not always know the exact causative organism of the infection and wants to wipe it out completely. The second reason is that these combinations of antibiotics have been shown to be more effective than just using one specific antibiotic.

An example of synergistic drugs having an unwanted effect is the combination of multiple blood thinners, such as Coumadin and aspirin. In some patients' cases, the combination of the two drugs may be warranted and helpful, while in others it could have a devastating effect on the patient, resulting in a massive bleed.

Antagonistic drug interactions are ones in which the two co-administered substances cancel each other out or greatly decrease each other's potential action.

A nurse who is well versed in pharmacological knowledge, including drug side effects, adverse effects, contraindications, and interactions, will be able to better serve and protect their patients from harm.

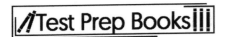

Examples of different types of drug interactions and examples within each type are described below:

- Drug-Disease Interactions:

  - NSAIDS and Peptic Ulcers: NSAIDs including aspirin, ibuprofen, naproxen, and indomethacin can cause stomach irritation and can aggravate peptic ulcer symptoms. Therefore, NSAIDs should not be used by patients with peptic ulcers or GERD. If NSAIDs are used by patients with hyperacidity, gastro-protective agents, such as proton pumps inhibitors (e.g., omeprazole, pantoprazole, lansoprazole, etc.), should also be used.

  - Diuretics and Diabetes: Diuretics are used to treat hypertension and edema. Hydrochlorothiazide is a commonly prescribed diuretic that can cause glucose intolerance and hyperglycemia. Therefore, if a patient with type 2 diabetes is prescribed a diuretic, blood sugar control becomes difficult, so routine monitoring of blood sugar is required. If blood sugar is not properly controlled, dose adjustments of the anti-diabetic medication or alternative diuretics should be considered.

- Drug-Food and Drug-Nutrient Interactions:

  - Statins and Grapefruit Juice: Statins (e.g., pravastatin, simvastatin, atorvastatin, and rosuvastatin) are used to treat hypocholesteremia. Patients taking this medication should avoid drinking grapefruit juice or consuming large amounts of grapefruit because this juice decreases the metabolism of statins, resulting in a buildup of statins in the body. The risk of serious side effects is increased when statin buildup occurs, with possible resultant muscle or liver damage. Pharmacists should counsel patients about avoiding grapefruit juice while on statins. Although increasing statin dosage may seem to benefit the patient, the liver can only process so much. Accumulation of a statin in the body can cause muscle damage, pain, and rhabdomyolysis—a serious and potentially lethal side effect. In rhabdomyolysis, the skeletal muscle is rapidly catabolized. Patients taking statins should undergo routine blood tests and notify their doctors immediately about symptoms of muscle pain or fatigue. Undetected and unmanaged rhabdomyolysis can result in death.

  - MAOIs and Tyramine: Monoamine oxidase inhibitors (MAOIs) are used to treat chronic depression that does not respond to other medications or treatments. Due to side effects and drug interactions, MAOIs are not commonly prescribed. Examples of MAOIs are phenelzine (Nardil®), selegiline (Emsam®), and tranylcypromine (Parnate®). MAOIs can cause serotonin syndrome. There are many medications and foods that can lead to severe side effects when combined with MAOIs. Foods like wine, cheese, certain meats, and pickled foods carry tyramine, which leads to spikes in blood pressure, if co-administered with MAOIs.

- Drug-Laboratory Interactions:

  - Antibiotics and Bacterial Cultures: Treatment with certain medications can affect laboratory results. For example, the blood or urine sample collected from a patient taking an antibiotic for one infection might yield a false antibiotic sensitivity or culture report for a second infection. The lab work should, therefore, be scheduled after the wash-out period of the first antibiotic.

- Drug-Drug Interactions:

  - Warfarin and NSAIDs: Warfarin is a commonly prescribed blood thinner, indicated to prevent blood clots in various cardiovascular diseases. Patients on warfarin should not take other prescription/OTC/herbal medications without consulting with their prescriber and pharmacist.

126

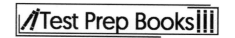

For example, commonly available OTC NSAIDs can cause an increase in the blood-thinning effect of warfarin and result in internal hemorrhage. The following medications can interact with warfarin:

- Aspirin
- Acetaminophen (at high doses)
- Ibuprofen
- Naproxen
- Celecoxib
- Diclofenac
- Indomethacin
- Piroxicam

- Oral Contraceptives and Antibiotics: Antibiotics can decrease the effect of hormonal oral contraceptives thus increasing the possibility of pregnancy even while taking the contraceptive. Non-hormonal back-up methods, such as condoms, should be used while a woman taking an oral contraceptive is prescribed an antibiotic. Other medications that can affect the efficacy of oral contraceptives include anti-fungals, a few anti-seizure medications, certain HIV medications, and a few herbal preparations, like St. John's Wort.

- Nitroglycerin and Erectile Dysfunction Medications: Nitroglycerin is a vasodilator that is often used to treat episodes of angina. To prevent recurring angina, the extended-release capsules of nitroglycerin are taken daily, whereas in cases of non-frequent occurrence, sublingual tablets or sprays can be used. Medications to treat erectile dysfunctions, such as sildenafil, tadalafil, and vardenafil, should not be taken with nitroglycerin. These medications augment the vasodilatory effect of nitroglycerin and can lead to irreversible hypotension and fatality. Emergency care should be sought immediately if this combination accidentally happens. The symptoms of hypotension include dizziness, fainting, and cold, clammy skin.

- Drug-OTC Interactions

  - Antihypertensives and Decongestants: Pseudoephedrine and phenylephrine are used as decongestants in different OTC cough and cold medications. These medications have sympathomimetic effects and can cause elevated blood pressure. Therefore, if a decongestant medication is taken by patients on antihypertensive medication, it reduces the blood pressure control of the antihypertensive agent. Hypertensive patients should avoid taking OTC medications containing sympathomimetic agents.

  - Antihistamines and Sedatives: OTC antihistamines, such as diphenhydramine and chlorpheniramine, are used to treat various allergic conditions. Antihistamines can cause sedation and drowsiness, which can potentiate the side effects of sedatives and hypnotics. Patients taking sedatives—such as diazepam, lorazepam, alprazolam, and midazolam—should be cautious when taking an OTC antihistamine.

- Drug-Alcohol Interactions

  - Alcohol should be avoided while patients are on prescription medications. Consumption of alcohol with medications can cause nausea, vomiting, fainting, loss of coordination, or extreme drowsiness. More severe reactions can lead to heart problems, internal bleeding, and difficulty breathing. Certain medications, when combined with alcohol, can cause toxicity. As alcohol is a strong CNS depressant, combining it with other depressants, like benzodiazepines or sleeping

127

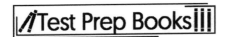
medications, can be dangerous and can cause respiratory failure. If alcohol is combined with a high dose of acetaminophen, there is potential for serious liver damage. Additionally, if alcohol is consumed while taking metronidazole, the patient can experience significant side effects including nausea, vomiting, abdominal pain, cramps, facial redness, headache, tachycardia, and liver damage.

OTC Medications

Some OTC medications impose significant risks with certain disease conditions. A few OTC medications can lead to an increase in blood pressure, so these may be contraindicated in patients with hypertension. The following medications are known to cause problems for patients with hypertension:

- NSAIDS (ibuprofen and naproxen)
- Decongestants like pseudoephedrine
- Migraine formulations with caffeine

Patients with high blood pressure should talk to a pharmacist or a physician before taking OTC medications or herbal supplements.

Age

In elderly adults, there can also be significant changes in pharmacokinetics and pharmacodynamics of a medication. Geriatric populations often have comorbid conditions, including cardiovascular disease, diabetes, and renal insufficiencies. Aging can decrease the body's clearance of a medication, resulting in buildup and manifesting in unwanted effects. Routine blood work and dose adjustments may be necessary in the geriatric population.

Pregnancy

During pregnancy, medications should be prescribed carefully, to prevent harm to the developing fetus. For some medications, there might not be enough data available regarding safety during pregnancy, and therefore, must be used cautiously after weighing the benefits versus the risks. Many medications are contraindicated during pregnancy, as they have teratogenic effects and can cause birth defects. If a patient is on a teratogenic medication prior to pregnancy, the medication should be stopped upon conception. A few examples of medications that are contraindicated in pregnancy include ACE inhibitors (e.g., ramipril, enalapril, lisinopril, etc.), ARBs (losartan, candesartan, irbesartan, etc.), isotretinoin, tetracycline antibiotics, hormonal therapies, and immunosuppressants (e.g., methotrexate).

Adverse Effects

With all medication administration, the nurse must be mindful of the drug's potential adverse effects. As far as pharmacology has come in the past century, no drug has been perfected to the point of not having any potential adverse effect. An **adverse effect** is defined as a negative response to a medication that is not part of the desired effect. The chemical structure of the drug is what usually triggers these adverse effects. Adverse effects are greatly minimized by appropriate dosing for the individual patient.

The administration of any drug is associated with the potential for **adverse effects**. The adverse effects of commonly prescribed drug classes are predictable in some situations. However, the route of administration, ethnic differences related to the pharmacotherapeutic reaction, and patient adherence and comorbidities can all affect the expression of the adverse effects in an individual patient. The medical-surgical nurse will also assess possible drug interactions among the patient's prescribed drugs and all OTC drugs and herbal supplements. Continuing surveillance of the incidence of adverse effects is necessary. According to practice guidelines a new adverse effect should first be considered as an adverse drug reaction (ADR). **Hypersensitivity reactions** are most often time sensitive, which means that the timing of the reaction can be associated with the administration of the drug; IV administration

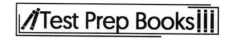
results in the most rapid reaction. Drug-to-drug reactions commonly are delayed; they manifest themselves in changes in the patient's physical condition.

The nurse is aware that adverse drug reactions (ADRs) are more likely with drugs that are lipophilic, due to the increased absorption rate. Some of these reactions are well documented, however, other reactions are less predictable and may result from an identified reaction among the patient's prescription drugs. Additional risk factors for ADRs include polypharmacy, genetic alterations in pharmacodynamics and pharmacokinetics, age, gender, and comorbidities. ADRs are categorized according to response time. **Immediate adverse drug reactions (ADRs)** occur within the first hour after administration of the drug. **Delayed ADRs** occur after the first hour. However, the expanded view of response time identifies six specific categories of reactions: rapid, first dose, early, intermediate, late, and delayed.

Rapid reactions that occur during or immediately following the administration of a drug are generally believed to be due to administration errors. For instance, the incorrect administration of a vancomycin infusion can result in "red neck syndrome," which is manifested by erythema, flushing, and pruritus of the upper body. **First dose** reactions occur with the initial dose of the medication and may or may not occur with repeated doses. **Early reactions** occur after the first few doses, and this effect can often be avoided if the therapy is begun with the lowest therapeutic dose and then titrated according to the incidence of demonstrated reactions. **Intermediate reactions** occur after the repeated administration of the drug and are most common in susceptible patients. For instance, hyperuricemia secondary to furosemide administration is an intermediate reaction that warrants close observation and intervention. **Late** and **delayed reactions** occur at various times following administration of the drug. In most instances, these reactions are predictable and can be controlled by removing the drug from the treatment plan or altering the dosage.

The FDA categorizes ADRs as serious when the outcome of the therapy is death or results in permanent disability, birth defects, or prolonged hospitalization. Reactions that meet any of these criteria must be reported to the FDA MedWatch program. More commonly, adverse reactions are designated as mild, moderate, or severe.

Some drug side effects are quite obvious. Take, for example, warfarin. Warfarin, or Coumadin, is used to thin out the blood in patients at risk for forming deadly blood clots, such as those with atrial fibrillation. However, if inappropriately dosed and under-monitored, warfarin can cause serious hemorrhaging because of its effect on the body's clotting mechanisms and ability to achieve hemostasis. Patients taking warfarin should be carefully monitored for overdosage and signs of bleeding.

At times, a drug may cause an adverse effect when it is co-administered with some other substance that affects its chemical structure or its ability to be absorbed by the body. Narcotics, for example, should not be taken while drinking alcohol. Alcohol, a depressant, exacerbates the effect of the narcotic, also a depressant, to the point that the patient's drive to breathe and their consciousness may be completely knocked out, causing death.

Another type of adverse effect is an allergic reaction. Depending on the patient's unique makeup of the immune system, some drugs may cause the immune system to kick into overdrive, decreasing the desired effect and adding a lot of unwanted effects. Common signs of an allergic reaction include mild reactions such as itching and rash, escalating all the way to a severe reaction such as anaphylactic shock. **Anaphylaxis** involves an inflammation and narrowing of the patient's airway. This makes breathing difficult and presents a life-threatening situation.

The nurse should be aware of common contraindications for a certain drug's use. A **contraindication** is a situation in which it is inappropriate to administer a drug. For example, if a patient is taking a potassium-sparing ACE inhibitor for the management of heart failure, supplementation of potassium should be avoided or only carefully done under the management of the attending physician or nephrologist. This is because the ACE inhibitor causes the body to excrete *less* potassium than it normally does, meaning supplementing potassium puts the patient at risk for

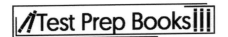

hyperkalemia, a life-threatening condition that can cause heart rhythm abnormalities and dysfunction. Another common contraindication to be mindful of is the administration of Coumadin, or warfarin, with another blood thinner such as aspirin. The concurrent usage of these two medications aimed at decreasing the body's own hemostatic response can result in a life-threatening hemorrhage in the patient and should be avoided.

If the nurse ever suspects that the administration of a drug is contraindicated by the usage of another, they should always raise their concern with the ordering physician, the pharmacist on staff, and/or nursing management to confirm. It is a patient safety issue that is worth the extra time to investigate to prevent patient harm.

Adverse effects and contraindications are some of the rarer occurrences in day-to-day pharmacological therapies that the nurse will encounter. More commonly, the nurse will encounter milder, unwanted effects of drug administration called **side effects**. Most drugs have side effects or undesirable effects of administration. For example, a patient put on antibiotics for a respiratory infection may experience gastrointestinal (GI) upset such as stomachache, excessive flatulence, and diarrhea. Antibiotics destroy the native GI tract bacteria as part of their mechanism of action, which is what causes these side effects. Side effects are usually mild enough that the patient can either bear with them until they are finished taking the medication for the original cause, or the doctor may prescribe a counter drug to lessen the side effects of the original drug. As each additional drug carries with it the potential for more side effects, use of more medications should be weighed carefully as to their potential for helping the patient. The clinical judgment of the doctor and nurse and the patient's preference are all considered in these decisions.

Routes of Administration

The two most common routes of medication administration the nurse will encounter are oral and intravenous. Oral medications are delivered via the alimentary canal. This can include medications given in a nasogastric tube or a gastric tube, buccal medications that are absorbed when placed between the gums of the teeth and the cheek, and sublingual medications that are absorbed after being held under the tongue.

There are, of course, other routes of medication administration that the nurse will need to be knowledgeable and competent in performing. A drug may be administered parenterally, which means any other route than the alimentary canal, and includes intradermal, subcutaneous, intramuscular, and intravenous routes.

Intramuscular injections are the preferred route for vaccinations such as the pneumococcal and influenza vaccines. The deltoid muscle is preferred for most vaccines, but other sites the nurse may use, if necessary, include the ventrogluteal, dorsogluteal, and vastus lateralis sites. One important aspect of intramuscular injection is the Z-track technique. In this technique, the nurse pulls the skin downward or upward, injects the medication at a 90-degree angle, and then releases the skin. This creates a "zigzag," or Z-shaped, track that prevents the injected fluid from leaking backward into the subcutaneous tissue. Backward leakage of tissue may cause tissue damage. The nurse must avoid massaging the site, as this may cause leakage and irritation.

The intradermal route of delivery is often used for specific tests such as allergy tests or tuberculosis testing.

Subcutaneous medication administration is the preferred route for many insulin injections in patients with diabetes, as the small amount of the drug is perfect for glucose management as well as being nonirritating in such a low volume.

Other routes of administration may include drugs that are applied topically to the skin and absorbed. Transdermal patches may be used to slow the release of a drug over a longer period of time, such as days or weeks.

Patients with respiratory ailments greatly benefit from inhaled drugs, which travel directly to the lung tissue they are intended to target. Types of respiratory drugs include metered-dose inhalers (MDIs), nebulizers, and certain inhalable, effervescent, dry powders.

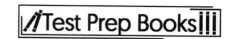

Parenteral/Intravenous Therapies

Clients requiring intravenous therapies will need to be assessed for the appropriate vein to be used. Selecting the best vein is crucial to ensuring the medication can be delivered safely and effectively. The nurse should always go farthest away from the center of the patient's body first. It may be tempting to go for a thick, juicy vein near the patient's inner elbow first, but using distal veins first is proper procedure. This is because if a vein is blown toward the center of the patient's body, it cannot be used again distally. The only time it is appropriate to use a more proximal vein, such as the antecubital (AC) (located in the fold of the elbow), is in emergent cases. The AC is also a frequent blood draw site for quick draws on stable patients. It is also preferred that the nurse select the patient's nondominant arm. If the patient is left-handed, for example, the right arm is preferred for an IV site.

When selecting an IV site, the nurse should avoid the side of the body where a dialysis catheter is, a side that is paralyzed, and a side where a mastectomy has been performed, if possible.

Education will be needed for the patient who is to receive intermittent parenteral fluid therapy. Fluids are often required for the sake of client hydration and electrolyte needs. An IV is often obtained for this purpose so that it is available when needed.

The patient should be educated about signs of IV infiltration that they will need to report to the nurse. An infiltrated IV is one in which the catheter has dislodged outside of the vein or the vein has blown, and IV fluids and medications are leaking into the interstitial space. Signs of IV infiltration include swelling, coldness, and pain around the IV site. The nurse will not be able to pull back any fluid or blood from the IV catheter as it is dislodged from the correct site of insertion.

Other complications of IV therapy include hematoma around the insertion site; extravasation of a toxic drug into the surrounding tissue; embolus or clot formation; fluid overload in the patient from overadministration; phlebitis, or swelling and inflammation of the vein; and infection around the IV site.

The nurse oversees IV pump function for correct and accurate delivery of IV fluids and medications. IV pumps are prone to breakdown and failure and thus will need close nurse supervision. The nurse monitors the fluid and medication bags above the pump and ensures that the measurements on the machine match up with the actual delivery.

Medications

Medications Acting on the Nervous System

Antidepressants and Anxiolytics

Antidepressants are used to treat different mood disorders including depression, anxiety, phobias, and obsessive-compulsive disorder (OCD). Treatment for depression includes various medications, in addition to cognitive behavioral therapy (e.g., counseling).

Antidepressants exert their therapeutic effects by modulating the release or action of various neurotransmitters in the brain. Neurotransmitters are chemical messengers that transmit signals from one neuron to another. The common side effects of antidepressants are serotonin syndrome (headache, agitation, tremor, hallucination, tachycardia, hyperthermia, shivering and sweating), sexual dysfunction, weight changes, gastric acidity, diarrhea, sleep disturbances, and suicidal ideation.

Commonly prescribed antidepressant medications include the following:

- Sertraline
- Fluoxetine

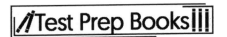
- Paroxetine
- Citalopram
- Escitalopram
- Venlafaxine
- Desvenlafaxine
- Duloxetine
- Trazodone
- Bupropion
- Amitriptyline
- Nortriptyline

Benzodiazepines are a class of medications used for the short-term treatment of anxiety. They are often combined with antidepressants during initial treatment to increase treatment compliance. Benzodiazepines have the potential for significant physical dependence and withdrawal symptoms. These drugs can be used as sedatives and hypnotics and are also utilized as an add-on therapy with anti-convulsant medications. Benzodiazepines are often used to treat symptoms from alcohol withdrawal. The majority of benzodiazepines are labeled as Class IV controlled substances. The common side effects of these medications include physical dependence, sedation, drowsiness, dizziness, and lack of coordination.

The following are commonly prescribed benzodiazepines:

- Diazepam
- Lorazepam
- Clonazepam
- Alprazolam
- Midazolam
- Temazepam

Antipsychotics

Antipsychotics are used to treat psychosis, including schizophrenia and bipolar disorder. Psychosis is often characterized by a cluster of symptoms including delusions (false beliefs), paranoia (fear or anxiety), hallucinations, and disordered thoughts. The most common side effects of antipsychotics are dyskinesia (movement disorder), loss of libido or sex drive, gynecomastia (breast enlargement) in males, weight gain, heart diseases (QT prolongation), and metabolic disorders including type 2 diabetes.

The following are examples of commonly prescribed antipsychotics:

- Chlorpromazine
- Fluphenazine
- Haloperidol
- Aripiprazole
- Olanzapine
- Risperidone
- Ziprasidone
- Clozapine

Stimulant Medications

Stimulant medications are also called sympathomimetic agents, as they work by augmenting the sympathetic neurotransmitter activity (e.g., epinephrine and norepinephrine). These drugs are often used during emergencies to treat cardiac arrest and shock. Stimulant medications are also commonly used to treat attention-deficit

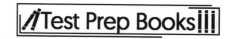
hyperactivity disorder (ADHD). The common side effects of such medications include irritability, weight loss, insomnia, dizziness, agitation, headache, abdominal pain, tachycardia, growth retardation, hypertension, cardiovascular disturbances, and death.

The following are examples of sympathomimetic drugs that are used in the treatment of ADHD:

- Methylphenidate
- Dextroamphetamine
- Lisdexamfetamine
- Mixed salts of amphetamine
- Atomoxetine

Anticonvulsant Medications

Anticonvulsants are also called antiepileptic or anti-seizure medications. They are used in the treatment of epileptic seizures. They suppress excessive firing of neurons and therefore prevent the initiation and spread of seizures. This class of medications is often used to stabilize mood in bipolar disorder or for the treatment of neuropathic pain. The common side effects are dizziness, sedation, weight gain, hepatotoxicity, hair loss, blood disorders, etc. Anticonvulsants are teratogenic and can cause significant harm to a fetus and result in birth defects. Therefore, female patients on anticonvulsant therapy should consult with their physicians before planning pregnancy.

The common medications in this class include the following:

- Carbamazepine
- Oxcarbazepine
- Phenytoin
- Valproic acid
- Divalproex
- Levetiracetam
- Lamotrigine
- Topiramate
- Clobazam

Medications Acting on the Cardiovascular System

Lipid-Lowering Medications

Lipid-lowering medications are used for the treatment of high blood lipids (hyperlipidemia), including high cholesterol (hypercholesterolemia) and high triglycerides (hypertriglyceridemia). Although a patient with hypercholesterolemia typically will not experience symptoms, the condition leads to the accumulation of fatty deposits in the blood vessels and liver, called atherosclerotic plaques. As time progresses, the deposits slow, impede, or block the flow of blood through the vessels. When blood flow is compromised to the heart muscle, ischemic heart disease can result. If the blood flow to the brain decreases, there is a possibility of ischemic stroke. Compromised blood supply in peripheral tissues and limbs can cause the development of peripheral vascular diseases (PVD). Lifestyle changes, such as a healthy diet and regular exercise, can significantly reduce the risk of hypercholesterolemia, even in the presence of predisposing genetic risk factors. Total cholesterol is determined from two components: high-density lipoproteins (HDL) cholesterol, considered the "good" cholesterol, and low-density lipoproteins (LDL) cholesterol, considered the "bad" cholesterol. Although it is helpful to keep a lower total cholesterol level for health and reduced disease risk, it is more critical to keep the ratio of HDL to LDL elevated.

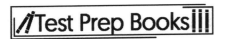

Examples of lipid-lowering agents include the following:

- Statins: pravastatin, simvastatin, atorvastatin, rosuvastatin
- Cholesterol absorptions inhibitors: ezetimibe, cholestyramine, colestipol
- Fibrates: Gemfibrozil, fenofibrate

Antihypertensive Medications

Antihypertensive medications are used to treat high blood pressure. Although hypertensive individuals generally do not have symptoms, some people experience headaches, blurred vision, and dizziness. When high blood pressure is left untreated, it can lead to different clinical conditions including coronary artery disease, heart failure, kidney failure, or stroke. There are two values that comprise a blood pressure measure. The top number is the systolic pressure (the pressure on the arterial walls when the heart muscle contracts) and the bottom number is the diastolic pressure (the pressure on the arterial walls when the heart muscle relaxes). Normal, healthy blood pressure in adults should be a systolic reading less than 120 mmHg and a diastolic reading less than 80 mmHg.

There are three stages of high blood pressure, as outlined below:

- Prehypertension is characterized by systolic pressure between 120-139 mmHg and diastolic pressure between 80-89 mmHg.

- Stage 1 hypertension is characterized by systolic pressure between 140-159 mmHg and diastolic pressure between 90-99 mmHg.

- Stage 2 hypertension is characterized by systolic pressure of 160 mmHg and higher and diastolic pressure of 100 mmHg and higher.

ACE Inhibitors (ACEIs)

"ACE inhibitors," or angiotensin-converting enzyme inhibitors, are used to treat hypertension and cardiovascular diseases. The most common side effect of ACE inhibitors is a chronic dry cough, which, in many cases, is so annoying for a patient that it results in switching the medication to a different class. Other frequent side effects are low blood pressure (hypotension), dizziness, fatigue, headache, and hyperkalemia (increased blood potassium levels).

Examples of some ACE Inhibitors include the following:

- Ramipril
- Enalapril
- Lisinopril
- Captopril
- Quinapril
- Perindopril

ARBs

Angiotensin Receptor Blockers (ARBs) have similar therapeutic effects as ACE Inhibitors; however, they tend to have better compliance due to their lower incidence of persistent cough. They block the effect of angiotensin at the receptor site and are widely used for hypertension and cardiovascular disease. The common side effects are hypotension, fatigue, dizziness, headache, and hyperkalemia.

Examples of ARBs include the following:

- Losartan
- Irbesartan

134

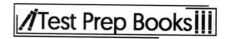
- Valsartan
- Candesartan
- Telmisartan
- Olmesartan

CCBs

Calcium Channel Blockers (CCBs) work by decreasing calcium entry through calcium channels. By regulating the movement of calcium, contraction of vascular smooth muscle is controlled, which causes blood vessels to dilate. This reduces blood pressure and workload on the heart, so this type of medication is used to treat hypertension and angina and to control heart rate. Common side effects of CCBs include dizziness, flushing of the face, headache, edema (swelling), tachycardia (fast heart rate), bradycardia (slow heart rate), and constipation. In combination with other medications that treat hypertension, calcium channel blocker toxicity is possible. Combinations, like verapamil with beta-blockers, can lead to severe bradycardia.

The following are examples of common calcium channel blockers:

- Amlodipine
- Nifedipine
- Felodipine
- Verapamil
- Diltiazem

Beta Blockers

Beta blockers are an important class of antihypertensive medications and are widely used to treat hypertension and cardiovascular disease. Some of them are also used to treat migraines, agitation, and anxiety. The side effects of beta blockers include hypotension, dizziness, bradycardia, headache, bronchoconstriction (trouble breathing), and fatigue.

Commonly prescribed beta blockers include the following:

- Atenolol
- Metoprolol
- Propranolol
- Sotalol
- Nadolol
- Carvedilol
- Labetalol

Vasodilators

Vasodilators cause blood vessels to dilate, lowering resistance to flow and reducing the workload on the heart. Vasodilators are used to treat hypertension, angina, and heart failure. The common side effects associated with their use include lightheadedness, dizziness, low blood pressure, flushing, reflex tachycardia, and headache. Vasodilators should not be combined with medications for erectile dysfunction, as this interaction can cause a fatal drop in blood pressure.

Examples of common vasodilators include the following:

- Nitroglycerin (available as sublingual tablets, sprays, patches, and extended-release capsules)
- Isosorbide mononitrate
- Isosorbide dinitrate

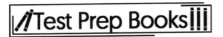

- Hydralazine
- Minoxidil (limited use)

Alpha-1 Receptor Blockers

Alpha-blockers decrease the norepinephrine-induced vascular contraction, causing relaxation of blood vessels and a resultant reduction in blood pressure. This type of medication is used to treat high blood pressure and benign prostatic hyperplasia (BPH). The common side effects of this class of medications include hypotension, dizziness, headache, tachycardia, weakness, and nausea.

Examples of alpha blockers include the following:

- Prazosin
- Doxazosin
- Terazosin
- Tamsulosin (primarily used to treat BPH)
- Alfuzosin (primarily used to treat BPH)

Diuretics

Diuretics are used alone and in combination with other medications to treat hypertension. They are often used to eliminate excess body fluid to treat swelling/edema. Diuretics inhibit the absorption of sodium in renal tubules, resulting in increased elimination of salt and water. This action increases urine output, decreases blood volume, and lowers blood pressure. Side effects of diuretics include hypotension, dizziness, hypokalemia, dehydration, hyperglycemia, polyuria (frequent or excessive urination), fatigue, syncope (fainting), and tinnitus (ringing in ears).

Examples of commonly prescribed diuretics include the following:

- Furosemide
- Bumetanide
- Hydrochlorothiazide
- Spironolactone
- Amiloride
- Triamterene

Hematologic Pharmacology

Anemia is a general term for the reduction of RBCs circulating within the body or the decrease in hemoglobin that helps transport oxygen to the tissues. The goal of anemia treatment is to increase the number of RBCs and raise the hemoglobin levels. There are different types of anemias, and supplemental medications are necessary to correct the deficiencies. **Iron-deficiency anemia** is the lack of sufficient amounts of iron used for hemoglobin synthesis. The most cost-effective medication to treat iron-deficiency anemia is **ferrous sulfate (iron)**. Practitioners should expect to see blood levels return to normalcy after approximately 2 months of use. Patients should be instructed to take ferrous sulfate on an empty stomach and informed that milk products and antacid medications interfere with the absorption of iron. **Pernicious anemia** is the insufficient production of hydrochloric acid in the stomach.

The intrinsic factor found in the gastric mucosa that is necessary for the absorption of **vitamin B12** in the small intestine is decreased in pernicious anemia. Replacement of vitamin B12 in parenteral form is preferred and will increase the regeneration of RBCs. Patients should be encouraged to eat vitamin B12–rich foods such as animal proteins and eggs. **Folic acid deficiency anemia** is due to a decrease in folic acid levels that interferes with the DNA synthesis and maturation of RBCs. Pharmacological treatment is aimed at increasing folic acid levels. **Oral folate** is recommended. Serum folic acid levels should increase within a period of 3 to 4 months. **Aplastic anemia** results from bone marrow dysfunction. RBCs, WBCs, and platelets are produced in the bone marrow. Decreased levels of erythrocytes, leukocytes, and platelets is termed **pancytopenia**. Autoimmune disorders are a prevalent cause of

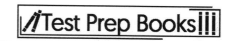
aplastic anemia. Pharmacological treatment is aimed at reducing the immune response. Immunosuppressants such as **cyclosporine** can help prevent further damage to the bone marrow. **Hematopoietic growth factors** stimulate the production of WBCs and RBCs. **Filgrastim (Neupogen®)** is a colony-stimulating medication. Common side effects involve the musculoskeletal system and can cause muscle and bone pain.

Medications Acting on the Respiratory System

Antiasthmatics

Antiasthmatics are used to prevent and treat the acute symptoms of asthma, which is a disease characterized by wheezing, cough, chest tightness, and shortness of breath. Acute asthma can be life-threatening and needs to be treated promptly. Asthma is caused by inflammation and constriction of the airways, which results in difficulty breathing. Acute asthma may be exacerbated by certain triggering factors including environmental allergens, certain medications (e.g., aspirin), stress or exercise, smoke, and lung infections. It is important to avoid the triggering factors to prevent acute symptoms. The common side effects of antiasthmatics are cough, hoarseness, decreased bone mineral density, growth retardation in children, mouth thrush, agitation, tachycardia, and a transient increase in blood pressure.

There are two categories to asthma medications that can be used alone or in combination:

- Bronchodilators (dilate the airway to ease breathing):
    - Salbutamol
    - Formoterol (generally used in combination with inhaled corticosteroids)
    - Salmeterol (generally used in combination with inhaled corticosteroids)
- Anti-inflammatory agents:
    - Fluticasone (inhaled corticosteroid)
    - Budesonide (inhaled corticosteroid)
    - Beclometasone (inhaled corticosteroid)
    - Montelukast
    - Zafirlukast

COPD Treatment

Chronic Obstructive Pulmonary Disease (COPD) is an obstructive airway disease that is characterized by coughing, wheezing, shortness of breath, and sputum production. COPD is a progressive disease that worsens over time. COPD is a combination of two common conditions: chronic bronchitis and emphysema. Chronic bronchitis is inflammation of the smooth lining of bronchial tubes. These tubes are responsible for carrying air to the alveoli, which are the air sacs in the lungs responsible for gaseous exchange between the lungs and blood. Emphysema results from alveolar damage, reducing the ability for healthy gas exchange. These two pathologies cause breathing difficulties in patients with COPD. The contributing factors for the development of COPD include smoking, environmental pollutions, and genetic risk factors. The side effects of COPD medications are similar to that of antiasthmatics.

The medications commonly used to treat COPD include the following:

- Bronchodilators (dilate the airway to ease breathing):
    - Salbutamol
    - Formoterol (generally used in combination with inhaled corticosteroids)
    - Salmeterol (generally used in combination with inhaled corticosteroids)
- Anti-inflammatory agents:
    - Ipratropium (Atrovent)
    - Tiotropium (Spiriva®)
    - Fluticasone

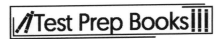

○ Budesonide

Medications Acting on the Digestive System

Gastric Acid Neutralizers/Suppressants

Gastric acid neutralizers/suppressants either neutralize stomach acid or decrease acid production and, therefore, provide relief of symptoms associated with hyperacidity. They are also used to treat gastroesophageal reflux disease, or GERD. In GERD, the lower esophageal sphincter does not close properly, which causes the contents of the stomach to back up into the esophagus. This leads to irritation, which is why the common symptoms of GERD include heartburn, coughing, nausea, difficulty swallowing, and a strained voice. There are many factors that can cause or exacerbate GERD including obesity, pregnancy, eating a large meal, acidic foods, a hiatal hernia, and smoking. Lifestyle modifications such as avoiding trigger foods, losing weight (if obesity is a component), decreasing meal size, and trying not to lie down immediately after eating, can reduce symptoms.

The medications used to treat hyperacidity in the stomach include the following:

- Antacids (e.g., calcium carbonate)
- Ranitidine
- Famotidine
- Omeprazole
- Esomeprazole
- Lansoprazole
- Rabeprazole
- Pantoprazole

Medications Acting on the Endocrine System

Anti-Diabetic Medications

Anti-diabetic medications are used to treat diabetes, which is a chronic metabolic disease in which the body cannot properly regulate blood sugar levels. This dysregulation is caused by either inadequate or absent insulin production from the pancreas (Type 1 diabetes) or inadequate action of insulin in peripheral tissues (insulin resistance in Type 2 diabetes). Type 1 diabetes usually occurs in early childhood and is typically treated with insulin injections or medications. Type 2 diabetes generally develops later in adolescence or adulthood and is related to poor diet, lack of physical activity, and obesity. Diabetes often does not to cause daily symptoms, but symptoms do arise when blood sugar is either too high (from inadequate control) or too low (from inappropriate dosing of hypoglycemic (antidiabetic) agents, including insulin). A few of the symptoms of diabetes include increased thirst and hunger, fatigue, blurred vision, a tingling sensation in the feet, and frequent urination.

Examples of some antidiabetic medications include the following:

- Insulin
- Metformin
- Acarbose
- Gliclazide, glyburide, glimepiride
- Rosiglitazone and pioglitazone
- Sitagliptin and saxagliptin

The most effective way of treating Type 2 diabetes is to combine both drug and non-drug therapies. As a part of the treatment, drug therapy can stimulate the pancreas to produce more insulin or help the body better use the insulin produced by the pancreas.

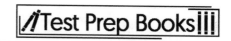

Female Hormones

Hormonal medications are generally used as oral contraceptives to prevent pregnancy. Female hormonal medications are also used to treat premenstrual symptoms (PMS), post-menopausal symptoms, acne, and endometriosis. They are also used as emergency contraceptives to prevent unwanted and accidental pregnancy. Oral contraceptives can provide hormones (estrogen and/or progestin) that suppress the egg maturation and ovulation process. Additionally, hormonal contraceptives prevent the endometrium from thickening in preparation to hold the fertilized egg. A mucus barrier is created by progestin, which stops the sperm from migrating to the fallopian tubes and fertilizing the egg.

There are many side effects associated with oral contraceptives, including increasing the risk of fatal blood clots, especially in women older than 35 or in women who smoke. More common and less severe side effects include the following:

- Nausea and stomach upset
- Headache
- Weight gain
- Spotting between periods
- Mood changes
- Lighter periods
- Aching or swollen breasts

More serious side effects that need immediate emergency care include the following:

- Chest pain
- Blurred vision
- Stomach pain
- Severe headaches

Examples of some commercially available brands of contraceptive include the following:

- Yasmin®
- Ortho Tri-Cyclen®
- Sprintec
- Ovcon®
- Plan B® (emergency contraceptive)

Medications Acting on the Immune System

Antivirals

Antivirals are used to fight viruses in the body by either stopping replication or blocking the function of a viral protein. They are used to treat HIV, herpes, hepatitis B and C, and influenza, among other viruses. Vaccines are also available to prevent some viral infections. Side effects of antivirals include headache, nausea, blood abnormalities including anemia and neutropenia (low neutrophil count), dizziness, cough, runny or stuff nose, etc.

Some examples of disease-specific antivirals include the following:

- Acyclovir, valaciclovir (Valtrex®): Herpes simplex, herpes zoster, and herpes B
- Ritonavir, indinavir, darunavir: Protease inhibitor for HIV
- Tenofovir (Viread®): Hepatitis B and HIV infection
- Interferon: Hepatitis C

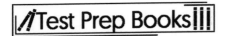
- Oseltamivir (Tamiflu): Influenza

Antibiotics

Antibiotics are antimicrobial agents that are used for treatment and prevention of bacterial infections. The mechanism of action of an antibiotic involves either killing bacteria or inhibiting their growth. Antibiotics are not effective against viruses, and therefore, they should not be used to treat viral infections. Antibiotics are often prescribed based on the result of a bacterial culture to ascertain which class of antibiotic(s) the respective strain will respond to. The common side effects of antibiotics include allergies, hypersensitivity reactions or anaphylaxis, stomach upset, diarrhea, candida (fungal) infections, and bacterial resistance (superinfection, in which a strain of bacteria develops resistance to broad classes of antibiotics).

Commonly prescribed antibiotics include the following:

- Penicillin V
- Amoxicillin (with or without clavulanic acid)
- Ampicillin
- Cloxacillin
- Cephalexin
- Cefuroxime
- Cefixime
- Tetracycline
- Doxycycline
- Minocycline
- Gentamicin
- Tobramycin
- Ciprofloxacin
- Levofloxacin
- Erythromycin
- Azithromycin
- Clarithromycin
- Clindamycin

Antimetabolites

Antimetabolites are used to treat diseases including severe psoriasis, rheumatoid arthritis, and several types of cancer (breast, lung, lymphoma, and leukemia). The most commonly used medication of this class is methotrexate, which suppresses the growth of abnormal cells and the action of the immune system. Methotrexate is widely used to treat rheumatoid arthritis. This medication is typically prescribed as a once per week dose, and it should not be prescribed for daily dosing because overdosing can be lethal. Pharmacists should be alerted to any prescriptions for daily methotrexate, as the doctor must be contacted to confirm and correct the dosing.

The following are the potential side effects of methotrexate:

- Dizziness
- Drowsiness
- Headache
- Swollen gums
- Increased susceptibility to infections
- Hair loss

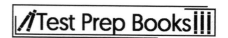

- Confusion
- Weakness

Steroids

Steroids are used to treat allergies, asthma, rashes, swelling, and inflammation. These medications are available in different forms, such as oral tablets, nasal sprays, eye drops, topical creams and ointments, inhalants, and injections. The common side effects of steroids include insulin resistance and diabetes, osteoporosis, depression, hypertension, edema, glaucoma, etc.

The following are examples of commonly prescribed corticosteroids:

- Prednisone
- Hydrocortisone
- Fluticasone
- Triamcinolone
- Mometasone
- Budesonide
- Fluocinolone
- Betamethasone
- Dexamethasone

Medications Acting on the Genitourinary System

UTIs occur within the urethra, kidney ureters, or bladder. UTIs that travel can extend into the kidneys and cause pyelonephritis. UTIs are caused by bacteria. Pharmacological treatment includes antibiotics. A culture and sensitivity test should be performed to determine the type of bacteria for proper antibiotic selection. **Trimethoprim-sulfamethoxazole (Bactrim DS®)** may be prescribed to non-pregnant females with no comorbidities over a period of 3 days. Patients should be informed that the most common side effects of Bactrim include GI disturbances such as nausea and vomiting. Another antibiotic commonly used in treating UTIs is **nitrofurantoin (Macrobid®)**. Common side effects include nausea, vomiting, and headache. UTIs may cause a burning sensation when urinating.

Phenazopyridine HCL (Pyridium®) is a pain reliever that targets the lower urinary tract. Pyridium helps relieve bladder spasms. Patients should be alerted that Pyridium causes orange discoloration of the urine and may stain surfaces and clothing. BPH is the age-related enlargement of the prostate gland in males. BPH can constrict the urethra and alter the flow of urine. Patients with BPH can have urinary retention, urethral obstruction, and bladder distention. Pharmacological treatment includes decreasing the volume of the prostate and lowering the resistance of the bladder outlet. Medications that decrease the resistance of the bladder outlet include alpha-adrenergic blockers. A common medication is **tamsulosin (Flomax®)**. Headache and dizziness are very common side effects, and patients should be instructed to change positions slowly. Other common symptoms include stuffy nose and abnormal ejaculation. Medications such as **finasteride (Proscar®)** reduce dihydrotestosterone serum levels that decrease the volume of the prostate. Proscar may cause impotence and is a reason for discontinuation by patients. Medications that decrease the volume of the prostate may take 6 to 12 months for a full response.

Medications Acting on the Reproductive System

Erectile dysfunction (ED) is a condition in male patients that prevents them from achieving or sustaining an erection during sexual intercourse. Many factors influence ED, including spinal cord injuries, psychological distress, diabetes, and medications such as beta-blockers. There are several medications that can treat ED. The **corpus cavernosa** is a region of erectile tissue that fills with blood during an erection. Medications that dilate the corpora cavernosa are used to treat ED. These medications are known as **PDE5 inhibitors**. A common PDE5 inhibitor is **sildenafil (Viagra®)**. Viagra relaxes the blood vessel walls and increases blood flow to specific areas of the body. Due to blood vessel

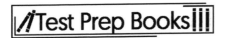
relaxation, Viagra can cause a sudden decrease in blood pressure. Common side effects include flushing of the skin and headache. Other PDE5 inhibitors used for the treatment of ED include **vardenafil (Levitra®)** and **tadalafil (Cialis®)**.

PCOS is an endocrine hormone disorder that affects the reproductive system in females. PCOS is characterized by high levels of androgen hormones, dysfunction in ovulation, and cysts within the ovaries. Excess insulin is a possible factor for PCOS development. Increased insulin levels can lead to an increase in androgen production. **Metformin (Glucophage®)** is often used to treat PCOS. Glucophage decreases insulin resistance and can assist with weight loss and prevent the development of type 2 diabetes. Obesity is part of the metabolic syndrome that often accompanies PCOS. Common side effects of metformin include diarrhea, nausea, vomiting, and loss of appetite. **Birth control medications** that contain estrogen and progestin will reduce the production of androgen hormones. Blood clots are a possible side effect of **oral contraceptives**, and careful examination of the patient's health history should be considered. Excessive hair growth on the face and chest is a manifestation of PCOS. Medications such as spironolactone (Aldactone) help block the effects of androgen hormones on the skin. **Aldactone** is a potassium-sparing diuretic that prevents the loss of potassium from the body. Patients should be educated on avoiding potassium supplements and excessive ingestion of potassium-rich foods. Common side effects are fatigue, headaches, nausea and vomiting.

Patient Medication Education

Any time a new medication is administered, the nurse should first educate the patient about the medication and any potential side effects. Nurses should be able to relay how the medication works in the body, the intended effect of the medication and why it is being prescribed, and the potential adverse reactions. Patients have the right to be informed of their medications and to refuse them.

Another important aspect of medication education is explaining how to use a medication. For example, inhalers should be shaken and primed before use. The patient should be taught the proper technique for inhaling as they depress the canister. The patient should also be taught to rinse their mouth out afterward to avoid oral ulcers. Nitroglycerine is another great example. Patients should take one tablet of nitroglycerine and rest at the first sign of angina. If the symptoms are still present after five minutes, the patient should take another dose and call EMS. Then, they should wait five more minutes and take a third dose for a maximum of three doses. These are very complex instructions that the nurse is in the prime position to teach and have the patient repeat back to gauge understanding.

Polypharmacy

Polypharmacy occurs when a patient takes multiple medications to treat different medical conditions. This happens mostly in elderly patients who are being treated for several medical conditions. Polypharmacy can cause serious drug interactions. Polypharmacy also tends to happen when a patient sees multiple doctors to treat separate conditions. Pharmacy technicians can help to prevent adverse consequences of polypharmacy by alerting pharmacists to drug interactions.

Safe Drug Management and Disposal

Stewardship
Stewardship can take many forms, including programs for common diseases like diabetes or harm-reduction programs that provide clean needles to reduce the spread of HIV. When following safe disposal practices, nurses should always put sharps in red sharps containers. Never re-cap a needle used on a patient. A common example of safe drug management is antibiotic stewardship. Educating patients that only bacterial infections need antibiotics reduces antibiotic resistance and antibiotic-resistant super infections.

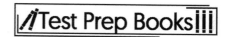
Regarding home medication management, nurses should ensure patients know all their medications and the correct way to take them. This is especially true for patients with polypharmacy who are on multiple medications that are often taken more than once a day. Pill planners are an excellent tool for these patients because the planners allow them to sort their medications day by day. For disposal of at-home and over-the-counter medications, patients should discard the medications in specialized medication disposal bins often found at pharmacies. Unused medications should not be left in medicine cabinets, as children or other family members could misuse the medication. If a medication take-back option is not readily available, some medications can be flushed according to the FDA Flush List. If a medication is not on the flush list, it can be disposed of in a sealable container in the regular trash.

Adherence to Pharmacotherapeutic Plan

Ongoing monitoring of the effectiveness of the pharmacotherapeutic plan also requires an accurate assessment of the patient's **adherence** to the plan. Adherence may also be identified as **compliance**, but however it is defined, there is evidence that up to 50 percent of all patients who take five or more drugs rarely demonstrate 100 percent adherence to the prescribed regimen. The result is the sub-optimal treatment of a chronic disease that can progress to a more acute form of the condition. Nurses should understand that there are several contributing factors for this finding, including the cost of the drug, the complexity of the pharmacotherapeutic plan, and the adverse effects associated with the prescribed drugs. Factors that enhance adherence include comprehensive patient education, a cooperative relationship with the nurse, and provider attempts to limit drug costs. The nurse is aware that in addition to the use of generic drugs, many national pharmaceutical providers have a lower cost formulary that can provide an alternative to the newer but more costly drugs.

Patient outcomes can be positively affected by clear communication between the patient and provider as to the goals of the drug regimen. There is also clear evidence that comprehensive communication increases the patient's health literacy, which can enhance the patient's level of adherence, which can improve patient outcomes. In contrast, the number of drugs that is included in the drug plan or the patient's lack of understanding of the possible actions and reactions associated with the prescription drugs are inversely proportional to the patient's level of adherence and resulting outcomes. Self-monitoring programs that use technology such as phone applications or paper and pencil instruments have demonstrated limited effect in changing patient adherence; however, there is evidence of positive outcomes with self-monitoring in patients who are taking prescription drugs for the first time. There is also a significant relationship between patient adherence and the expected adverse effects of the prescribed drugs.

Advanced Access Devices

Ports, central lines, and epidurals are all **advanced access devices** used to deliver medication. Each is placed by a trained doctor, anesthesiologist, or certified registered nurse anesthetist with the assistance of a nurse. It is extremely important for the nurse to verify the route of administration for drugs when using advanced access devices. Some medications can be fatal if given via the wrong access device.

Ports are central venous access devices surgically planted under the skin, typically on the anterior chest wall below the clavicle. Once the site has healed, the skin acts as a protective barrier against infections. Ports are used when there is a long-term need to administer medications, such as with chemotherapy. A port is made up of a self-sealing septum that covers a reservoir attached to tubing, which goes into the central vein. Accessing the port for medication administration, flushing, or withdrawing blood is a sterile procedure.

Central lines are inserted into the right atrium of the heart via the central venous superior vena cava, subclavian, or jugular veins. Central lines are used when the patient does not have suitable peripheral veins, when the patient is receiving multiple therapies such as chemotherapy and parenteral nutrition, or when the patient needs access for an extended period, such as with chemotherapy. Some catheters have up to three lumens, which makes access for

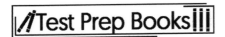

multiple therapies easier. The nurse should inspect the site for infection or infiltration and perform a sterile dressing change every twenty-four hours.

Epidurals are the administration of pain medication into the epidural space of the spine. It can be used for surgery, labor, trauma, and in some cases for long-term cancer patients. Common complications with epidurals include bradycardia and hypotension, which can be mitigated with IV fluids and medication management.

Financial Implications to Patients

Nurses should screen for social determinants of health when asking if patients are compliant with taking their medications. Patients may not be able to afford their medications and, therefore, may not be taking them or may be spreading out the doses to last longer. For example, if a patient can only afford one vial of insulin a month, they may inject every other day instead of daily. The nurse can work with a social worker, the pharmacy, and the prescriber to try to find less expensive, alternative medications. The nurse can also refer the patient to an insurance specialist to make sure their insurance plan provides the best coverage for their medications. Elderly patients often face this dilemma due to being on a fixed income. Providing them with alternative resources can ensure they are receiving the medications they need, reducing morbidity and mortality.

Pain Management

Pain

Pain is a subjective symptom. Every person will experience pain in different proportions. It is estimated that more than 60 percent of people who experience acute pain will not receive adequate pain management. Up to 75 percent of people who have chronic pain throughout their life span will suffer from partial or total disability that can become permanent. A person's perception of pain varies. The pain threshold is influenced by social and environmental factors. **Pain tolerance** is a person's ability to endure pain. Tolerance can be influenced by gender, sociocultural background, and age. **Acute pain** is characterized by a sudden onset that is localized and usually temporary. Acute pain will last 6 months or less and has an identified cause, such as surgery, infectious process, or trauma. Physical symptoms include elevated heart rate, dilated pupils, pale skin, diaphoresis, and increased blood pressure and respirations.

Chronic pain is present for more than 6 months and is not always linked to a direct cause. Medical treatment is difficult and may not provide relief to the patient. Chronic pain is usually dull and aching. Conditions that can cause chronic pain include back pain, cancer, and postoperative pain. It is important for practitioners to educate patients on pain intensity rating scales. One of the most common pain assessment tools is the numeric rating scale. This scale measures pain from 0 to 10 and is commonly used in clinical settings. Pediatric patients and patients who are cognitively impaired may use the face, legs, activity, cry, consolability (FLACC) and FACES scales. The FLACC scale is based on observation of activity and body movement, and the FACES scale provides a pictorial perception of pain. Practitioners should attempt to determine the etiology of the pain and treat the disease process. When a cause cannot be found, treatment is aimed at controlling pain. Pharmacological treatment includes nonsteroidal anti-inflammatory drugs (NSAIDs), opioid analgesics, topical anesthetics, and nerve block injections. Complementary therapies can enhance the patient's quality of life. Alternative therapies include herbal medications, meditation, imagery, music, and aromatherapy.

Pain Assessment

Pain is a subjective topic that varies by patient; therefore, healthcare professionals have a responsibility to combine clinical knowledge, personal expertise, and patient involvement in developing a safe and effective pain management plan. Unmanaged pain can lead to reduced quality of life and the inability to complete basic tasks like eating, can affect mood, and often leads to prolonged depression. In complex surgical cases, unmanaged pain can lead to poor

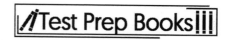
recovery outcomes, including increased rates of infection and hormonal disruption. Pain management plans can employ a number of different techniques depending on the severity of the case.

Preoperative Pain Assessment

Preoperative pain can be assessed in a number of ways, including visual and physical assessments, obtaining reports from the patient, and administering formal pain measurement scales. Visual and physical pain assessments may include noticing any conditions or injuries a patient has (for example, patients with a noticeable degree of kyphosis in their backs are expected to report a significant degree of muscular pain and tension along the spine) or noticing the intensity of pain that occurs with certain movements.

Patient self-reports of pain should be noted and taken seriously; however, patients who have previous prescriptions for narcotics or appear to desperately want them should be treated with extreme caution.

Finally, formal pain measurement instruments include numeric rating scales and verbal rating scales that patients work through with their healthcare providers to determine pain intensity. For preoperative patients, medical teams may choose a specific instrument with the patient prior to the procedure. During the preoperative period, medical teams may choose to review the instrument in detail with patients to ensure that they know how to properly report their pain levels. The selected instrument should then be utilized to continuously assess pain during the recovery period.

Medications for Pain Management

Pain is the most commonly seen symptom. However, since cases often vary widely in scope and every patient will have a different personal threshold for pain tolerance, best practices are difficult to develop when it comes to pain management. It is often done on a case-by-case basis. However, when a patient's pain is not managed in a way that seems appropriate to that individual, it can cause patient and family dissatisfaction in the healthcare organization. As a result, medical staff must try to provide effective and safe pain management options that can make the patient comfortable at the present time, but that also do not cause harm over time. In some cases, like a sprained muscle, ice therapy and time can provide adequate pain management. More serious cases, defined as pain that does not subside after an objectively reasonable period of time for the injury, may require topical, intramuscular, or oral pain medication. These can include stronger doses of common over-the-counter pain medications, or prescription pain medications.

Prescription pain medications, especially opioids and muscle relaxers, are known for causing debilitating addiction, so when prescribing them to a patient, the lowest dose and dosing frequency necessary should be utilized. Additionally, patients should be closely monitored for their reactions to their pain medications. Finally, some individuals who are addicted to prescription pain killers and muscle relaxers may feign injuries in order to receive another prescription. Therefore, all patients' medical histories should be thoroughly evaluated to note their history of pain medication usage. Patients should also be assessed for showing any signs of drug abuse history and withdrawal symptoms (such as damaged teeth, shaking, and agitation).

Procedural sedation allows patients to remain somewhat alert during medical procedures that may be uncomfortable but not unbearably painful, such as resetting bones. Unlike general anesthesia, where patients are completely sedated and do not feel any sensations, procedural sedation allows patients to be somewhat conscious and aware of bodily functions. It can be utilized with or without pain-relieving medications. Practitioner awareness is crucial when administering procedural sedation, especially when pain relief is also utilized. Recently, overuse and improper use of common procedural sedation agents, such as propofol, and common pain relief medications that are often used in conjunction, such as fentanyl, have caused high profile deaths.

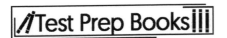
Analgesia, Narcotics, NSAIDS, and Opioids

Analgesics is an umbrella term for a variety of pain-relieving pharmaceuticals that can include mild over-the-counter medications as well as prescription-strength medications that require close monitoring by a medical professional. Different categories of analgesics work by targeting different pathways to pain.

Nonsteroidal anti-inflammatory drugs (NSAIDS) include commonly recognized medications such as ibuprofen; prescription strength doses are simply much more concentrated than versions that can be bought over the counter. NSAIDS work by targeting areas of inflammation in the body that result in pain; consequently, they are most effective for pain situations involving muscles or soft tissues.

Opioids, a type of narcotic, are prescription-only medications that work by targeting nociceptors in the brain to reduce pathway signaling that result in the physical perception of pain. While these medications are often able to eliminate pain quickly, they can also cause extremely uncomfortable side effects, like severe nausea and dizziness, in some patients. Additionally, most narcotics are highly addictive, and an opioid epidemic is well-documented in the United States. These types of prescriptions should be carefully prescribed and monitored if they are required in patient treatment plans. As patients near the end of their prescription, they may need tailored treatment to avoid withdrawal symptoms.

Multimodal Chronic and/or Acute Pain Management

Multimodal pain management refers to using pharmacological, non-pharmacological, and alternative medicine to treat pain. Pharmacological management includes everything from over-the-counter (OTC) pain medication to anesthetics. Non-pharmacological pain management refers to modalities such as heat, ice, compression, and physical therapy. Alternative medicine, or complementary and alternative medicine (CAM), is often viewed as a more natural or non-westernized type of medicine. This includes treatments such as meditation, yoga, supplements, massage, and chiropractic therapy. These pain management types can each be used separately or in combination. CAM is becoming more and more popular in the United States, and patients often ask about non-pharmacologic or alternative treatments. Nurses are in an excellent position to educate patients on all their choices.

Acute mild pain is generally treated with OTC pain medications and non-pharmacologic modalities such as the RICE (rest, ice, compression, and elevation) technique for musculoskeletal injuries. Acute, moderate-to-severe pain is often treated with a short course of powerful, pharmacologic pain medications such as opioids. If pain lasts for longer than three months, it is considered chronic pain. Chronic pain is multi-factorial and often requires a combination of the three different types of treatment.

Patient Pain Management Expectations

Patients often expect to be pain-free after receiving pain treatment. Managing this expectation can have a considerable impact on the patient's outcome. Asking the patient what a positive outcome would be for them can give the nurse insight into their expectations. If a patient expects to be pain-free, the nurse can educate on how the goal is to make the patient comfortable, not necessarily free of pain. Educating the patient that some pain is normal and means the body is healing can help manage expectations as well. Understanding a patient's thoughts, perceptions, and goals around pain can help the nurse form an individualized plan to best meet that patient's needs.

The opposite is also true. If a patient is terrified of a procedure due to fear of the pain, the nurse can set realistic expectations on the level of pain they may experience. It is important to be truthful when describing the level of pain that a patient might face during a procedure. The nurse should not underplay the pain and let the patient be caught off guard during the procedure. Be truthful and the patient will enter the procedure with the right mindset regarding pain.

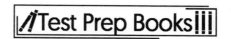
Patient Advocacy

Nurses are the patient's advocate to receive proper pain management. During rounding, a nurse should ask about a patient's pain level. If the patient's pain is not controlled with the current treatment, it is the nurse's duty to bring that to the attention of the provider and advocate for why the patient's treatment needs to be adjusted. Uncontrolled pain can lead to increased heart rate and respiratory rate, decreased appetite and sleep, and an overall decrease in quality of life. Due to the opioid epidemic, some providers are hesitant to prescribe opioid pain medications even in warranted situations. The nurse must advocate on behalf of the patient to receive the best care, whether that is with pain medication or non-pharmacologic or alternative treatments. The reverse is also true. If a nurse assesses signs of opioid dependence in the acute setting, it is their responsibility to advise the provider of these findings. The provider may alter the treatment in the best interest of the patient.

Non-Pharmacological Interventions

Nonpharmacological Interventions

Non-pharmacological interventions can also manage pain. **Contemporary and alternative medicine (CAM)** include health and wellness practices that can occur in tandem to conventional medical care. CAM practices, such as massage, yoga, meditation, acupuncture, and tailored diets often support conventional care or provide a way for patients to manage unpleasant, yet unavoidable, side effects of conventional care. It is important to know if patients engage in CAM modalities, as these should be taken into consideration when preparing for surgical procedures. Additionally, some CAM modalities may be recommended to the patients during the recovery period. It is important to note that not all CAM therapies are evidence-based, as CAM is an emerging field that requires more clinical research.

Herbs

Herbs and herbal medications are a component of CAM, although some conventional practices utilize them (or pharmaceuticals derived from them) as well. Noting whether or not a patient takes any herbal supplements is a vital part of the preoperative process. Many herbal supplements are not regulated by the United States Food and Drug Administration (by standards that conventional pharmaceuticals are); therefore, it is difficult to know what concentration of herbs are actually in these products. Certain levels of common herbal modalities can interfere with anesthetics and other conventional pharmaceuticals, rendering them ineffective or causing unpleasant symptoms in the patient.

Medical Marijuana

Medical marijuana is an alternative medicine used primarily by patients with chronic pain, anxiety disorders, and altered neuromuscular conditions. Marijuana, or cannabis, is often used recreationally. Many patients may deny its use for fear of judgement. Medical marijuana must be prescribed by a healthcare provider for a specific disease or medical condition. Although prescribed, marijuana used for medical purposes will still exert the same effects as recreational cannabis. The main ingredient in marijuana, delta-9-tetrahydrocannabinol (THC), causes euphoria and decreased coordination while slowing motor activity. The use of medical marijuana may interfere with other prescribed pharmacological treatments and should be included in the medication reconciliation of operative patients.

Repositioning

Repositioning a patient who is feeling uncomfortable may be the first step in relieving a cramp or excessive pressure. This may involve getting the patient in or out of bed, sitting in a chair, or ambulating if appropriate. The nurse may also use pillows to prop and position the patient into a more comfortable position in the bed.

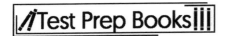
Some of the common patient positions are as follows:

High Fowler's Position: The head of the patient's bed is raised sixty to ninety degrees and the knees are either flexed or extended out straight.

Fowler's Position: The head of the patient's bed is raised forty-five to sixty degrees.

Semi-Fowler's Position: The head of the patient's bed is raised thirty to forty-five degrees.

Supine: The patient is lying on their back.

Lateral: The patient is lying on their side.

Prone: The patient is lying on their stomach, with their head turned to the side.

When positioning a patient in bed, always raise the entire bed high enough to avoid bending over while assisting the patient. Be sure to lower the head of the bed to its lowest position before leaving the patient.

Bony areas of the body should always be padded. These can include the head, elbows, tailbone, and heels. The illustrations below show the pressure points on the body in three positions: sitting, lying on the back, and side lying.

While lying down, the lower back often feels better when the knees are elevated with a pillow. The head of the bed should be raised per the patient's comfort.

When a patient is lying on their back (**supine**), the following actions may be done for their comfort:

- Place pillows under the head, knees, lower arms, and heels.
- Elevate the head of the bed per needs of patient.
- Make sure water, nurse call button, and personal items are within reach.
- Raise all of the side rails on the bed if the patient is unable to get up without assistance.

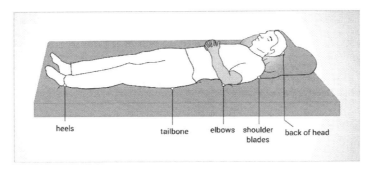

Side-lying position:

- Place a pillow under their head.
- Tuck a pillow under the back to keep the patient from rolling onto their back.
- Put pillows between bent legs, knees, and between ankles.
- Place a pillow between arms.
- Elevate the head of the bed, per comfort.

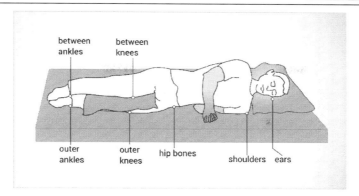

Seated position (in a wheelchair, lounger, or chair):

- Place a cushion or pillow under the patient's bottom if the chair is hard.
- Make sure there is no extra pressure behind the knees. A folded blanket could be used for padding.
- Place folded blankets under the patient's forearms if the arms of the chair are not padded.

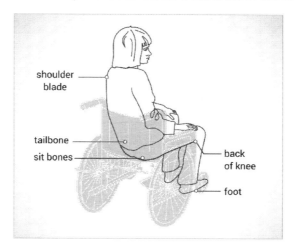

Heat and Cold

The nurse can use heat and cold in even more targeted approaches to relieve pain. Application of heat, such as warm washcloths, electric blankets, and warm baths will increase blood flow to the painful area, reduce muscle spasms, slow down peristalsis, relax the smooth muscles, and even decrease stomach acid production.

Cold application, on the other hand, cannot only decrease the spasmodic activities of muscles but also cause vasoconstriction in the areas where it is applied. The application of cold items such as an ice pack, cool washcloth, and ice cubes can decrease inflammation and increase peristalsis. The application of cold items may have a longer-lasting effect than the application of heat in some patients.

Therapeutic Touch

The nurse should not feel uncomfortable offering therapeutic touch where and when appropriate. Most nursing schools train their students in at least the most basic of massage techniques that the nurse may use on patients experiencing muscle tension. Massage should only be applied with the patient's consent and in an appropriate manner. The nurse may use lotion or oil if appropriate to relieve areas of muscle tension. Common areas that become tense include the neck, shoulders, and lower back. By massaging these areas, the nurse may be able to

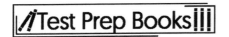

promote healthy blood flow, decrease tension, and maybe even relieve achiness that the client may be experiencing.

Spiritual Comfort

Some clients may request alternative therapies for spiritual needs. The nurse may refer the client to the appropriate entity for these interventions. For example, most hospitals offer a clergy that will come to the patient and talk with them. Patients may have spiritual issues they may want to discuss. The clergy and spiritual staff available at the hospital can address those needs, talk with the patient, and pray with them.

Psychological Modalities

The nurse may use certain psychological modalities for relieving a patient's pain or discomfort. Distraction such as music therapy can be helpful in moving the patient's focus off the discomfort, as pain is perceived in the mind and can sometimes be overcome there as well. The nurse may educate the patient about a topic that is troubling them, thus relieving any anxiety they may feel. Simple strategies aimed at relaxation such as controlled, deep breathing may assist a patient in pain. Deep breathing causes the body to take in far more stress-reducing oxygen and release the waste product carbon dioxide, thus making the patient immediately feel better. Breathing techniques are a hallmark of natural childbirth, as the woman focuses on her breathing to work her way through each contraction. Sometimes the simple act of listening to the patient as they voice their concerns may be all it takes to alleviate their apprehension, working through the inner conflict.

Relaxation Strategies

There are certain relaxation strategies that may be used on patients when muscle tension is present. These fall mainly into the categories of progressive muscle relaxation, autogenic training, and biofeedback. Progressive muscle relaxation techniques will have the patient alternately tighten and then relax different muscle groups. Autogenic training involves the patient training their body to respond to verbal commands, often targeted at the breathing rate, blood pressure, heartbeat, and temperature of the body. Biofeedback often includes breathing exercises. The goal of all of these relaxation strategies is to promote relaxation and reduce stress.

Whichever nonpharmacological technique the nurse chooses should be selected very carefully, using critical thinking and sound nursing judgment to best serve the patient's need and alleviate their discomfort.

Surgical/Procedural Nursing Management

Informed Consent

Once the physician performing the procedure explains the procedure, risks and benefits, and alternative treatments and provides opportunity for the patient to ask questions, the consent form may be signed. Types of consents obtained preoperatively are surgical, blood, anesthesia, and photography/video consents. These consent forms may be separate, or they may be combined, depending on the health care facility. For example, consent for blood products may be discussed and included in the **surgical consent** document. The nurse may have the consent form signed by the patient once consent is obtained by the physician. If the patient is eighteen years old or older, capable of decision making, and awake, alert, and oriented, the consent form should be signed by the patient. If the patient is incapable of signing the consent form due to impaired mental status or if the patient is incapacitated, the next of kin or power of attorney (POA) should sign it. Additionally, the consent form must be witnessed by another person; this person is usually another nurse or professional who is employed by the operating facility.

The surgical team may not proceed with a procedure if consent isn't obtained; performing a procedure the patient (or next of kin or POA) hasn't consented to can be considered assault. The exception to this is an emergent procedure, where the physician deems the patient's life or limb is in jeopardy unless the procedure is performed. In

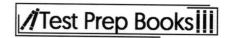
emergent situations, consent is not required, but the surgeon must document in the medical record the nature of the case and an explanation as to why consent is bypassed.

Preoperative Medication Reconciliation Protocol

Preoperative review of the current medication regimen is imperative to patient safety and optimal patient outcomes. The **medication reconciliation** process includes a review of all medications, including the name, dosage, route, frequency, and last dose taken. All medications should be recorded; this includes prescription and over-the-counter medications, as well as vitamins, supplements, and herbal remedies. Use of alcohol, tobacco, caffeine, and recreational drugs should also be documented. This information can be obtained through patient and/or family recall or the medication administration record if the patient is from a health care facility. Any medications that are deemed contraindications to the procedure should be promptly reported to the healthcare provider. For example, a patient taking daily warfarin is at a high risk for bleeding. Patients undergoing surgical or invasive procedures would need further considerations from the healthcare provider. The medication reconciliation should be reviewed by the surgeon and anesthesiologist preoperatively. If certain medications are not stopped prior to the procedure, the surgery may not proceed as planned. For example, if a patient was instructed to stop Plavix seven days prior to the procedure and the medication reconciliation process revealed the patient took Plavix yesterday, the surgeon may deem the surgery unsafe for the patient at this time.

Recreational Drug Use

Nurses must assess a patient's use of recreational drugs during the preoperative assessment. Illicit drugs may cause interactions with the anesthetic agents and alter the effects of intraoperative or postoperative medications. The interactions and effects are specific to the type of substance used. For example, patients who inject heroin may have hardened veins, making it difficult to obtain IV access. Cocaine and amphetamines are central nervous system stimulants, which can increase blood pressure and precipitate cardiac arrest. Hallucinogens, or psychedelics, such as LSD and "shrooms" produce an altered state of consciousness and can interfere with perioperative medications, increasing the risk of hallucinations, anxiety, and paranoia.

Preoperative Medications

Patients are often prescribed preoperative medications to prevent pain, decrease anxiety, and manipulate gastrointestinal effects. Commonly ordered medications include sedatives such as lorazepam. These medications decrease anxiety and prevent patients from having a recollection of the surgical experience. Narcotics, such as fentanyl or morphine, help with the patient's sedation and can decrease the amount of anesthetic agent needed during the procedure. Anticholinergic medications, such as atropine, decrease respiratory secretions and prevent laryngospasms. Gastric acid production and acidity can be decreased by histamine-2 receptor blockers, such as ranitidine. These medications prevent side effects such as regurgitation and vomiting.

The nurse should also review the **pharmacology**, or the action created by a drug, of the patient's current medications. Knowing the pharmacological effects of these medications and those of the scheduled preoperative medications can help keep the patient safe. If the patient is hypotensive and bradycardic and scheduled to receive a beta-blocker drug as a standing preoperative order, the nurse, understanding the potential pharmacological effects of the beta-blocker, would know to hold the drug and consult the physician. The nurse should have access to online drug references and the capability of consulting with a pharmacist, if needed.

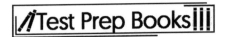

Perioperative Checklists

Perioperative checklists are an excellent method to validate the execution of processes and procedures and are an essential pathway for communication among multiple disciplines. They enable health care professionals to adhere to standards and identify potential trends that may impact operational procedures, decrease adverse events, reduce medical errors, address unusual occurrences, and affect the overall quality of care. The arrangement of data on a checklist appears in a format that is easier for staff to process. Some organizations have chosen to adopt the World Health Organization's (WHO's) Surgical Safety Checklist in an effort to increase patient safety while further enhancing documentation standards.

The World Health Organization (WHO) published a surgical safety checklist to serve as a baseline for all medical facilities that offer surgeries. It accounts for periods that are at risk for increased or significant medical errors during the perioperative period and encourages medical facilities to adapt the guidelines as needed while still addressing these critical timeframes. This document provides a standardized list of actions that should be performed in order to keep surgery patients safe.

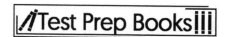

Surgical Safety Checklist

Before induction of anaesthesia ▶

SIGN IN

☐ Patient has confirmed
- identity
- site
- procedure
- consent

☐ Site marked/not applicable

☐ Anaesthesia safety check completed

☐ Pulse oximeter on patient and functioning

Does patient have a:

Known allergy?

☐ NO

☐ YES

Difficult airway/aspiration risk?

☐ NO

☐ YES, and equipment/assistance available

Risk of >500 ml blood loss (7 ml/kg in children)?

☐ NO

☐ YES, and adequate intravenous access and fluids planned

Before skin incision ▶

TIME OUT

☐ Confirm all team members have introduced themselves by name and role

☐ Surgeon, anaesthesia professional and nurse verbally confirm
- patient
- site
- procedure

Anticipated critical events

☐ Surgeon reviews:

What are the critical or unexpected steps, operative duration, anticipated blood loss

☐ Anaesthesia team reviews:

Are there any patient-specific concerns?

☐ Nursing team reviews:

Has sterility (including indicator results) been confirmed?

Are there equipment issues or any concerns?

Has antibiotic prophylaxis been given within the last 60 minutes?

☐ YES

☐ Not applicable

Is essential imaging displayed?

☐ YES

☐ Not applicable

Before patient leaves operating room

SIGN IN

Nurse verbally confirms with the team:

☐ The name of the procedure recorded

☐ That instrument, sponge and needle counts are correct (*or not applicable*)

☐ How the specimen is labelled (*including patient name*)

☐ Whether there are any equipment problems to be addressed

☐ Surgeon, anaesthesia professional and nurse review the key concerns for recovery and management of the patient

153

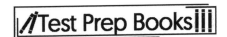

Preoperative Tasks

In preparing the patient for the operative phase of care, the nurse completes tasks to promote optimal patient outcomes and patient safety. The following text describes routine preoperative tasks:

- Before treatments, medication administration, or transfer of care, the nurse verifies patient identity using two patient identifiers. This is usually done by reading the patient's identification band and asking the patient to state their name and date of birth.

- The nurse verifies the procedure by asking the patient what surgery is being done and by reading the surgical consent and comparing it to the physician order. The nurse also ensures the surgical site is marked, per Universal Protocol.

- The following steps are taken by the nurse to assess the patient's health status:

  - Data is collected, analyzed, and prioritized. The nurse obtains vital signs, performs a pain assessment, reviews allergies and medication intolerances, analyzes lab values, reviews pertinent medical and surgical history (including current and previous medical conditions and family history), reviews the chart, and verifies NPO status.

  - Verbal and nonverbal communication is done utilizing an age-based competency model. This is done during the patient interview process and physical assessment. The nurse should consider the patient's cultural preferences while formulating the plan of care. A common example of this in the preoperative phase is in the Jehovah's Witnesses community, as these patients may not wish to receive blood or blood products.

  - Medication reconciliation occurs prior to surgery. This includes review of the patient's current medication regimen, also noting the use of herbal remedies, vitamins, and supplements. The nurse also notes use of tobacco, alcohol, caffeine, and recreational drugs.

  - Physical assessment is completed; this includes documentation of impaired skin integrity, mobility limitations, and presence of body piercings or implanted foreign objects.

- After collection and review of data, the nurse formulates patient-specific diagnoses. Nursing diagnoses are formulated based on subjective, objective, and psychosocial assessments. These diagnoses provide the foundation for focused nursing care plans. Additional nursing diagnoses are identified along the care continuum, and the nursing care plans are modified accordingly. The nurse may use nursing diagnoses approved by NANDA and PNDS, for instance.

- The nurse's preoperative patient assessment is documented in the medical record. It should be easily retrievable by the interdisciplinary team in order for optimal patient care to take place. Electronic medical records (EMRs) are effective in providing fast, easy access of the preoperative assessment to all members of the health care team. Documentation of the preoperative assessment is imperative for identification of deviations from baseline assessment.

Universal Protocol

The Joint Commission is an agency that accredits healthcare facilities based on their regulatory compliance. **Universal Protocol**, enacted by The Joint Commission (TJC) in 2004, is designed to prevent errors involving wrong procedure, wrong patient, and wrong site surgery. The nurse must ensure that all universal protocol activities are documented and stored in the patient's medical record according to facility policy.

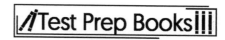
This protocol is divided into three categories: patient identity, site marking, and time-out. During the patient identity phase, the nurse uses two patient identifiers—typically, the patient's name and date of birth. The patient's medical record number may also be used. Prior to entering the operating room, the nurse asks the patient to state their name and date of birth while the nurse views the patient's identification band. The nurse verifies the patient's stated information on the patient's ID band with the surgical consent and other documents, if applicable. The nurse must ensure that the patient is able to confirm their identification verbally. If the patient is not conscious, other methods must be used to confirm identity, such as the medical record number. Other verification items include completed laboratory and diagnostic tests, blood products, implants, and special equipment that will be needed for the procedure.

The surgical site must be marked prior to starting the procedure. Surgical site marking occurs if the procedure involves differentiation of right or left side or multiple structures, such as fingers or toes. The surgeon who will be present during the procedure must identify the anatomical location and physically mark the skin with a tool that is consistently used throughout the facility. The marking tool must be able to withstand skin preparation and draping. The operative surgeon completes this prior to induction of anesthesia, involving the patient in the process. To promote clarity, the site is marked with either the surgeon's initials or with "yes," depending on the protocol of the surgical institution. Marking the operative site with an "X" can be ambiguous and should be avoided. Site marking is performed with a skin marker that remains visible after skin prep. Also, it should be done as close to the surgical site as possible and be visible after the patient is draped.

Immediately prior to the procedure, the surgical time-out is performed. The time-out consists of verification of patient identity, procedure, site, position, and availability of implants (if indicated). This occurs after the patient is prepped and draped and when all team members are engaged. All healthcare providers involved in the surgery, such as the surgeon, circulating nurse, anesthesiologist, and operating room technician, must be present for and participate in the time-out. If the case doesn't involve general anesthesia or deep sedation, the patient may participate. The time-out ensures that everyone agrees with the procedure to be performed, confirms the identity of the patient, and verifies the correct surgical site. Each member of the team has the opportunity to ask questions and address concerns during this time. It is imperative that the entire surgical team verbally concurs with the time-out, and the procedure may not begin until this happens. If a patient will be having multiple procedures during the surgery, a time-out must be performed before making each designated incision. The time-out is documented by the nurse and placed in the patient's medical record.

Frequent Monitoring

After completion of the procedure, the provider and/or surgeon will give orders for the patient to be transferred to the next level of care. The determination of where the patient is transferred is dependent on several factors, including intraoperative complications, patient acuity, and hemodynamic stability. Medical-surgical nurses must anticipate a post-surgical transfer to the intensive care unit (ICU) or post anesthesia care unit (PACU).

Any patient who has received anesthesia during surgery must be monitored postoperatively in a unit equipped to perform frequent assessments and emergency interventions. Priority assessments in the PACU include oxygenation, level of consciousness, and cardiovascular status. The patient's respiratory status must be assessed continuously to ensure an intact airway. Assessments include respiratory rate, depth, rhythm, breath sounds, and oxygen saturation levels. Level of consciousness includes the patient's alertness and ability to follow commands. Cardiovascular status is assessed via vital signs, cardiac monitoring, and temperature. The nurse observes trends, compares them to the patient's baseline, and reports any deviations from the norm. Patient criteria for transfer out of the PACU is often included in hospital protocols. Once the patient meets the criteria, they can be transferred safely to an inpatient

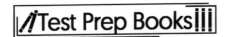

unit or be discharged home. Most patients transferred to the PACU remain on the unit for approximately one hour postoperatively.

In some instances, the patient will become unstable during the procedure and require a transfer to the ICU. Other patients have extensive surgeries or medical conditions requiring constant monitoring. Patients who are unstable or need to remain intubated benefit from ICU care. The nurse must anticipate critical care orders by the provider. For example, if a patient was unable to spontaneously breathe on their own after general anesthesia, the patient will remain intubated. The patient will require mechanical ventilation in the immediate postoperative period. The patient would be transferred to ICU for continued care.

Wound Healing

Wound healing occurs in stages from the immediate postoperative period, lasting up to a few years after surgery. The medical-surgical nurse should understand the factors that affect wound healing and identify opportunities for patient education to promote proper wound healing and decrease the risk of SSI. Patient conditions that may adversely influence the body's wound healing capability are malnutrition, hyperglycemia, obesity, smoking, and respiratory compromise. These conditions contribute to lack of blood and nutrient supply to tissue, therefore decreasing wound healing capability.

There are three stages in wound healing: inflammation, proliferation, and remodeling. The inflammation phase begins in the immediate postoperative period and lasts about six days. During the inflammation phase, hemostasis occurs. After hemostasis, phagocytosis takes place. In phagocytosis, the white blood cells "clean up" the area by eliminating foreign particles. **Edema** also occurs in the inflammation phase. Edema, or swelling at the surgical site, is a result of the immunological system signaling blood flow to the area to promote wound healing. Proliferation occurs around one to two days postoperatively and continues for approximately three weeks. During proliferation, the wound tissue appears reddened; this is from the formation of granulation tissue. Blood vessels of surrounding tissue are replenished, and scab formation begins. The final phase of wound healing is the remodeling phase. The remodeling phase begins at about three weeks after surgery and can last for two years postoperatively. During remodeling, collagen fibers connect together, and scar tissue eventually forms.

There are three methods for facilitating wound healing. These are primary union, granulation, and delayed primary closure. Each of these three methods involves inflammation, proliferation, and remodeling, to some degree. Primary union happens in surgical cases with aseptically made wounds with little or no tissue damage. Primary union occurs in ideal surgical conditions, and it is the preferred method for wound healing. Granulation is the second way wound healing may be achieved. The wound is left open and heals from the inside out. Infected wounds are often left open after debridement for granulation to occur. Delayed primary closure is used in contaminated or traumatic cases with a high risk of infection. The wound is typically packed with gauze and monitored for infection and drainage. On postoperative day three to five, the wound is closed. Delayed primary closure may be used in cases of compartment syndrome, where swelling is highly anticipated.

Intraoperative factors that influence the wound healing process are sterile technique, length and direction of incision, hemostasis, wound moisture, presence of necrotic tissue, the material used to close the surgical wound, tension applied by the surgeon in wound closure, and stress on the wound after surgery. When the perioperative team uses proper sterile technique, the chance for microorganisms to enter the surgical wound is decreased. Keeping the surgical wound free of these microorganisms helps to promote proper wound healing.

Maintaining Wound Dressings

Incisions created during surgery increase the patient's risk of infection. Postoperatively, the nurse will manage various wound dressings and products that prevent contamination of the wound. The type of dressing is dependent on the location, size, and depth of the wound or surgical incision. Regardless of the type of dressing, the nurse must

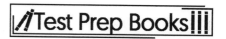

look for signs of bleeding, dehiscence, and evisceration postoperatively. Any indication of hemorrhage or wound complications should be reported to the healthcare provider or surgeon immediately. The nurse must also ensure that patients are premedicated with analgesics prior to performing a dressing change to ensure adequate pain management.

Laparoscopic surgeries are minimally invasive. The incisions are typically small and do not require staples or sutures to keep them approximated. The types of wound dressings used for these incisions are transparent films or adhesives to allow for visualization of the incision. Hydrocolloid dressings are occlusive or semi-occlusive and prevent wound contamination. However, these dressings are not absorbent and are typically used for wounds with light drainage.

Foam dressings covered with hydrophilic polyurethane film are used for surgical wounds that are expected to produce light to heavy amounts of drainage. These dressings can remain in place for 3 to 7 days, depending on the amount of exudate. Skin graft surgeries will be covered with antimicrobial dressings or collagens to protect and prevent infection to the graft or donor site.

Complex surgical wounds or wounds that become complicated postoperatively may have negative pressure wound therapy applied. Negative pressure therapy provides high absorbency of drainage, decreases bacterial colonization, and stimulates the formation of granulation tissue. Negative wound therapy requires a sponge over the incision that must be exchanged every 2 to 3 days depending on the amount of exudate collected.

Pertinent Potential Complications and Management

Whenever a procedure is performed on a patient, there is a potential risk of complications. If these complications occur, the nurse should be prepared with the knowledge of how best to manage them. Some potential complications involve mistakes made by the healthcare team, such as performing the procedure on the wrong patient or the wrong body part. This can be avoided by ensuring that a proper time-out is performed prior to the procedure. During a time-out, the physician and the rest of the team confirm that they are performing the right procedure on the right patient and that all safety and monitoring equipment is in place prior to starting the procedure. Whenever possible, this is conducted prior to sedation so that the patient can also confirm that the time-out is accurate.

Other complications may occur during the procedure that are simply based on how the patient's body reacts to the procedure and the procedural sedation. Many sedating medications can cause a decrease in respiratory rate and oxygenation. This should be monitored through capnography and managed with supplemental oxygenation. If the patient's respiratory rate becomes too low, the nurse should notify the physician so that interventions such as using a bag valve mask or intubation can be performed. The patient's airway may also be impaired by secretions or vomiting, which should be managed with positioning and suctioning to prevent aspiration. Some medications may also lower a patient's blood pressure. This is generally managed by administering a bolus of IV fluid but may be escalated to needing vasopressors if the IV fluid is not enough. Finally, while most medications administered during procedural sedation have a short half-life, some patients may have difficulty metabolizing them and may struggle to return to their baseline mental status following their administration. Because of this, the nurse may need to administer a reversal agent, or continue to manage symptoms until the patient is awake enough to be on their own.

Preoperative Fasting

Preoperative fasting is a preventive measure taken before surgery in order to reduce procedural complications that may occur from a full stomach (such as regurgitation) and the influence of increased metabolic hormones (such as insulin) in the body. This process involves the patient abstaining from food and water for a pre-determined period of time before a procedure. Current research is inconclusive on the length of preoperative fasting that is most effective, but in practice, patients normally fast for a period of two to eight hours based on age and surgery type.

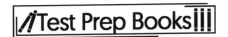

Fluid Replacement

Fluid replacement is the practice of replacing specific fluids that have been lost due to trauma, pathology, environmental factors, or surgical complications. It is most commonly needed in situations of excessive heat, gastrointestinal disease, or malnutrition and dehydration. Fluid can be replaced orally or intravenously. Dehydrated patients often need solutions containing water and an electrolyte mix based on the substances in which the patient is deficient. Comparatively, patients who have lost blood or plasma will need blood transfusions to replace the lost fluid.

Rapid Sequence Intubation

Rapid sequence intubation is an advanced airway management technique for emergency cases. In this procedure, patients are sedated to the point of unconsciousness and intubated with an endotracheal tube. This is most commonly used in critical cases where time is of the essence, such as in anaphylactic patients or those who need ventilation yet are unable to receive it through bag valve mask techniques. Rapid sequence intubation is also utilized in patients who are at risk of aspiration. This technique should not be used in patients who are already unconscious from their injuries.

Cricoid Pressure

Cricoid pressure is a safe practice utilized when rapid sequence intubation is required. The technique is most commonly practiced in emergency surgeries. In these cases, patients are not scheduled for the surgery and therefore have not taken the necessary preoperative precautions, such as fasting. Any gastrointestinal contents present the risk of regurgitation into the lungs and consequent asphyxiation when the patient is anesthetized. The application of pressure at the location of cricoid tissue creates an internal esophageal seal, blocking the pathway to the lungs and mitigating asphyxiation risk. Intubation occurs after this takes place.

Advanced Cardiac Life Support

Advanced cardiac life support (ACLS) refers to standardized procedural guidelines to rapidly treat emergency cardiac cases like heart attacks and heart failure, as well as situations that arise from cardiac embolisms, such as strokes. Only certain medical personnel, including registered nurses and nurse practitioners, are allowed to administer the protocols of ACLS. These protocols include analyzing heart rhythms, administering medication intravenously, or performing emergency surgery. Protocols are updated every five years; the most recent version was published in 2020. The 2020 guideline updates include the following: the adult bradycardia algorithm increased the atropine dose to 1 mg; physiological parameters such as arterial blood pressure or end-tidal CO2 can be used to monitor CPR quality; for pregnant patients while they are supine, relief of aortocaval compression through left lateral uterine displacement should be provided; given the opioid epidemic, do not wait to see the effects of naloxone before beginning ACLS.

DIC

Disseminated intravascular coagulation (DIC) is a rare but serious condition in which blood clotting becomes abnormal and overactive. This leads to the buildup of clots within the body that can cause blood vessel obstructions. In other instances, the clots promote continuous internal bleeding. DIC is commonly seen as a secondary condition in cancer patients, in cases where blood transfusions are rejected by the recipient, in patients with organ infections, in patients with severe tissue injury, and in septic patients. It can come on unexpectedly, and up to 50 percent of patients who experience DIC die. Patients who survive may experience permanent organ damage.

The main treatment of DIC is to treat the underlying cause, such as a transfusion reaction or infection. Sepsis protocols can also be implemented to provide respiratory and hemodynamic stability. If the patient is experiencing clotting, heparin may be used. If the patient is bleeding, then plasma, platelets, FFP, or red blood cell transfusions may be needed.

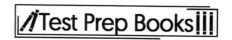

Malignant Hyperthermia

While **malignant hyperthermia (MH)** is rare, it is a life-threatening disorder that can be chaotic for an unprepared surgical team. Susceptibility to MH is hereditary, and it can be triggered by commonly used succinylcholine and anesthetic gases. Early signs of MH may include jaw clenching, unexplained tachycardia, muscle rigidity, and an increase in EtCO2. If untreated, the patient's core body temperature can rise to a dangerous level. During an MH crisis, immediate, aggressive treatment is essential. Dantrolene is the first line of treatment for MH, and the initial recommended dose is 2.5 mg/kg. Other common drugs used during an MH crisis include insulin in a glucose solution and calcium chloride. Calcium channel blockers should not be used. While MH may be somewhat unpredictable, all of the surgical team should be aware of their roles and responsibilities in an MH crisis to ensure prompt treatment.

It is imperative that patients be screened preoperatively for MH. Patients may not refer to the condition by name, but the circulator should be suspicious if the patient mentions unspecified anesthesia complications from a previous surgical procedure or in their family's surgical history. If MH is suspected, the circulator is responsible for making the surgical team aware of the potential for this emergency and preparing for a potential crisis. The anesthesia team should be notified immediately so that they can prepare the anesthesia machine and drugs appropriately. Emergency equipment and drugs, typically stored on an MH treatment cart, should be readily available. It is recommended that thirty-six vials of dantrolene be available at all times.

In the event of an MH crisis, the circulator should initiate the call for help and request assistance from any available personnel. The anesthesia team will need to focus on the treatment protocol, and the circulator should assist as needed. For example, dantrolene will need to be reconstituted with 60 milliliters of sterile water, and the circulator and other nurses can perform this duty while the anesthesia team concentrates on the patient. A Foley catheter should be placed if not already present. If the patient's core body temperature rises, the circulator (or delegated personnel) may need to provide ice to cool the patient directly and/or chilled IV solutions for infusion, irrigation, and catheter irrigation.

Anaphylaxis

Another rare but dangerous condition that may prevent itself in the operating room (OR) is anaphylaxis. **Anaphylaxis** is a severe allergic reaction that, outside of the OR, typically presents as a rash, swelling of the throat, hypotension, and/or shortness of breath. However, in the OR, detection of anaphylaxis can be difficult because the patient cannot complain about their symptoms and may be covered in drapes. The most common trigger for an anaphylactic reaction during surgery is exposure to latex. Other triggers include many of the drugs most commonly used in the OR: penicillin, succinylcholine, rocuronium, propofol, isosulfan blue, and iodine contrast dye. Immediate treatment of anaphylaxis is to remove the suspected source, if possible. As the cause may be an administered drug, treatment should focus on Basic Life Support (BLS) protocols, administration of epinephrine, airway management, and fluid administration.

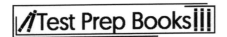
Again, one of the most common causes of anaphylactic reactions during surgery is exposure to natural latex rubber. Patients should be assessed preoperatively for a potential latex allergy. As it can be hereditary, the circulator should ask about the patient's allergies along with any family members' allergies to latex. In particular, if a patient is allergic to bananas, they may also be allergic to latex. When a potential latex allergy is suspected, the circulator is responsible for alerting the surgical team and ensuring the room is prepared appropriately, including using only latex-free supplies and latex-free gloves.

Alert Band

Latex Allergy

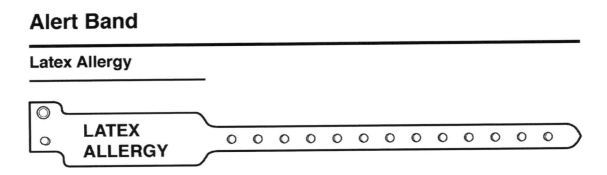

In the event of an anaphylactic reaction, the circulator should initiate the call for help and request assistance from available personnel. Again, the anesthesia team will need to concentrate on prompt treatment, which may include drug and fluid administration. The circulator should assist and delegate as needed.

Surgical Site Infection

Infection prevention and control are paramount objectives in providing safe healthcare. Patients in the perioperative environment are at increased risk of hospital-acquired infection (HAI) as compared to those not undergoing surgery. The surgical incision creates a way for pathogens to be introduced into the body. Evidence-based guidelines for prevention of surgical site infection (SSI) are adopted by all accredited healthcare institutions.

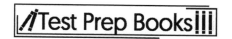
Measures in prevention of SSI are laid out by organizations such as the **Centers for Disease Control and Prevention (CDC)**, the Institute for Healthcare Improvement (IHI), and The Joint Commission (TJC). Infection prevention and control must be viewed from a multifactorial viewpoint in perioperative nursing. Standard precautions are used in the perioperative setting as a method to reduce infection rates. Standard precautions include hand hygiene, the use of **personal protective equipment (PPE)**, and environmental control.

Surgical Site Infections Risk Factors

Patient Factors

Age	Diabetes	Nicotine or Steroid Use
Altered Immune Response	Malnutrition or Obesity	Preoperative colonization with Staph. aureus
Prolonged Preoperative Stay		

Cardiopulmonary Arrest

Cardiopulmonary arrest is a life-threatening emergency characterized by the sudden unexpected cessation of heart function, breathing, and consciousness caused by a disturbance in the electrical conduction of the heart. Immediate basic life support (BLS) followed by current advanced cardiac life support (ACLS) protocol is the treatment. Defibrillation is the treatment choice for cardiopulmonary arrest caused by ventricular tachycardia or ventricular fibrillation. The time between patient collapse and initiation of resuscitation efforts is the most important factor in patient survival.

The brain is the first organ impacted by loss of blood flow and oxygenation. Cardiac arrest lasting longer than 8 minutes has poor survival rates. A diagnostic work-up during and after stabilization will include an ECG, arterial blood gases (ABGs), troponin counts, CBC, electrolyte counts, and renal function labs.

Blood Loss

Large amounts of blood loss can cause severe complications, including shock, cardiac failure, and/or death. These situations most commonly occur as a result of trauma, illness, or surgical complications. Blood loss can occur by blood leaving the body through an external wound, or it can occur internally. Internal bleeding can quickly become

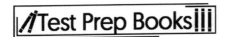

fatal as it is less obvious until symptoms become critical. To treat blood loss, medical professionals can transfuse blood from a safe, compatible source; however, this can cause unwanted side effects such as hemolysis, kidney damage, infection, or allergic reactions if the source of transfused blood is tainted or the wrong blood type for the recipient. If the patient has already progressed to shock or cardiac events as a result of blood loss, they may need to be resuscitated through defibrillation, administered medication, or have fluid imbalances addressed.

Classes of Hemorrhage

Hemorrhage refers to any instance where extreme blood loss occurs. It can occur anywhere in the body and can refer to both external and internal cases of blood loss. Hemorrhage cases can be categorized into three classes of severity. Class 1 cases are mild and often do not require medical care. Class 2 cases are more moderate, with patients' bodies trying to compensate for the blood loss. These patients will show symptoms of elevated heart rate and pale skin. Class 2 cases are often easily treated through intravenous fluids. Class 3 cases are severe, with patients losing 30–40 percent of total volume. Patients are likely to experience shock and require blood transfusions. Class 4 cases are the most critical and the most likely to result in death. They include cases where over 40 percent of total blood volume has been lost; immediate blood transfusions and other medical interventions are usually necessary in these cases.

Transfusions

Transfusions refer to replacements of blood, plasma, platelets, lymph, or specific blood cells. Patients may need transfusions in situations of extreme blood loss, in instances of blood disorders, or in instances of blood infections. While safeguards to ensure blood donations are tested for blood type and disease, recipients of transfusions may still experience complications such as hemolytic reactions, allergic reactions, rejection, lung injury, sepsis, or contraction of a disease.

The potential need for a blood transfusion during surgery must be assessed in the preoperative phase of surgery. In collaboration with the healthcare provider, the nurse must review laboratory results and identify medical conditions that may necessitate a blood transfusion. Some medical conditions to screen the patient for include anemias, blood clotting disorders, and medications that may increase the risk for bleeding such as anticoagulants or antiplatelet medications. Laboratory results that indicate a low platelet count, low hemoglobin, or a prolonged bleeding time should also be taken into consideration.

The nurse must also anticipate a blood transfusion for specific surgeries that may result in significant blood loss, such as trauma surgeries. Ruptured organs, compound fractures, and traumatic tissue injuries can all result in excessive blood loss intraoperatively. The nurse must ensure that the patient has preoperative laboratory work drawn to facilitate a blood transfusion. Blood typing and crossmatching are required to safely identify the patient's blood type and donor compatibility.

As part of the health history, nurses must identify any contraindications to blood transfusions. Patients may refuse blood products due to religious and cultural beliefs. Any surgical patient that is identified as having a contraindication must be given alternative options.

When a patient is identified as a risk for significant blood loss or when prevention of exposure to allogeneic blood is preferred, a blood salvage may be ordered. A blood salvage, also known as autotransfusion, reinfuses the patient's own blood after it is processed (separated, washed, and concentrated) intraoperatively. The benefits of autologous blood infusion are that it eliminates the potential for infection or rejection, due to the patient's body recognizing the blood as its own. It also prevents accidental infusion of contaminated blood, such as from another patient with a blood disease. Blood may be collected before a patient has a surgery (up to 6 weeks prior), during surgery, or after surgery. Postoperative blood salvage is most commonly ordered for major orthopedic surgeries, such as joint replacements. The blood is collected in a specialized surgical drain that is designed for performing an autologous blood transfusion. As with any blood transfusion, the nurse must be cautious to observe for any signs of fluid

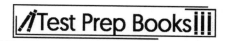
overload, infection, and emboli. The patient may be at risk of anemia or collection and labelling error; autologous blood infusions are also costlier than other forms of blood transfusion.

Deep Vein Thrombosis

Deep vein thrombosis refers to a clot that forms in a deep vein (as opposed to a superficial vein). Deep veins are responsible for critical deoxygenating processes; therefore, clots in these veins can cause serious complications, such as blockages. Deep vein thrombosis is characterized by swelling, pain, and warmth. It most commonly occurs in the lower legs.

Embolus

An embolus is a mass found in blood vessels. Most often, it is a clot composed of fatty acids, cholesterol, or blood. However, they also can be bubbles of air or gas. Emboli can block passageways and prevent adequate blood circulation from occurring. Fatty acids, cholesterol, and blood embolisms normally result from the build-up of these substances over time, which then break off and travel through the body's extensive blood vessels until they are snagged by vessel walls or otherwise unable to pass. Air embolisms occur from wounded or punctured vessels, while gas embolisms most commonly occur in deep sea divers who dive or resurface too quickly. In these situations, air pressure imbalances cause gas bubbles inside the divers' blood vessels.

Hypertension

Hypertension refers to elevated systolic or diastolic blood pressure. It is generally defined as a systolic reading of 140 or higher, or a diastolic reading of 90 or higher. Prolonged periods of hypertension are considered a critical condition that can potentially lead to seriously adverse outcomes, such as heart attack, aneurysms, stroke, or metabolic disorders. This is due to the constant burden on the walls of the blood vessels that ultimately makes it difficult for blood to circulate adequately.

Hypotension

Hypotension refers to low systolic or diastolic blood pressure. It is generally defined as a systolic reading of 90 or lower, or a diastolic reading of 60 or lower. Some endurance athletes may be prone to hypotension without any serious consequences. Other adults may have chronic hypotension with mild dizziness, but no debilitating symptoms. Elderly patients or patients who are at risk of going into shock are considered critical if they appear hypotensive, as this can indicate that oxygenated blood may not be circulating to crucial organs, such as the brain.

Shock

Shock refers to instances of extremely low blood pressure resulting in inadequate blood circulation. This is considered an emergency situation. Shock can occur from infection, extreme blood loss, spinal cord injury, or a severe allergic response. Patients may appear unresponsive and feel cold to the touch. Based on the type of shock, patients will be treated with fluid replacements, antibiotics, and/or immobilization.

Thrombus

A **thrombus** is a clot of blood. It most commonly occurs in autonomous wound repair to slow bleeding and support wound healing. In pathologic cases, clotting occurs at levels that can cause blockages in blood vessels. Some people, such as those with congenital heart diseases or leukemia, are predisposed to this condition and must be monitored for even minor injuries.

Local Anesthetic Systemic Toxicity (LAST)

Local anesthetic systemic toxicity (LAST) is a serious complication that can occur after the injection of local anesthetics such as ropivacaine, bupivacaine, and lidocaine, which are used to numb the tissues surrounding the surgical area. Nerve blocks numb the area around the nerves to decrease pain. Local anesthesia is meant to be administered in a precise location. However, if the medication reaches the systemic circulation, the risk of toxicity is

163

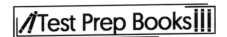

increased. Systemic involvement will result in adverse effects, likely observed immediately post injection. Some adverse effects are delayed depending on the patient's weight, medical history, and concentration of the medication.

Mild LAST is characterized by symptoms involving the central nervous system, such as perioral numbness, confusion, dysarthria, tinnitus, and agitation. The patient may also report a metallic taste in the mouth. Signs and symptoms of moderate LAST include dizziness, blurred vision, drowsiness, and headache. The most severe form of LAST involves the cardiovascular system, resulting in cardiac dysrhythmias, hypotension, bradycardia, and respiratory or cardiac arrest.

The first intervention that should occur if the patient is experiencing symptoms of LAST is to stop the local injection. If mild, the central nervous system effects may subside. The nurse should monitor vital signs and ensure that the patient's airway is intact. Oxygen administration may be indicated if the patient's respiratory system is compromised. If the patient experiences a severe reaction, seizure control is indicated. The nurse should anticipate administering medications such as benzodiazepines. Should the patient proceed to respiratory arrest, ventilatory support is needed. The pharmacological management of LAST involves a lipid emulsion. Lipids bind to the molecules of the anesthetic medication, preventing their systemic effects and reversing the toxicity.

Scope of Practice Related to Procedures

Scope of practice refers to the tasks and responsibilities that fall within a particular role. Within nursing, the specific scope of practice may vary somewhat depending on where the nurse practices and what resources are available. This is especially true with procedures involving procedural sedation. However, there are universal responsibilities that are considered a part of the scope of practice for all nurses that are expected to be performed. Additionally, nurses must understand the scope of practice for others on the team during the procedure to ensure that the procedure is performed safely and to know who needs to be brought in as a specific resource and who can be delegated to for certain tasks.

Perioperative Nursing Process

The preoperative patient assessment includes obtaining subjective and objective data and is essential in formulating the patient's plan of care. Each step of the **nursing process** (assessment, diagnosis, planning, implementation, and evaluation) is used during the preoperative assessment.

During the initial step, the nurse performs subjective, objective, and psychosocial assessments. During the subjective assessment, the nurse allows the patient the opportunity to ask questions and evaluates the patient's knowledge of the procedure and what to expect during the process. The objective assessment is the data collection piece (lab values, vital signs, physical assessment, etc.). A psychosocial assessment addresses the patient's support systems (family, friends, and economic) as well as the patient's feelings. Common feelings patients have during this time are anxiety, fear, anger, hopelessness, worry, and feeling overwhelmed by their disease process. Sometimes the nurse can alleviate these feelings by explaining what to expect in the preoperative, intraoperative, and postoperative phases of care. The nurse should speak to the patient in terms the patient can easily understand. If the patient expresses a strong fear of death related to the surgery, the nurse should inform the surgeon. Because the patient's emotional state influences the body's stress response, the surgeon may choose to do the surgery at another time or cancel it altogether.

During the diagnosis phase, the nurse uses the assessment data and formulates nursing diagnoses. The diagnoses guide the planning phase, where the nurse develops next steps in care. These steps involve nursing actions but may include steps to be taken by interdisciplinary team members. For example, if one diagnosis is knowledge deficit related to the surgical procedure, the nurse may ask the surgeon to review the plan with the patient and family again.

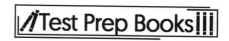

Once the nurse completes the planning process, implementation begins. Implementation often begins with educating the patient on the plans, expected outcomes, and how the patient can be involved in the plan of care. For example, if the nurse is implementing a postoperative pain management plan, the nurse should explain this to the patient during the preoperative phase, while the patient is (presumably) at their baseline. With the agreement of a negotiated pain level and the plan for postoperative pain medication and nonpharmacological pain management measures, the patient is more likely to achieve desired pain control.

The final phase of the nursing process is evaluation; however, evaluation happens across the continuum of the nursing process, not just at the end. The nurse frequently evaluates the effectiveness of care plans, adjusts as necessary, and reevaluates.

Assessment
Relevant Patient Data
The nurse uses multiple techniques in performing the **preoperative health assessment**; these include the patient interview, screening tools to identify potential risk for complications, collection of objective data values, and review of the medical record. During the preoperative period, the nurse's data collection should include vital signs, height and weight, review of allergies, NPO (nothing by mouth) status, current pain assessment, skin integrity, presence of implants and body piercings, presence of tubes (such as drains, chest tubes, urinary catheter, percutaneous endoscopic gastrostomy tube, or nasogastric tube), vascular access catheters, and immobilization devices (cast, surgical boot, sling, etc.).

The patient should understand the importance of NPO for surgery because noncompliance compromises the patient's safety by creating risk for aspiration and a compromised airway. Pain should be assessed preoperatively for patient comfort and also to establish the patient's postoperative pain goal. If skin breakdown is present, this must be documented in the medical record as being present on admission. Skin integrity, including risk for impaired skin integrity, is taken into consideration during surgical positioning. Measures such as extra padding with pillows and foam and use of alternate positioning may be utilized to prevent further impairment of the skin. An alternate type of **electrosurgical unit (ESU)** dispersive electrode may be considered in patients with high risk for skin breakdown.

Physical assessment data, along with a review of medical and surgical history, form a picture of the patient's **health status**. The patient interview provides useful information and can also provide insight into potential issues including anxiety, financial worry, discharge planning needs, and psychosocial issues such as domestic abuse. The nurse should consult with interdisciplinary teams when indicated. Focused assessments may be conducted based on initial assessment findings. Screening tools are standards of care and are utilized in the preoperative assessment. The nurse implements plans based on abnormal screening tool findings. For instance, the patient who scores above the desired score upon Obstructive Sleep Apnea screening is automatically referred to the anesthesiologist for follow-up assessment of respiratory risk during surgery. Abnormal assessment findings must be reported to the physician and documented in the medical record.

Laboratory Results
Senior patients almost always require laboratory screening to determine whether or not chronic disease exists, while most other patients will only require laboratory screening if their physical assessment or medical history shows a risk factor for cardiovascular or respiratory disease. These two types of disease, at any stage, can make surgery of any kind a riskier process for the patient; therefore, preparatory measures allow the medical team to provide the safest treatment. Commonly ordered laboratory tests for these conditions include blood counts, electrolyte counts, glucose tests, electrocardiographs, and chest radiographs.

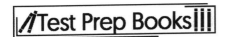

Pathophysiology

Pathophysiology refers to changes in the body due to a disease process. The patient's history of chronic and acute disease is discovered during the preoperative patient interview and chart review. Understanding the pathophysiology of the patient's disease process (or processes) empowers the nurse to know if assessment findings are congruent with the disease process or if findings are indicative of something else.

For example, if a patient has 2+ pitting edema with a history of CHF, the nurse may suspect the edema is secondary to a CHF exacerbation and investigate further by auscultating lung sounds and consulting with a cardiologist. It is also important for the nurse to consider the pathophysiological processes associated with the patient's scheduled procedure. The nurse should note that although the scheduled procedure may be minor, the patient's diagnosis may be quite serious. If the patient is having a PowerPort insertion, the surgery process is minor. However, the patient may have a diagnosis of stage IV lung cancer, and this is quite serious. Understanding this, the nurse may allow more time for the patient to verbalize feelings and provide emotional support for the patient.

Anatomy and Physiology

The nurse must have an understanding of basic anatomy and physiology concepts in order to conduct an accurate patient assessment. Each patient, at minimum, requires an assessment of the cardiac, respiratory, and renal systems prior to surgery. Knowledge of cardiac anatomy is necessary in order to auscultate heart sounds, including an apical pulse. **Electrocardiograms (ECGs)** are routinely performed preoperatively, and in order to accurately obtain an ECG, the nurse must correctly place the leads. Without a basic understanding of cardiac anatomy, the nurse can't perform this task.

Understanding anatomy of the respiratory system is essential in auscultating breath sounds accurately. If the nurse isn't sure where the right upper lobe of the lung is located, accurate assessment of breath sounds isn't possible.

In performing the renal assessment, the nurse should understand what lab values are associated with acute or chronic renal insufficiency. Also, if the nurse needs to perform a post-void bladder scan, they need to know which area of the lower pelvic region to place the ultrasound probe. If the patient is complaining of severe pain in the right flank area, the nurse should be aware that this could be related to a kidney issue.

Abnormal findings in any of these three categories warrant further investigation to ensure the patient is safe for surgery. The nurse's knowledge of anatomy and physiology enables the nurse to discern findings that deviate from the norm. Documentation of anatomical and physiological assessments provides a baseline for comparison postoperatively.

Focused Assessment

Prior to the surgical or invasive procedure, the nurse must perform a focused physical assessment. The focused assessment is dependent on the type of procedure being performed. However, an overview of the patient's health status will include an assessment of all major body systems.

For example, a patient undergoing abdominal surgery will require a focused gastrointestinal assessment. This may include inspecting the abdomen for distention, auscultating bowel sounds, and inquiring about the last meal and bowel movement. A focused integumentary assessment includes inspecting the skin for lesions, color, and hydration. Immobility during the perioperative period is a factor to consider for patients at risk for skin integrity issues. Respiratory assessments evaluate breath sounds, ease of breathing, and chest characteristics. A cardiovascular assessment will help determine the patient's ability to perfuse major organs. Assessments include inspection for jugular vein distention or edema and auscultation of heart sounds for rate and rhythm. Musculoskeletal assessments test muscle strength and ability to ambulate. Postoperative care includes early ambulation and mobility, so it is important for the nurse to assess a patient's range of motion and ability to perform activities of daily living.

166

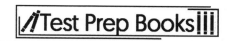
A neurological assessment is imperative in the preoperative phase. A patient's level of consciousness, orientation, and speech pattern help determine their overall physical and mental state. Sensory and motor function should be documented and compared to postoperative findings. Intraoperative medications can alter a patient's coordination and response time. Any changes from the patient's baseline assessment should be promptly reported to the healthcare provider.

After a patient undergoes a procedure and is in the recovery phase, it is important to assess readiness for discharge from the post-anesthesia care unit (PACU). The nurse will use various tools to perform focused assessments. A commonly used instrument is the Aldrete scoring system. The Aldrete score ranges from 0 to 10, with 10 being the ideal score for discharge. The total score is determined by individual areas of assessment. The highest score for each assessment area is 2 points. Areas of assessment include consciousness, mobility, circulation, breathing, and color (oxygenation).

Hemodynamics

A crucial part of patient assessment and monitoring is their hemodynamic profile. Hemodynamics are the forces that cause blood to circulate throughout the body, originating in the heart, branching out to the vital organs and tissues, and then recirculating back to the heart and lungs for reoxygenation and pumping. There are at least three different aspects of hemodynamics that can be focused on: the measurement of pressure, flow, and oxygenation of the blood in the cardiovascular system; the use of invasive technological tools to measure and quantitate pressures, volumes, and capacity of the vascular system; and the monitoring of hemodynamics that involves measuring and interpreting the biological systems that are affected by it.

Hemodynamics can be assessed using noninvasive or invasive measures. Noninvasive measures would include the nurse's assessment of the patient's overall presentation, heart rate, and blood pressure. Invasive measurements would include inserting an arterial blood pressure monitor directly into an artery or the insertion of a Swan-Ganz catheter. The Swan-Ganz catheter, also known as a pulmonary artery catheter (PAC) or right-heart catheter, is threaded into the patient's subclavian vein, down the superior vena cava, right up to the PA. This type of catheter is used quite commonly in ICU patients. PACs give information about the patient's cardiac output and preload. Preload is obtained by estimating the pulmonary artery occlusion pressure (PAOP). Another way to assess preload is determining the right ventricular end-diastolic volume (RVEDV), measured by fast-response thermistors reading the heart rate. There is some question as to whether the use of PACs helps patients or not. Some studies suggest that the use of PACs does not reduce morbidity or mortality but rather increases these occurrences. Their use, therefore, should be weighed carefully according to the physician's discretion.

There are many different parameters to consider when assessing a patient's hemodynamics. Blood pressure is the measurement of the systolic pressure over the diastolic pressure, or the pressure in the vasculature when the heart contracts over the pressure when the heart is at rest.

Mean arterial pressure (MAP) shows the relationship between the amount of blood pumped out of the heart and the resistance the vascular system puts up against it. A low MAP suggests that blood flow has decreased to the organs, while a high MAP may indicate that the workload for the heart is increased.

Cardiac index reflects the quantity of blood pumped by the heart per minute and per meter squared of the patient's body surface area.

Cardiac output measures how much blood the heart pumps out per beat and is measured in liters.

Central venous pressure (CVP) is an estimate of the RVEDP, thus assessing RV function as well as the patient's general hydration status. A low CVP may mean the patient is dehydrated or has a decreased amount of venous return. A high CVP may indicate fluid overload or right-sided heart failure.

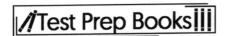

Pulmonary artery pressure measures the pressure in the PA. An increase in this pressure may mean the patient has developed a left-to-right cardiac shunt, they have hypertension of the PA, they may have worsening complications of COPD, a clot has traveled to the lungs (pulmonary embolus), the lungs are filling with fluid (pulmonary edema), or the left ventricle is failing.

The pulmonary capillary wedge pressure (PCWP) approximates the left ventricular end-diastolic pressure (LVEDP). This number, when increased, may be a result of LV failure, a pathology of the mitral valve, cardiac sufficiency, or compression of the heart after a hemorrhage, such as cardiac tamponade.

The resistance that the pulmonary capillary bed in the lungs puts up against blood flow is measured via pulmonary vascular resistance (PVR). When there is disease in the lungs, a pulmonary embolism, hypoxia, or pulmonary vasculitis, this number may increase. Calcium channel blockers and certain other medications may cause the PVR to be lowered because of their mechanism of action.

A hemodynamic measurement used to assess RV function and the patient's fluid status is the RV pressure. When this number is elevated, the patient may have pulmonary hypertension, failure of the right ventricle, or worsening congestive heart failure.

The stroke index measures how much blood the heart is pumping in a cardiac cycle in relation to the patient's body surface area.

Stroke volume (SV) measures how much blood the heart pumps in milliliters per beat.

The systemic vascular resistance parameter reflects how much pressure the vasculature peripheral to the heart puts up to blood flow from the heart. Vasoconstrictors, low blood volume, and septic shock can cause this number to rise, while vasodilators, high blood levels of carbon dioxide (hypercarbia), nitrates, and morphine may cause this number to fall.

The following is a list of commonly measured hemodynamic parameters and their normal values:

- Blood pressure: 90–140 mmHg systolic over 60–90 mmHg diastolic
- Mean arterial pressure (MAP): 70–100 mmHg
- Cardiac index (CI): 2.5–4.0 L/min/m^2
- Cardiac output (CO): 4–8 L/min
- Central venous pressure (CVP) or right arterial pressure (RA): 2–6 mmHg
- Pulmonary artery pressure (PA): systolic 20–30 mmHg (PAS), diastolic 8–12 mmHg (PAD), mean 25 mmHg (PAM)
- Pulmonary capillary wedge pressure (PCWP): 4–12 mmHg
- Pulmonary vascular resistance (PVR): 37–250 dynes/sec/cm^5
- Right ventricular pressure (RV): systolic 20–30 mmHg over diastolic 0–5 mmHg
- Stroke index (SI): 25–45 mL/m^2
- Stroke volume (SV): 50–100 mL/beat
- Systemic vascular resistance (SVR): 800–1200 dynes/sec/cm^5

Diagnosis

Nursing diagnoses are formulated after collecting assessment data, reviewing the medical record (including current medications), and interviewing the patient. Several **North American Nursing Diagnosis Administration (NANDA)** and Perioperative Nursing Data Set (PNDS) approved nursing diagnoses apply to the preoperative patient population. Common preoperative nursing diagnoses are anxiety regarding risks (including impaired skin integrity and mobility as well as death) and a lack of knowledge regarding the surgical procedure. Different age groups create an inherent risk for certain problems. Elderly patients are more at risk for impaired skin integrity, hypothermia, and

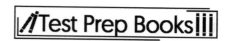
dehydration. Using the nursing diagnoses, assessment findings, and collaboration with the interdisciplinary team, the plan of care is implemented to best meet the patient's needs. Evaluation of the plan of care occurs during the preoperative, perioperative, and postoperative phase, depending on the criteria being evaluated.

The diagnostic procedures performed depend on the planned surgical procedure, patient's history, risk factors, and best practice standards. Examples of diagnostic procedures include computerized axial tomography (CT), electrocardiogram (ECG), hemoglobin and hematocrit, pregnancy test for a female patient of childbearing age, type and screen, international normalized ratio (INR), blood glucose, and chest x-ray. These can be done in various settings, such as a physician's office, laboratory, outpatient clinic, or hospital. If a diagnostic procedure shows a deviation from the patient's baseline, such as an ECG change, more tests may be ordered to clear the patient for surgery. In this example, the patient may undergo a cardiac catheterization to determine cardiac risk for surgery.

At this point, the surgeon and cardiologist discuss risks and benefits based on diagnostic data. Occasionally, diagnostic procedures reveal incidental findings that render a patient ineligible for surgery, such as an abdominal aortic aneurysm. In order for nursing diagnoses and medical plans to be formulated, the results of the diagnostic procedures must be documented in the patient's medical record and reviewed prior to surgery.

Preoperative Planning

Using the nursing process, a plan of care is created that reflects the goals, interventions, and expected outcomes set by the nurse. Steps involved in planning the care of the preoperative patient are modeled by evidence-based guidelines and surgical core measures:

- An individualized plan of care is developed considering the following criteria:

  - The nurse anticipates the physiological responses of the patient and formulates diagnoses that reflect identified risks and needs. Commonly identified risks in the preoperative patient are risk of infection, altered thermal response, and impaired skin integrity. Interventions related to these risks are incorporated in the plan of care.

  - Current Surgical Care Improvement Project (SCIP) measures are implemented by the surgical team preoperatively. These include preoperative antibiotic prophylaxis, administration of beta-blocker drugs in certain patients, and application of antiembolism stockings and/or compression devices.

  - The nurse prepares the patient for safety needs unique to preoperative patients. The patient may be exposed to radiation and lasers during the procedure; measures are taken to minimize exposure to the patient and operative personnel. Fire safety measures include a fire extinguisher in the room and normal saline or sterile water on the sterile field if electrosurgery is used. Patient positioning is carefully examined, and the nurse ensures that proper anatomical alignment and padding are used.

  - The nurse identifies behavioral responses of the patient and family. Measures are taken to reduce anxiety and fear. Cultural and spiritual needs are met as appropriate. Comfort measures are used as much as possible. Pain management, including pain medication administration, may also be considered.

  - Age-specific needs are incorporated in the care plan as needed. This may include temperature regulation, alternative positioning methods, selecting smaller instruments (pediatric or neonatal patient), providing a tangible comfort item (blanket, toy), or consoling a crying or extremely fearful patient.

  - The nurse arranges for an interpreter to be present if a language barrier exists. If cultural or religious needs are identified, the nurse incorporates these into the plan whenever possible.

169

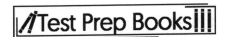
- o Ethical and legal guidelines are upheld according to professional standards. The nurse provides nonbiased, competent, safe care and practices within guidelines per institutional policies and procedures.

- o Interdisciplinary teams are used in providing evidence-based care. IDTs in the surgical setting can include radiology personnel, ultrasound technicians, pharmacists, laboratory staff, and consulting physicians.

- The nurse uses a patient-centered care model in practice. Patient-centered care dimensions include patient preferences, emotional support, physical comfort, information and education, continuity and transition, coordination of care, access to care, and family and friends. These aspects are considered on an individual basis. The nurse uses the patient-centered care model throughout the nursing process.

- Expected patient outcomes are identified by the nurse, and the plan of care is reflective of these. When deviations from the expected outcomes are identified, the nurse modifies the care plan and associated interventions.

- Standard precautions are adhered to by the nurse and the operative team to decrease the risk of hospital-acquired infection. Performing hand hygiene at the appropriate times is the number one measure healthcare professionals can take to minimize infection risk. PPE should be available at all times for the health care team's use.

Individualized care plans for perioperative patients should focus on existing disease processes, as applicable. A medical history will help determine what actual or potential problems the nurse should address throughout the surgical experience. For example, a patient with history of diabetes mellitus is identified as having a risk for infection or delayed wound healing after surgery due to altered glycemic control. The nurse would establish interventions that aim to control the patient's serum glucose. Additionally, patient education regarding postoperative care and glucose control are imperative. As with any other nursing process, an evaluation of the interventions must be performed to ensure that the outcomes were successfully met.

Intervention

Nurses must identify actual or potential problems that a patient may experience. A nursing diagnosis should have related risk factors and defining characteristics that serve as evidence of an actual or potential problem. Nursing interventions will be aimed at preventing or correcting existing problems. For example, in the preoperative phase, the patient may be at risk for infection due to their medical history and physical assessment. Risk diagnoses typically do not have defining characteristics since the chosen diagnosis is a potential problem. A patient at risk for infection would have the following nursing diagnosis according to NANDA (an international organization responsible for standardizing terms used in diagnoses): risk for infection related to alteration in skin integrity, obesity, and history of smoking. The related factors would be specific to the patient's disease process. Nursing interventions would emphasize teaching about early mobilization, prepping the skin for surgery, and providing adequate hygiene and hydration.

Acute pain is a primary nursing diagnosis for a patient in the postoperative stage. The surgical procedure and intentional injury to the skin will result in physiological changes. The patient may experience an increase in blood pressure, pulse, and respirations. Facial grimacing and guarding behaviors are additional defining characteristics. Prompt recognition of signs and symptoms along with adequate pain management are key nursing interventions in the recovery period.

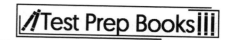
Evaluation

Successful evaluation of the plan of care is determined by the completion of patient outcomes. Care plans differ at every stage of the perioperative experience. The expected outcomes are based on the patient's ability to reach the goals and the nurse's ability to implement all interventions.

In the preoperative phase, a common goal for patients is an understanding of the procedure and subsequent recovery expectations. A patient is deemed prepared for surgery when they are able to consent to the procedure, understand the risk and benefits, verbalize the expected outcomes, and demonstrate the ability to perform postoperative activities. When a goal is not achieved, the nurse must ensure that any deficiencies in patient knowledge are addressed prior to advancing to the intraoperative phase.

Postoperative evaluation of goals and expected outcomes can be short or long-term. A patient in the recovery phase of a procedure can achieve an expected outcome immediately, or it may take days, weeks, months, or even longer to observe results. Many facilities have nurse advice lines that follow up with patients postoperatively to ensure they are meeting their expected outcomes. For example, a patient undergoing cataract surgery may demonstrate an immediate improvement in vision after the procedure. The patient's goal of improved sensory perception can be evaluated immediately after treatment. However, a patient who has a repair of a lower extremity fracture will require several weeks of rehabilitation before the goal of intact mobility can be evaluated.

Alterations in Body Systems

Physiological response refers to surgery-specific reactions produced by individuals who undergo a medical procedure or related trauma. This response appears to take the same course across most individuals and includes temporary nervous, endocrine, and metabolic system changes. Immediately upon a traumatic event (such as surgery), the body produces stress hormones (such as cortisol, adrenaline, and catecholamines), excess growth hormones, and excess insulin. This creates systemic inflammation in the body. In the ensuing days, the body's metabolic system shows an ebb-and-flow effect through cyclic decreases and increases in cardiac output, oxygenation, and glucose consumption until the body is able to return to a state of homeostasis. Post-surgery, homeostasis is supported through medical interventions of nutritional supplementation (especially of glucose and amino acids), electrolyte rebalancing, and pharmaceuticals to decrease the metabolic stress on the body.

Nurses must have the ability to assess a client for alterations in their body systems. This is an inevitable occurrence, as a body system alteration is precisely the reason the client is at the hospital in the first place. The nurse will identify the body system alteration and draw up a plan of care based on their findings.

Intake and output are items that are closely monitored by the nurse to discover if an alteration in a body system has occurred. There are several types of drainage a client may experience that fall into the category of input and output. The nurse measures the drainage where appropriate and notes its appearance. Color, quantity, consistency, and any other notable characteristics are observed and documented. Types of drainage the nurse may encounter in client care include feeding tube drainage, respiratory secretions, drainage from a chest tube, rectal tube output, and urinary catheter output.

Clients with cancer may be put on radiation therapy to target and destroy cancerous tumors. This client may develop alterations in certain body systems as a result. The client is likely to become quite fatigued, as their energy is sapped by the intensity of the therapy. Weakness often accompanies fatigue. They may experience skin reactions such as a rash. The skin may become red, looking like a sunburn. The skin above the targeted location for radiation absorbs a bit of the radiation, which is why the reaction occurs. Other radiation therapy side effects may be specific to the area in which the therapy is targeted. If therapy occurs near the stomach or abdomen, for example, stomachache, nausea, vomiting, and diarrhea may occur.

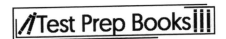

If the nurse is caring for a woman who is pregnant, they will be mindful of certain body alterations associated with the prenatal period. One such complication is high blood pressure during pregnancy, called *preeclampsia*. The woman's blood pressure is carefully monitored during the prenatal period to watch for the development of this condition, which could lead to complications for both the mother and the baby. Gestational diabetes is another prenatal complication of which the nurse is mindful. Somewhere between twenty-four and twenty-eight weeks, pregnant women are screened for gestational diabetes by performing the oral glucose tolerance test (OGTT). This glucose screening will identify if the woman is at risk, and treatment will follow if necessary.

Patients who are developing an infection will often have some telltale symptoms that the nurse will be watchful for. The classic signs of a localized infection on the outer surface of the body will be redness, inflammation, heat, and swelling. If the infection is systemic, within the body, the patient may have a fever, increased WBC count (or decreased if the infection has been prolonged), prodromal malaise, fatigue, chills, elevated heart rate, and an altered level of consciousness and orientation. Some infections will have specific symptoms related to the organ or tissue of the body affected. For example, a urinary tract infection (UTI) will cause the patient to have pain or burning while urinating, called *dysuria;* possibly have blood in the urine; and have frequent urges to void. A respiratory infection, on the other hand, will have respiratory-specific symptoms such as cough, difficulty breathing, and adventitious breath sounds on lung auscultation.

Having a basic knowledge of how an infection works, from start to finish, is advantageous to the nurse when trying to understand what is going on within the client's body. The causative organism must enter the body through some entryway: respiratory tract, break in the skin, urinary tract, IV access, GI tract, and so on. The organism then goes through what is called the "incubation period," which refers to the time that elapses between the organism entering the body and when symptoms actually begin occurring. During the incubation period, the organism is usually multiplying until it starts to have a noticeable effect on the body. Some pathogens will have a longer incubation time, while others will have shorter. Depending on the pathogen, there may be some communicability of the disease involved, in which the disease can be spread from one person to another. Therefore, observing universal precautions is vital to prevent the spread of disease. Meticulous handwashing by the nurse and all members of the health-care team, as well as patients and family, is vital.

A full-blown infection occurs when the body's natural defenses cannot overcome the organism effectively and symptoms occur, compromising overall body function. The patient may have an elevated WBC count on the CBC, indicating the body is bolstering its immune defenses to try and overcome the infection. The final stage of the infection is when the body's immune system plus the help of medication and therapeutic interventions destroy the organism, restoring the body to natural, normal functioning ability.

Behavioral Responses Regarding Surgery

Not only does the surgical process have physiological effects on the body, but it also induces **behavioral responses**. Behavioral responses to surgery include, but are not limited to, the following: anxiety, fear, agitation, depression, noncompliance, altered body image, stress, and disturbances in eating and sleep patterns. The fear of dying is one of the most common causes of preoperative anxiety. Patients often verbalize being afraid of not waking up from surgery. Anticipating postoperative pain and not knowing if it will be controlled adequately can certainly promote anxiety and fear. This is one reason the nurse performs a preoperative pain assessment and education on the postoperative plan for pain management. Allowing the nurse and patient to negotiate a tolerable pain level together gives the patient a sense of ownership and control in the care plan, helping to decrease anxiety and fear.

A patient may also experience postoperative anxiety and fear awaiting biopsy results, as this can be life changing for the patient and their family. The patient may feel a loss of control overall, and this contributes to agitation, noncompliance with treatments set forth by someone other than himself/herself, and sometimes anger with the health care team or with everyone in general. Depression may be a behavioral response. For instance, a cardiac transplant recipient often suffers from depression as a result of internalizing the fact that the transplant was able to

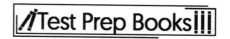

take place because a person lost their life. The patient may feel undeserving of the gift that has been received: a second chance at life. For this reason, a cardiac transplant workup consists of a psychiatric evaluation. Some patients respond to the stress of the surgical process with eating and sleeping disturbances. Recognizing the patient's individual behavioral responses and incorporating these responses into the plan of care helps provide holistic patient care.

Anesthesia

During a procedure, patients may choose general anesthesia or localized anesthesia to mitigate potential pain. **General anesthesia** will place the patient into a fully sedated and unconscious state. This is most often used in major surgeries involving large muscle groups, organs, or other contexts that can be painful or otherwise cause patients the inability to remain still (as movement can cause critical surgical complications). Localized or **regional anesthesia** numbs sensation in a specific area but allows patients to remain alert and conscious. After surgical procedures are over, patients may experience a great deal of pain which can be managed through non-pharmacological mechanisms or prescription medications, including patient-controlled analgesia (PCA), where the patient controls a device that administers pain relief as needed.

Moderate or procedural sedation is a form of sedation that involves administration of medications that are meant to control pain and reduce psychological trauma (usually through memory loss). While the patient remains unaware of what is happening during the procedure due to the sedation, the patient may still be able to follow simple commands and respond to certain stimuli. The patient should also be able to maintain their airway without intubation or ventilation. Because of these factors and the relatively short half-life of the medications administered, procedural sedation is often used for sedation in procedures that are relatively quick to perform and less invasive than those that would require a deeper form of sedation. Examples of these relatively quick procedures include initial reduction of a broken limb, cardioversion, chest tube placement, and endoscopy. Since these procedures are generally lower risk, a nurse under the supervision of a doctor may be asked to perform the procedural sedation.

PSA

Procedural sedation and analgesia (PSA) allows patients to remain somewhat alert during medical procedures that may be uncomfortable but not unbearably painful, such as resetting bones. Unlike general anesthesia, where patients are completely sedated and do not feel any sensations, PSA allows patients to be somewhat conscious and aware of bodily functions. It can be utilized with or without pain-relieving medications. Practitioner awareness is crucial when administering procedural sedation, especially when pain relief is also utilized. Progressive care nurses who will assist with PSA must be well trained, ACLS certified, and know their related facility policies. Prior to a patient having procedural sedation, the nurse should confirm that the patient has informed consent on the chart and that pre-procedure vital signs and rhythm strips have been obtained. If procedural sedation is to be done at the bedside, the nurse should make sure that airway management devices are within reach of the bedside for the provider to use and the patient is being appropriately monitored with continuous oxygen saturation, heart rate and rhythm, respiratory rate, and end tidal carbon dioxide monitoring. During the procedure frequent blood pressure readings should be obtained. Any abnormalities should be immediately reported to the practitioner. The nurse should make sure meds for ACLS as well as reversal medications, such as naloxone and flumazenil, are available if needed and that the patient has patent IV access. Most hospital policies require 1:1 nursing care for the patient during procedural sedation and for 30 minutes after, provided the patient has returned to pre-procedure baseline.

Depending on the practice setting, the medical-surgical nurse may administer certain intravenous moderate sedation medications and provide moderate sedation monitoring. Regional anesthesia may be used alone or in combination with moderate sedation. Regional anesthesia is achieved when local anesthetic is injected along a nerve pathway. Regional anesthesia is a good option for patients who are deemed too high risk for undergoing general anesthesia. Types of regional anesthesia are spinal, epidural, and Bier block. The type of anesthesia is selected after patient assessment, history and physical, and diagnostic tests. Other factors that determine the type

173

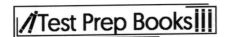
of anesthesia used are patient preference, age, length of surgery, surgeon preference, and the **American Society of Anesthesiologists (ASA)** classification.

ASA classification is a method of assessing patient health status prior to surgery. The patient is given an ASA value of I through VI:

- ASA I indicates a healthy patient. The ASA I patient is at low risk for complications based on health status.

- ASA II is given to a patient with mild systemic disease. Pregnancy, obesity, controlled diabetes, and controlled hypertension put the patient into ASA II status.

- The patient with severe systemic disease that is not incapacitating is an ASA III. Patients with uncontrolled diabetes, poorly managed hypertension, chronic obstructive pulmonary disease (COPD), end stage renal disease (ESRD), remote history of cerebrovascular accident (CVA), or remote history of myocardial infarction (MI) can be classified as ASA III.

- ASA IV indicates the patient has severe systemic disease that is a constant threat to life. Examples of this are recent history of MI or CVA, cardiac ischemia, significant heart valve dysfunction, and ejection fraction below twenty percent.

- ASA V describes the patient who is near death and is not expected to survive without the operation. The patient with a ruptured abdominal aortic aneurysm (AAA), acute cardiac tamponade, or intracranial bleed can be categorized as ASA V.

- The patient who has been declared brain dead and is being kept alive for the purpose of organ recovery is classified as ASA VI.

- In addition to ASA classes I through VI, the procedure is given an "E" after the class designation if it is an emergency procedure. The patient with a ruptured abdominal aortic aneurysm can be designated an ASA "VE."

Scope of Practice

The exact scope of the nurse during a procedural sedation has not been standardized and can vary from state to state, from hospital to hospital, and even between departments and specialties within a hospital. For example, some hospitals may only allow nurses in certain specialties with specific training to perform procedural sedation. Departments such as the intensive care unit, the emergency department, the gastrointestinal lab, and interventional radiology may be more likely to perform procedural sedation, and nurses in those departments are more likely to be trained in how to administer it. Additionally, depending on the hospital or on laws put in place by the state, nurses who are allowed to perform procedural sedation may be limited in which medications they can administer themselves and which require physician administration. For example, in some areas, nurses may administer IV push ketamine and midazolam but must hand off IV push propofol administration to the physician. Whatever situation the nurse may be in regarding performing the sedation and their specific involvement in the procedure, all nurses involved in that patient's care should understand what to expect in a patient who has had said procedure and what to expect following the sedation.

While certain specifics in a nurse's scope of practice during a procedure may vary, there are universal responsibilities that are expected of all nurses caring for the patient receiving procedural sedation. First, any nurse caring for the patient should be assessing them. During and after the sedation, the nurse should be monitoring the patient's airway, breathing, heart rate, oxygenation, and blood pressure. These can all be affected by sedation medications. The nurse should also assess the patient's level of sedation during and after the procedure. This is

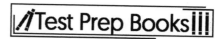

necessary in order to know when it is safe for the patient to do things like walk unassisted, take anything by mouth, and eventually be discharged. The second responsibility of the nurse is to advocate for the patient and the patient's safety. The nurse must ensure that the physician has obtained informed consent from the patient prior to the procedure. The nurse should also ensure that the proper equipment is available for the procedure, including monitoring devices and resuscitation supplies in case of emergency. If needed, the nurse should also ensure that additional resources are available during the procedure, such as respiratory therapy, a pharmacist, and additional staff if more assistance is needed. Finally, the nurse is responsible for ensuring the patient (and possibly their family or caregivers) are provided with adequate education. While the physician may be responsible for educating to ensure informed consent, the nurse can provide additional information to educate the patient on what to expect during and after the procedure. The nurse should also educate any caregivers on potential monitoring and care required after the procedure.

In addition to understanding their own scope of practice during a procedure, nurses must understand the scope of practice of others on the team who may be involved in the procedure and procedural sedation. The physician's scope includes diagnosing the need for the procedure, performing the procedure, obtaining informed consent prior to the procedure, ordering medications and interventions, and, in some cases, administering sedation medications. A respiratory therapist may also be present to assist in assessing the patient's airway and breathing, provide interventions such as oxygen administration and airway management (suctioning or positioning), and potentially assist in emergent intubation if indicated. If a pharmacist is present for the procedure, their role is to advise the physician on medications and their dosages and also to assist in drawing up or mixing any administered medications. Ancillary staff may also be involved in the procedure, and their scope may depend on their particular specialty. For example, a technician in the emergency department may assist with splinting during a limb reduction, while a technician in the GI lab may assist with procedure setup. The nurse must understand the roles within the team to ensure that the patient is receiving the care they need during and after the procedure, to advocate for appropriate care, and to know what tasks should be delegated to which team member. When the procedural team works together well and within their designated scopes of practice, the patient will be more likely to have improved outcomes and avoid potential complications.

Supplies, Instruments, and Equipment

Surgical instruments are categorized by their purpose. Generally, instruments fall into three categories: cutting instruments, clamps, and graspers/holders. Cutting instruments are those used for cutting tissue. Knife handles are used for holding the surgical blade. The surgical blade may be used to make skin incisions, to incise or puncture a blood vessel, or to dissect a portion of tissue. To decrease the chance of sharps injury to the surgical team members, surgical blades with built-in safety devices should be used. The safety device is designed to cover the sharp while the blade is passed between the surgical team members. Two types of scissors are used in surgery: tissue and suture scissors. Tissue scissors are used for cutting tissue. Metzenbaum and Mayo are two types of tissue scissors. Suture scissors are used to cut sutures and other surgical supplies, such as paper and synthetic graft material. Bandage scissors and wire cutters are examples of suture scissors. Scissors are also used after skin incision to dissect tissue for exposure to the surgical area.

Clamps are used to hold areas together. The type of clamp used depends on the amount and type of tissue to be clamped together. Some clamps provide total occlusion, while others are used for partial occlusion of an area. A clamp has "teeth" that come together when the clamp is engaged. The teeth may be fine or robust, depending on the type of tissue the clamp is meant for. A commonly used surgical clamp is the hemostat. The hemostat is used to minimize blood loss by clamping vessels together. Hemostats come in a variety of sizes and may be straight or curved.

Graspers and holders are another category of instruments. They are designed to hold or grasp tissue and provide traction away from the surgical area. Graspers come in a multitude of styles and are selected by the surgeon

175

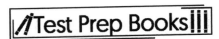

depending on the type and amount of tissue to be grasped. There are tissue holders as well as needle holders, or needle drivers.

Other surgical instruments include staplers, forceps, saws, scopes, and retractors. Staplers are used to wedge away organ tissue, such as lung tissue for biopsy. They are also used for stapling the skin closed at the end of the procedure. Forceps are used to pick up tissue. Saws can be used for sternotomy or cutting away bone in orthopedic procedures. Scopes are used for visualization in minimally invasive procedures such as laparoscopy and thoracoscopy. Retractors are used to separate tissue and provide visualization for the surgical area. Retractors come in a variety of sizes and may be used for retracting a small blood vessel or for retracting something as large as an entire abdomen.

In addition to surgical instruments, other supplies are needed to successfully perform a surgical procedure. Sutures are used to sew vessels together and to close the skin layers at the end of the procedure. Sponges, such as laparotomy and gauze, are used to absorb blood away from the surgical area. Sponges used in the surgical field have x-ray detectable material in them so they can be visualized on x-ray in the event of an incorrect surgical sponge count at the end of the case. Disposable knife blades are attached to knife handle instruments for making skin incisions or for incising vascular tissue. Surgical drapes are applied after skin prep is completed to maintain the sterile field integrity. Surgical gowns and gloves are worn by all members of the sterile field. Surgical implants are used in certain procedures, including aortic valve replacement, permanent pacemaker insertion, and lower extremity bypass graft. Surgical dressings are applied at the end of the procedure to protect the surgical area and minimize risk for surgical site infection.

Examples of anesthesia supplies are syringes, intravenous catheter access needles, intravenous tubing sets, ventilator circuits, endotracheal tubes, ambu bags, tongue depressors, alcohol pads, and tape.

Surgical equipment is used, along with surgical instruments and supplies, to perform the surgical procedure. Some equipment is standard for all surgical cases, while others are used for specific cases only. As technology changes and grows, new and different types of equipment are introduced into the perioperative environment. Robotic surgery, for example, has become very popular and requires a specific set of equipment.

In general, each operating room is equipped with the following: a monitor for patient vital signs, a surgical bed, a fire extinguisher, gas supply ports, vacuum ports for suction, suction canisters, an electrosurgical cautery machine, stools, tables for workspace and supplies, and extra tables for sterile set-up. Most surgical procedures require an anesthesia machine that is equipped with ETCO2 monitoring and a ventilator circuit. Some operating rooms contain a defibrillator, while others have a central location for the defibrillator and other emergency equipment. A monitoring tower, which includes gas supply, camera source, and light source, is used in minimally invasive cases for visualization. A pneumatic tourniquet is used in vascular and orthopedic procedures to reduce blood flow at the surgical site during critical points of the operation. X-ray equipment may be indicated to provide radiology imaging intraoperatively. A surgical laser is used in select cases for tissue ablation.

Implants and Explants

The term "surgical implant" refers to an item intentionally placed inside the body during surgery that will remain in place permanently or for a specified time frame, generally longer than twenty-one days or thirty days. This time frame is defined in the healthcare institution's policies and procedures. Documentation of the surgical implant includes the implant type, manufacturer brand and lot number, serial number, location of the implant, and expiration date. This implant information is documented in the patient's medical record. The surgical department also keeps record of all implants, along with the information that is documented in the medical record. This implant log can be referenced for tracking purposes in the event of a product recall. Surgical **explants** are documented in the same fashion as implants. The type of device that is explanted, along with as much other supporting information about the explant, is recorded in the medical record and on an explant log. The explant log is kept in the same area of the surgical department as the implant log for tracking purposes.

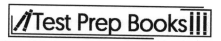

Types of surgical implants include prosthetic heart valves, synthetic grafts, medication ports, cardiac electrical devices, joint replacements, and spinal or orthopedic plates and screws. Prosthetic heart valves may be metal or biological. Biological sources come from pig, cow, or human donors. Synthetic grafts can be made from polyester or polytetrafluoroethylene (PTFE) and may even be impregnated with a blood thinner medication called Heparin. Medication ports are implanted in patients who require long-term intravenous access for blood draws, chemotherapy, or antibiotic therapy. The port accesses the subclavian or internal jugular vein and is implanted under the skin at the subclavian area. Cardiac electrical devices include permanent pacemakers and automatic implantable cardioverter-defibrillators. These both include a generator with leads attached to the heart. Joint replacement implants are used for knee and hip replacements. These may be made of stainless steel, titanium, or polyethylene. Metal plates and screws may be used in spinal and orthopedic surgeries, such as fusions and fractures.

A surgical implant is seen as foreign matter to the body and puts the patient at risk for infection at the implant site. Strict aseptic technique should be adhered to in surgical cases involving an implant. If infection does develop, the implant is surgically removed, unless it is deemed unsafe by the surgeon to do so. Antibiotic prophylaxis is administered to patients with surgical implants to decrease the infection risk.

Selection of Procedure-Specific Barrier Materials

Invasive procedures increase the risk of infection in patients. Intentional incisions created by the surgical instruments can facilitate the introduction of microorganisms into the patient's tissues. Strict infection control practices are crucial throughout the perioperative experience to prevent complications.

Barriers utilized pre and intraoperatively help decrease the risk of infection. The types of barriers used are dependent on the scheduled procedure. Preoperatively, the main barriers used to prevent infection are antimicrobial skin antiseptic solutions, specifically products containing chlorhexidine gluconate (CHG). Patients should be instructed to shower or bathe before the procedure with a CHG soap or solution. Special attention must be given to the area that will be exposed during the procedure. A three- step process of applying, lathering, and rinsing should be emphasized. Patients who are unable to bathe themselves should be assisted or given a bed bath with CHG microfiber cloths. The application of antiseptic solution leaves a film on the skin that acts as an initial barrier to microorganisms.

Surgical draping is one of the primary methods of intraoperative infection control. Surgical drapes are manufactured in various sizes and shapes to cover equipment, furniture, and the patient. A drape provides a physical barrier between the patient and microbes in the environment, thus decreasing the risk of infection. Drapes may be disposable, in the form of paper, or reusable cloths with appropriate sanitizing protocols.

The type of drape used is dependent on the anatomical location for the procedure. For example, a fenestrated drape is used when surgeries are to be performed on the abdomen, flank, or thoracic cavity. The fenestration (or window) allows for isolated exposure to the site. Other drapes allow enough room for the procedure to be performed while still providing a barrier to the rest of the body, such as abdominal or orthopedic drapes. Clear drapes are placed on surgical instruments and equipment, such as the da Vinci robot for laparotomies or a camera for endoscopic procedures. The clear drapes provide a barrier between the surgical instrument and the patient's body cavity.

Personal protective equipment such as gloves, gowns, masks, face shields, goggles, and shoe and hair covers are standard in the operating room. These barriers provide protection from microbes to the operating room staff as well as the patient. Additional equipment may be required for specific patients. For example, a procedure performed on a patient with tuberculosis requires specific airborne ventilation to prevent environmental contamination. These rooms require negative airflow to contain air particles within the operating room.

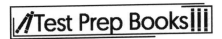
Barriers applied postoperatively help protect the patient from infection and injury. The type of protective barrier is dependent on the type of procedure performed. For example, a patient who had surgery to the eye will require a protective eye shield to prevent accidental injury. Patients treated surgically for burns may have antimicrobial ointments applied as a barrier to infection in the postoperative period.

Nutrition

Individualized Nutrition Needs

Many factors can affect a patient's dietary intake. Aging, injury, and health conditions can all impact a patient's ability to consume certain kinds or consistencies of food. For example, a patient who's suffered a stroke can have **dysphagia** (trouble swallowing) and be at risk for aspiration. Because of this, they might need a diet consisting of thickened liquids to prevent aspiration. The patient should be seated upright, fed slowly, and checked for complete swallowing with each bite. Patients at risk for aspiration should remain in an upright position for at least thirty minutes after eating.

Another example is an older patient with missing teeth who has a limited ability to chew and, therefore, requires a softened diet. There might also be patients who are unable to consume any food by mouth and require tube feedings.

Malnutrition is under- or overconsumption of food. Overconsumption can lead to obesity and type 2 diabetes, which puts a strain on all major body systems. Underconsumption can lead to poor development and vitamin and electrolyte deficiencies. It is important for the nurse to assess a patient's nutritional needs within twenty-four hours of admission. Vulnerable populations such as the elderly, children, people of low socioeconomic status, and people from undeveloped countries are at the highest risk for malnutrition. Other populations such as those with chronic diseases or cultural preferences also require specific nutritional needs, some of which are below.

Anorexia is an eating disorder that causes malnutrition and can be life threatening. Patients should be weighed daily with their back facing the scale. The nurse should monitor the patient during meals and one hour after to discourage purging.

Celiac disease is an autoimmune reaction to gluten, so clients cannot eat wheat, rye, or barley. Common symptoms include diarrhea and steatorrhea (fatty stools).

Cholelithiasis or gallstones occur when bile contains too much cholesterol or bilirubin. High-fat foods should be avoided.

Pancreatitis is inflammation of the pancreas. In the acute phase, patients should be on NPO to allow the pancreas to rest. If symptoms persist, a nasogastric tube may need to be placed. For chronic pancreatitis, patients should receive low-fat, high-carb, high-protein diets.

Nurses should provide culturally competent dietary education. This involves knowledge of ethnic considerations. While some generalizations can be made about specific groups, the best approach is to ask patients about their dietary preferences.

A kosher diet, which is part of the Jewish culture, has rules surrounding types of food that can be eaten and preparation of foods. In general, meat and dairy cannot be prepared or eaten together. Pork is not allowed. Mexican Americans and Native Americans have high incidences of type 2 diabetes, so carbs should be limited. Asian Americans should be educated to reduce salt to lower their risk of cardiac disease.

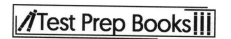

Therapeutic Diets

Therapeutic diets are prescribed for patients based on their physical condition, nutritional status, and possible upcoming procedures. The following are commonly ordered therapeutic diets:

- **Regular Diet:** No dietary restrictions

- **Nothing by Mouth (NPO):** Patient is not to have any food or drink when this diet is ordered. If a patient is ordered to have nothing by mouth (**NPO**) prior to surgery, and they consume something (including liquids), the surgery might have to be postponed or canceled.

- **Clear Liquid Diet:** Patient can consume clear liquids such as water, coffee, and tea (without milk or cream), as well as clear fruit juice, popsicles, gelatin, and clear broth.

- **Full Liquid Diet:** In addition to clear liquids, the patient can have any liquid that can be consumed through a straw. This includes pureed soups, ice cream, and meal replacement shakes.

- **Mechanical Soft Diet:** Patient is only given pureed foods.

Other commonly ordered diets are based specifically on a patient's individual nutritional needs as determined by a physician or dietitian. These include: diabetic, low sodium, low residue, high residue, heart healthy, low cholesterol, gluten free, and lactose free.

Monitoring patients' nutrition and hydration, based on their physician's recommendations as well as the patient's response to the therapy, is a critical part of patient care. Patients should have a variety of foods that can meet their specific dietary goals, as interesting and balanced meals increase the likelihood that patients will adhere to their prescribed nutrition therapy. Patients should also be monitored during their mealtimes to see if they need additional assistance with holding utensils and feeding themselves, or if they appear to not be eating or drinking well. Many health conditions increase the risk of patients not being able to accurately assess their hunger and thirst levels, leading to an increased risk of malnourishment and dehydration. Patients should regularly be monitored for signs of these issues, including sudden weight loss or weight gain, dry skin, dry mouth, a sunken appearance, and fatigue. Some patients may benefit from intravenous hydration support or nutrition supplementation through vitamins or liquid meals.

Nutrition Administration Modalities

Enteral nutrition (EN) provides nutrients to the GI tract (the stomach, duodenum, and jejunum); therefore, it requires a functioning gut. EN can be administered via several modalities, but the most common are nasogastric (NG) and percutaneous endoscopic gastrostomy (PEG). An NG tube can be placed by a nurse at the bedside, and a PEG tube is surgically placed in the OR. There are several indications for EN such as anorexia, chemotherapy, neurologic conditions, birth defects, orofacial fractures, and burns. Feeding tubes can be placed improperly, which allows the food to be administered to the wrong site of the body, such as the lungs. This poses an aspiration risk. To prevent this, the nurse should confirm proper placement of the tube via X-ray on initial placement. Afterward, the nurse should confirm the tube is still in place via aspirating stomach contents and ensuring a pH of <5. This should be done at every feeding or every eight hours for continuous feeds. The nurse should flush the tube with water before and after feedings, drug administration, and residual checks. Besides aspiration, common complications include vomiting, diarrhea, constipation, and dehydration. These can be mitigated by initial glucose checks, I/O, auscultating bowel sounds prior to feedings, daily weights, and tubing changes every twenty-four hours.

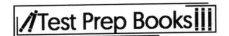

Total parenteral nutrition (TPN) is used in situations where a patient cannot orally ingest food or digest food through the stomach and intestines. In such cases, total parental nutrition is essential to maintain patient nourishment and to prevent wasting or malnutrition.

The clinical conditions requiring total parenteral nutrition include the following:

- Any cause of malnourishment
- Failure of liver or kidneys
- Short bowel syndrome
- Severe burns
- Enterocutaneous fistulas
- Sepsis
- Chemotherapy and radiation
- Neonates
- Conditions requiring full bowel rest, such as pancreatitis, ulcerative colitis, or Crohn's disease

Resources and Indications for Alternative Nutrition Administration

Hospitals should have a multidisciplinary nutrition support team, including gastroenterologists, dietitians, a specialist nutrition nurse, and other allied healthcare professionals such as speech and language pathologists (SLPs). SLPs are experts in oral anatomy and often perform swallowing tests at the bedside, as well as barium swallow tests for patients with dysphagia. Some signs and symptoms of dysphagia that would prompt a consultation with an SLP include difficulty chewing or swallowing, coughing or choking while swallowing, regurgitation of undigested food, drooling, and difficulty controlling food or liquid in the mouth. Dietitians' main roles are to conduct nutrition screenings and assessments, develop and execute a nutrition care plan, monitor the patient's response to the plan, and determine a care plan to transition or end nutritional support. The specialist nutrition nurse helps reduce complications for enteral and parenteral feedings and ensures nutrition protocols are being followed.

The main reason for alternative forms of nutrition administration is undernutrition defined as a BMI of less than 18.5 and unintentional weight loss greater than 10 percent within the last three to six months, or a BMI of less than 20 and unintentional weight loss greater than 5 percent within the last three to six months. Nutritional support should also be considered for people at risk of malnutrition, such as people with celiac disease, anorexia, short gut syndrome, and Crohn's disease. Specifically, there are several indications for enteral nutrition such as anorexia, chemotherapy, neurologic conditions, birth defects, orofacial fractures, and burns. Since parenteral nutrition is used when the GI tract is not functioning properly, its indications include GI obstruction, GI tract anatomical abnormalities, malnutrition, surgery or trauma, chronic diarrhea such as in Crohn's disease, or ulcerative colitis.

Practice Quiz

1. Which of the following is not a risk factor for falls in the elderly?
   a. Using a cane to walk
   b. Inadequate lighting in a room
   c. Muscle weakness
   d. Slower reflexes

2. What is the significance of a "pertinent negative" documented in the patient's EHR?
   a. The patient was unable to identify symptoms.
   b. The documentation of the physical assessment is incomplete.
   c. The assessment did not identify the symptoms commonly associated with a condition.
   d. The assessed manifestations are inconsistent with the patient's report.

3. Which of the following medications should not be taken in combination with nitroglycerin and what would be the result if they were taken together?
   a. Warfarin, excessive blood thinning
   b. Sildenafil, irreversible hypotension
   c. Allegra®, increased heart rate
   d. Sertraline, increased depression

4. According to the nursing theories of culturally sensitive practice, which of the following is the FIRST step?
   a. Cultural self-awareness
   b. Cultural skill development
   c. Cultural knowledge acquisition
   d. Cultural implementation training

5. What category of disinfectant is peracetic acid?
   a. High level
   b. Moderate level
   c. Intermediate level
   d. Low level

See answers on the next page.

Answer Explanations

1. A: Use of a cane is not a risk factor for falls in the elderly. A cane would actually benefit a person by giving them extra stability when walking. Poor lighting is a risk factor because it could cause someone to stumble over items on the floor or cause an imbalance by bumping into unseen furniture. Muscle weakness and slower reflexes are also risk factors for falls in the elderly.

2. C: The pertinent negative is a manifestation that is commonly associated with a condition, and the absence of that manifestation is an important consideration in the diagnosis of that condition. The remaining choices are not associated with the concept of the pertinent negative; therefore, Choices *A, B,* and *D* are incorrect.

3. B: Sildenafil and nitroglycerin should not be taken together, as both cause blood vessel dilatation, leading to the potential of irreversible hypotension. The other listed combinations do not have documented direct effects when taken in combination with nitroglycerin.

4. A: The first step to culturally sensitive practice is the assessment and acknowledgment of one's own biases and stereotypes. Without this self-awareness, the nurse's actions can be unduly influenced by these personal beliefs. Cultural awareness is necessary to gain the knowledge and skills needed to implement culturally competent patient care. Therefore, Choices *B, C,* and *D* are incorrect.

5. A: Peracetic acid is a high-level disinfectant. There are three categories associated with disinfectants: high level, intermediate level, and low level. Each category has different capabilities in which they destroy bacteria, microorganisms, viruses, or fungi. Peracetic acid can be useful in cleaning semicritical items.

Holistic Patient Care

Patient-Centered Care

Patient-Centered Care

Patient-centered care is an approach to healthcare and nursing care that recognizes and honors the unique preferences, needs, values, and experiences of the individual. It accomplishes this by addressing patient preferences, coordinating and integrating care, making information more available, approaching care holistically, encouraging patient and family participation, and increasing access. The resulting benefits are increased compliance, improved outcomes, decreased cost of care, and improved patient satisfaction.

Patient Preference

Patient preference is identified and incorporated at an organizational level in the location, layout, and operation of an organization. It impacts the service availability and culture of an organization. Departments implement and modify policies and procedures to address patient and family preference, such as the implementation of expanded visiting hours. Nurses and other individual care providers identify patient preferences regarding spirituality, culture, diet, learning style, and communication. Additionally, comfort, care, and general preferences are gathered during daily care. Nurses can promote the incorporation of patient preference through observing, asking questions, actively listening, and documenting preferences.

Care Management

Care management includes effective coordination of care, integration between services, and continuity of care during transitions. Strategies to improve care management include effective interdisciplinary communication and handoff (e.g., use of SBAR, bedside rounding), timely and accurate documentation, and interdisciplinary collaboration to provide a cohesive care experience.

Information and Patient Education

Patients have a right to timely, accurate, balanced information pertaining to their care. This can include timely communication of test results, ongoing discussions about care and discharge planning, discussion of treatment options, or supporting the patient's right to obtain a second opinion. Patient education needs to be geared to the learning level of the individual and be complete, unbiased, appropriate for the topic, and considerate of the learner's preference in communication and learning.

Holistic Approach to Care

Holistic care considers the emotional, physical, and spiritual health of the patient. Physical care includes safety and comfort. This is promoted through quality nursing care and purposeful rounding, which specifically addresses comfort needs. Emotional support is promoted with compassion, empathy, and active listening, and by addressing patient and family concerns rather than dismissing them. Spiritual support seeks to identify and support what brings hope and purpose in a patient's life. This can be a religious practice, a spouse, a child, a pet, nature, music, art, or anything that brings joy to the patient.

Spirituality

When developing a plan of care for a patient, the nurse must assess the patient's spirituality. **Spirituality** refers to a personal understanding and acceptance of one's role and meaning in the grand scheme of existence. It can be religious, faith-based, an energetic understanding, or a simple, personal reflection. A patient's faith and religious practices will influence how they perceive their health and well-being. Spirituality may play a positive role in patients' coping response. Patients who have a strong spiritual practice of any sort are associated with having more

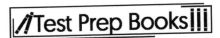

peaceful responses to their personal health, higher levels of stress control, less pain after surgical procedures, and easier recovery periods after medical procedures. Nursing interventions for the established care plan should be mindful of the patient's spiritual beliefs while also considering their physical well-being. For example, a patient may request frequent periods of privacy to perform a religious prayer. However, during the postoperative period, the nurse may need to assess the patient's vital signs frequently. Planning a timing strategy to achieve both outcomes would be the ideal goal. Spirituality can be another dimension for healthcare providers to investigate and utilize with patients as they prepare them for a surgical procedure or help them recover.

Patient and Family Participation

Shared decision-making is an approach to care planning that places high importance on active patient and family participation. This approach is a critical part in providing patient-centered care. Patients and families are informed and involved throughout the planning and implementation of treatment decisions as well as during discharge planning. Additionally, patient and family participation in goal setting has a profound impact on compliance, outcomes, and overall satisfaction. Family participation adds additional accountability and support, which improves the likelihood of ongoing participation upon discharge.

Access to Care and Resources

Access to care and resources can be impacted by location, disability, finances, access to transportation, support system, education level, and many other factors. These needs can be addressed with the building of rural care sites, home health services, community programs, financial assistance, and other social services.

Resources for Patient-Centered Care

Promoting patient-centered care requires a multifaceted approach. The following are examples of resources used to provide individualized patient care:

- Electronic Medical Record (EMR): Patient portals (EMR accessible to the patient) provide patients and their caregivers with increased access to health information. System features can include self-scheduling, messaging with providers, patient education resources, and various goal-setting and tracking applications.

- Communication boards: Inpatient communication boards, located in patient rooms, improve communication and patient/family involvement. They can contain names of providers, daily schedules, goals, and/or discharge planning information.

- Surveys: Surveys are utilized by organizations and departments to identify the patient and/or community preferences and needs. Results can impact business development and decision-making.

- Language services: Resources for facilitating increased access related to communication include language boards, picture boards or books, live interpreters, virtual interpreters, or telephonic interpreters.

- Social Services: Social Services is dedicated to providing information, resources, or referrals for patient resources (e.g., food, shelter, transportation, healthcare, childcare, community services, etc.).

- Discharge summary: Discharge summaries provide patients and caregivers with a concise review of a care interaction. Information can include diagnoses, new medications, modified or discontinued medications, test results, patient education materials, and referral information. These materials can also be utilized during transitions of care to promote continuity.

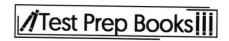

Patient Advocacy

The American Nurses Association (ANA) provides this definition of nursing practice: "The protection, promotion, and optimization of health and abilities, prevention of illness and injury, alleviation of suffering through the diagnosis and treatment of human response, and advocacy in the care of individuals, families, communities, and populations." The ANA also addresses the importance of advocacy in its Code of Ethics, specifically in Provision 3: "The nurse promotes, advocates for, and protects the rights, health, and safety of the patient." The ANA Code of Ethics further states: nurses must advocate "with compassion and respect for the inherent dignity, worth, and uniqueness of every individual, unrestricted by considerations of social or economic status, personal attributes, or the nature of health problems."

Advocacy is the promotion of the common good, especially as it applies to at-risk populations. It involves speaking out in support of policies and decisions that affect the lives of individuals who do not otherwise have a voice. Nurses meet this standard of practice by actively participating in the politics of healthcare accessibility and delivery because they are educationally and professionally prepared to evaluate and comment on the needs of patients at the local, state, and national level. This participation requires an understanding of the legislative process, the ability to negotiate with public officials, and a willingness to provide expert testimony in support of policy decisions. The advocacy role of nurses addresses the needs of the individual patient as well as the needs of all individuals in the society and the members of the nursing profession.

Advocacy is a key component of nursing practice. An **advocate** is one who pleads the cause of another; and the nurse is an advocate for patient rights. Preserving human dignity, patient equality, and freedom from suffering are the basis of nursing advocacy. Nurses hold a significant role that gives them the opportunity to care for patients in every way: caring for their needs, addressing any and all concerns, and ensuring that all outcomes are positive. More experienced nurses can aid in communicating with doctors and physicians while also serving as a guide through the complexities of the medical system. Nurses educate the patient about tests and procedures and are aware of how culture and ethnicity affect the patient's experience. Nurses strictly adhere to all privacy laws.

In clinical practice, nurses represent the patient's interests by active participation in the development of the plan of care and subsequent care decisions. Advocacy, in this sense, is related to patient autonomy and the patient's right to informed consent and self-determination. Nurses provide the appropriate information, assess the patient's comprehension of the implications of the care decisions, and act as the patient advocates by supporting the patient's decisions. In the critical care environment, patient advocacy requires the nurse to represent the patient's decisions even though those decisions may be opposed to those of the healthcare providers and family members.

Further, the patient has a right to privacy that sometimes seems a lesser priority. One practice that has become widely adopted is the covering of windows when the patient may be exposed. This provides additional privacy to the patient because personnel and visitors walking down the hallway will be prevented from observing the patient in a compromising position from outside the room. Covering the window is a simple way to treat the patient with dignity and respect.

Patient Satisfaction

Patient satisfaction is a term used in healthcare to describe an organization's ability to meet patient expectations. Hospitals have a duty to provide safe and effective care while also maintaining a favorable patient experience. This can be challenging to achieve, and the implications are significant. Not only does patient satisfaction have an impact on health outcomes, but it also impacts organizational business and financial success.

Patient satisfaction is a highly valued benchmark of healthcare quality. Data relating to patient satisfaction can be collected internally by a healthcare organization or through external institutions that focus on healthcare quality. In

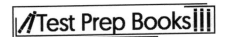
the business of healthcare, patient satisfaction often serves as the "demand" in a supply and demand economy. Higher patient satisfaction scores are associated with better patient health outcomes, and consequently associated with happier patients, patients who are more likely to return to and recommend a particular healthcare organization, higher quality of medical staff that the healthcare organization retains, increased level of outside funding that the healthcare organization receives, and fewer medical malpractice suits. Patients report higher satisfaction when they receive care that they find to be tailored to their needs, care that is safe yet efficient, and care that is accessible. In this regard, healthcare delivery requires a nuanced level of customer service; however, rather than delivering a tangible manufactured product, medical staff deliver a product that affects the patient's ability to live well and their long-term physical, mental, and emotional state.

Business and Financial Impact

Patient perception of experience is increasingly being used to measure hospital performance and reimbursement eligibility. The *Hospital Consumer Assessment of Healthcare Providers and Systems* (HCAHPS) survey, for instance, nationally collects and reports how patients perceive their healthcare experiences. The results, which are available to the public, can impact a hospital's image, marketability, and opportunities. Other federal initiatives, like the *Value-Based Purchasing* (VBP) *Program*, seek to put quality controls in place for hospitals receiving funding from the Centers for Medicare and Medicaid Services (CMS). A quality score—significantly tied to patient experience—is assigned to healthcare organizations and used to determine a small percentage of reimbursement as well as the provision of bonuses or penalties.

Management of Patient Satisfaction

Hospitals are extremely complex systems that handle a high volume of potentially sensitive and stressful patient interactions. Despite their best efforts at maintaining quality and patient satisfaction, hospitals inevitably will receive complaints and grievances. These concerns can be raised by anyone within or outside of an organization and can be received as an informal comment or a formal grievance filed with the organization or a regulatory body.

Nurses are in a unique position to intervene to recognize and possibly mitigate concerns raised within the care setting. When recognized and addressed early, development of serious grievances can sometimes be avoided altogether, and patient experiences can be improved. Nurses often directly and indirectly assist with the service recovery process (i.e., make things right) by being empathetic, helping to problem solve, escalating as required, or providing comfort and additional customer service measures to improve the experience of a disgruntled patient or family member. Nurses can also advocate for patient rights, such as the right to a second opinion, by providing information and discussing available resources.

Additionally, nurses are called—both professionally and ethically—to speak up when they identify an issue related to practice. A concern with an individual, ideally, would be addressed with the individual in a professional manner. However, nurses may also be required to escalate or report via additional channels, including supervisors, ethics committees, Human Resources departments, regulatory agencies, or even lawmakers.

Diversity and Inclusion

Culturally Sensitive Practice

Culturally sensitive practice requires identification of the diverse patient populations, assessment of cultural issues that affect healthcare delivery to those individuals, educational interventions to increase cultural awareness of all providers, and adaptation of services to meet the distinctive healthcare needs of all individuals. In addition to ethnic and racial groups, the plan of care must also be adapted to meet the needs of disabled children and adults, and LGBTQI patients. The medical-surgical nurse also recognizes that the essential components of patient adherence are closely related to the patient's cultural identity, which means that health beliefs, language preferences, and health

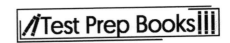

literacy must be assessed for all patients. The recommendations for culturally sensitive practice are consistent with the national standards for culturally and linguistically appropriate services (CLAS) in health care.

The specific language and communication support criteria include support for limited English proficiency, accommodation for any additional communication deficits, provision of all patient information sources in the patient's native language at the appropriate reading level, and the provision of skilled, professional interpreters. The medical-surgical nurse is aware that mandatory compliance is required for these support criteria by all federally assisted institutions to satisfy Title VI of the Civil Rights Act.

Nursing practice theories related to culture provide a framework for the study of the significance of cultural attributes of individual groups and the development of cultural competence in nurses. The theories assume that all providers have a need for the same patient information; however, the providers will use that information in different ways consistent with their scope of practice. The universal patient/family attributes that are consistent across all individual groups are identified. These include family roles, nutrition, customs associated with pregnancy and death, healthcare beliefs, and high-risk behaviors. Later models of cultural competence added the identification of "attitudes toward healthcare providers" as an additional universal attribute that can affect the patient/provider relationship. Providers are cautioned to consider self-awareness as the initial step toward culturally sensitive practice by identifying the effects of their own culture and biases on their behavior. Risks for inappropriate cultural care include stereotyping, which is most often an inaccurate viewpoint, that occurs when there is an assumption that all individuals of a specific group will exhibit the same behaviors, is also discussed.

Culturally appropriate care is not "one size fits all"; therefore, the medical-surgical nurse will assess the needs of individuals within and among cultural and ethnic groups by collecting **REAL data** that includes preferences for race, ethnicity, and language. The largest populations of ethnic minorities in the United States are Hispanic (16.3 percent), African American (13.6 percent), Asian American (5.6 percent), and Native American (1.3 percent).

When reviewing a patient's care plan, nurses must take into consideration the diversity of personal values. Subcultures are influenced by various factors such as occupation, family make-up, and social norms. Although a patient may identify as a particular race or ethnicity, the nurse must be careful not to assume certain practices or beliefs typically associated with the culture. For example, in Eastern medicine, an imbalance in nature is believed to cause illness and disease. Although this may be a common belief amongst people from certain regions, a patient may be accustomed to different health practices and beliefs based on their upbringing and lifestyle.

All patients, including Caucasian ones, may turn to alternative healers. Since it is important to know everything that a patient is taking, including herbs, the medical-surgical nurse should be aware of these other healers. Cultural competence demands the nurse not shame someone who has accessed alternative treatment. If the medical-surgical nurse is culturally insensitive, the patient might not open up and reveal needed information. Caucasians may treat their conditions by taking colloidal silver or avoiding foods in the "nightshade" family, on the advice of an alternative practitioner. A Hispanic or Asian American person may take herbs prescribed by a healer. Given such historical abuses of experimental protocol as the "Tuskegee Study of Untreated Syphilis in the Negro Male," African Americans may have reason to mistrust allopathic medicine, and some may access traditional folk medicine remedies (as do whites, Hispanics, and other people). Bear in mind, these are far from "rules," and people of any race may or may not turn to alternative or conventional treatments or carry fears about doing so.

At the organizational level, culturally competent care requires the recruitment and retention of a culturally diverse staff, the availability of professional interpreters that are well versed in the language and cultural preferences of the individual cultural groups, and coordination with traditional healers in the community. The development of a culturally competent staff relies on the provision of proper recruitment, career advancement opportunities, and educational interventions that support organizational standards for competent cultural practice by all providers. The skilled interpreters provide support for patient care staff and the patients and their families. Community liaisons

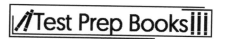

provide important connections with faith healers, medicine men, and other important individuals from ethnic and racial groups. These institutional efforts are also supportive of shared decision-making between the patient and the provider and culturally sensitive practice by the individual providers.

Culturally sensitive practice is an integral part of skilled nursing care that also benefits the patient and the healthcare institution. The focus on patient education allows the patient to put culturally or ethnically associated risk factors in perspective and to gain trust in providers who demonstrate cultural competence in care delivery. Providers have the satisfaction of delivering total care for their patients, and the ties to the greater community increase the availability of needed resources. Institutions benefit from staff and patient diversity and the potential increases in patient satisfaction.

Cultural/Ethnic Needs During Pre- and Post-Operative Period

A patient's perception of the surgical experience will be influenced by their cultural and ethnic background. It is important for the nurse to assess the patient's sociocultural needs during the preoperative period. The patient's background may require individualized nursing interventions to meet their needs. Some of those needs may include food preferences, translation services, and rituals performed pre- and post-surgery. For example, in the Chinese culture, yin (cold) and yang (hot) foods provide balance. In the immediate postoperative period, the patient may request specific foods to aid in recovery. Additionally, the nurse must always be prepared to request interpreter services for patients with a language barrier.

Implicit Bias

Implicit biases are the stereotypes and unconscious assumptions that influence how an individual views other groups of people. These automatic judgments, which can be positive or negative in nature, form the lens through which people see and behave toward and interact with other people. Within the context of the healthcare setting, this can—and does—lead to inequity in patient-care practices.

The formation of unconscious bias occurs through a complex combination of factors. Individual experiences create memories and impressions, and the brain uses this data to identify patterns that become judgments and beliefs. Beliefs are also greatly influenced by input from family, friends, social groups, communities, and media. Then, our brains process that information and categorize it with the intent of helping us effectively manage our environment.

Unfortunately, this process is not perfect. As mentioned previously, bias is largely formed by personal and social experiences; therefore, social groups can perpetuate inaccurate or problematic biases (e.g., racism, sexism, classism, religious extremism, etc.). Additionally, our brains are biologically wired to identify problematic stimuli as a survival mechanism. In doing so, we tend to overmeasure negative stimuli and undermeasure positive stimuli in our daily lives. Moreover, our brains have an automatic tendency toward confirmation bias, which means that our brains tend to interpret new data in ways that confirm our previously held beliefs. Our brains minimize—and sometimes even forcefully reject—information that does not line up with what we believe. This can be seen in political discussions, with religious beliefs, or in conversations about human rights and equality. Yet another way our brains can come to incorrect conclusions is by making conclusions based on their current level of knowledge and awareness. Children interpret and understand the world in a vastly different way than adults. People from different social and cultural backgrounds will see and interpret experiences and other people in vastly different ways based on their experiences.

Impact on Patient Care

When viewed in the context of healthcare, implicit bias can have devastating consequences for patient-care and health outcomes. In the United States, data has consistently shown that certain populations (e.g., non-white, female, non-English speaking, disabled, obese, non-heterosexual, history of drug abuse) are at an increased risk for

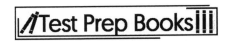
receiving suboptimal healthcare. This is an extremely complex and nuanced issue; however, healthcare provider bias is a major contributing factor to this inequity.

Provider bias can result in dismissal of patient concerns, which, in turn, can result in delayed or withheld treatment as well as worse health outcomes. One example of this would be delayed cancer diagnosis and treatment due to a female patient's reports of abdominal pain and changes in bleeding being dismissed by her male healthcare provider. Another example would be a nurse withholding ordering medications (without presence of contraindication) or not following up with the provider regarding inadequate pain management for a patient who has a history of drug use.

Minimizing the Adverse Impact of Implicit Bias

Consciousness accounts for just five percent of all of our total brain activity. This means that implicit bias is unavoidable. However, steps can be taken on an individual and organizational level to address and minimize its adverse impact on patient care.

On an organizational level, diversity in leadership and workforce is one strategy to manage implicit bias. This begins with hiring practices and promotion policies that value the input of individuals who represent different experiences, cultures, age groups, and interests. This helps to prevent biased decision-making or business practices.

On an individual level, caregivers must consciously begin to identify their own implicit biases by examining why they have these beliefs and critically examining their merit. This can allow individuals to recognize when subconscious thoughts are impacting their decisions and actions and can make them more accountable for their actions. Questioning our implicit biases and consciously focusing on the positive attributes of a situation or an individual can also begin to reprogram our subconscious belief systems, which can slowly impact those beliefs over time.

Education of Patients and Families

Health Maintenance and Disease Prevention

Facilitation of Learning

Facilitation of learning refers to the process of assessing the learning needs of the patient and family, the nursing staff, and caregivers in the community, and creating, implementing, and evaluating formal and informal educational programs to address those needs. Novice nurses often view patient care and patient education as separate entities; however, experienced nurses are able to integrate the patient's educational needs into the plan of care. Nurses are aware that the patient often requires continued reinforcement of the educational plan after discharge, which necessitates coordination with home care services.

As facilitators of learning, nurses may be involved in a large-scale effort to educate all patients over 65 admitted to the nursing unit about the need for both Prevnar 13® and Pneumovax 23® to prevent pneumonia. In contrast, nurses may provide one-on-one instruction for a patient recently diagnosed with diabetes. The first step of any teaching-learning initiative is the assessment of the learning needs of the participants. Specific needs that influence the design and content of the educational offering include the language preference and reading level of the participants. Nurses must also consider the effect of certain patient characteristics identified in the Synergy Model on the patient's capacity to process information. Diminished resiliency or stability, and extreme complexity, must be considered in the development of the educational plan. Nurses are also responsible for creating a bridge between teaching-learning in the acute care setting and the home environment. A detailed discharge plan, close coordination with outpatient providers, and follow-up phone calls to the patient may be used to reinforce the patient's knowledge of the plan of care.

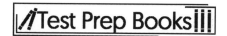

Successful learning plans for staff members and colleagues also consider the motivation of the participants to engage in the process. Successful facilitators include a variety of teaching strategies to develop the content and evaluate learning, in order to address adult learning needs and preferences, such as preferred language and reading level. Research indicates that when adults do not have a vested interest in the outcomes of the teaching/learning process, they may not participate as active learners.

The remaining element of successful facilitation of learning is the availability and quality of learning resources. There is evidence that individuals with different learning styles respond differently to various learning devices. The minimum requirements for successful facilitation of learning include the skilled staff to develop the educational materials, paper, a copy machine, and staff to interact with the patient in the learning session.

Barriers to the facilitation of learning must be anticipated and accommodated. Changes in the patient's condition commonly require reduction in the time spent in each learning session due to fatigue. Cognitive impairment can impede comprehension and retention of the information and will require appropriate teaching aids. The learning abilities of the patient's family members must also be assessed. Adequate instruction time might be the greatest barrier. Learning needs are assessed and discharge planning is begun on the day of admission; however, shortened inpatient stays require evaluation of the patient's comprehension of the plan of care.

Education on Body System Alterations

Patient education is an important aspect of care that the nurse diligently performs when body system alterations occur. Helping the patient understand what is going on in their body and answering their questions is an excellent way to reduce anxiety and promote calm and understanding. Anxiety, the nurse knows, only causes additional stress in the body, which will not be conducive to healing.

When educating the patient, the nurse will talk about the body system alteration they are experiencing, using their knowledge of pathophysiology, anatomy, and physiology as well as incorporating lessons about the pharmacological interventions being used on the patient. Discussion of risk factors related to the body alterations and side effects of medication is important to include. The nurse will discuss factors that will promote healing, such as the patient getting adequate rest and early mobility. The nurse will encourage the patient to call on the health-care team whenever a need arises, whether the need is for the nurse's aide, the nurse, or the physician. The patient should be encouraged to ask their questions and raise their concerns, as they are an important member of the health-care team. The nurse will include information about helpful resources that the client may access such as community groups for the client's specific condition or illness, social services, and community meal or ride programs.

Patient and Family Education Regarding Surgical Procedures

Patient and family education is a critical component of any operation. This allows patients and their families the opportunity to fully understand the procedure, voice questions or concerns, and empower them to play an active role in their health care. It can also foster rapport and a positive relationship between the patient party and the medical staff. Transparency, comprehensive education, and the sense of self-efficacy during medical procedures is often associated with better patient outcomes, increased patient satisfaction, and decreased complications during the recovery period.

Thanks to shorter hospital stays, the duration in which a nurse has to educate the patient about post-discharge care is also limited. Office-based medical-surgical staff, or those medical-surgical nurses who work in ambulatory facilities, provide education before and after surgery. Typically, education of the patient and family should take place in the days leading up to the surgery to reduce anxiety. Helping patients and families to understand what to expect the day of surgery and the days following surgery is valuable for the patient, the family, and the health care team.

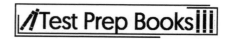

Family dynamics must be assessed to ensure successful recovery of the operative patient. During the preoperative phase, the nurse should assess the structure of the patient's family. Family patterns are diverse and can include two or more people that are related or unrelated to each other. Patients may consider significant others, friends, co-workers, or other members of the community to be part of their family. Not all family patterns are traditional, and it is important for nurses to determine the patient's capability to complete plan of care tasks successfully, whether individually or with family support.

Patient education before discharge is imperative, as studies show that timely discharge education contributes to the following:

- Reduction in readmissions
- Decrease in post-discharge complications
- Improvement in quality of care at the hospital and at home
- Increase in patient satisfaction
- Increase in adherence to self-care activities after discharge
- General reduction in the overall cost of care

Medical-surgical nurses managing patients who are undergoing procedures in which they discharge directly from a facility (as opposed to a unit) should prepare to educate patients and their families and provide for enough time to answer questions. Many organizations use a standardized set of education tools, and thus nurses should familiarize themselves with the content as well as be aware of those questions that patients and their families commonly ask.

Patients and patients' families who do not receive adequate education are at an increased risk for postoperative complications, poor symptom management, inadequate nutritional intake, substandard wound care, erratic sleep patterns, and limited activity. They may also suffer some psychological impact.

Education that the patients and families receive may vary nonetheless as a result of the procedure, the patient, and the anesthesia. Instructions should include content that concentrates on activities of daily living, such as walking, eating, lifting, fluid intake, and wound care. The following is an example of instructions given to a patient who will undergo lumbar spine surgery:

Written Postoperative Discharge Instructions for Lumbar Spine Surgery	
Nutrition	<ul><li>Return to your diet slowly.</li><li>Initially, you may want to avoid foods that are spicy.</li></ul>
Activity	<ul><li>Avoid strenuous activity for the next six weeks.</li><li>Avoid lifting objects greater than ten pounds for the next six weeks or twisting or bending.</li><li>Take short walks for the next four to six weeks that last ten to fifteen minutes in duration, and then slowly increase time until, by week six, you are walking upwards of one hour.</li><li>Avoid use of exercise equipment such as treadmills, stair climbers, or elliptical trainers unless cleared by your physician.</li><li>Discuss increasing your activity schedule with your physician.</li><li>You are permitted to shower the following day; however, cover the surgical site with plastic so that it stays dry.</li><li>Baths, pools, or Jacuzzis are not allowed.</li><li>Avoid sitting for greater than thirty minutes for meals.</li><li>Try to sit in a reclining position.</li></ul>

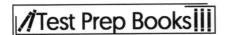
Written Postoperative Discharge Instructions for Lumbar Spine Surgery	
	• When lying down, a pillow between the legs may greatly increase your level of comfort. • Sexual activities may resume within the next seven days; however, your role should be passive. A side-lying or back position is best.
Getting out of Bed	• Ensure that you are lying flat, and then roll sideways, and push your body up.
Wound Care	• Do not remove your dressing until tomorrow. • If your dressing gets wet, remove it, and cover it with a dry dressing. • Change dressing daily. • Apply ice to the lower back region for ten to twenty minutes each day for four days. DO NOT PLACE ICE DIRECTLY ON SKIN. Cover the ice pack with a pillow slip. • Call the doctor if you see any drainage on the dressing.
Medications	• Be sure to take pain medications as prescribed for the first thirty-six to seventy-two hours to reduce risk of pain symptoms. • Stool softeners may be taken to prevent constipation. • Resume taking medications as prescribed by your physician. • Avoid taking any medications that contain aspirin for a minimum of four days.
When to Call the Doctor	Call the doctor if: • You have excessive drainage around the surgical site • You experience a temperature greater than 101 degrees (Fahrenheit) • You have any tenderness or swelling around the surgical site • You have unexplained shortness of breath, anxiety, or sweating • You have pain that is not relieved by medication

Side Effects

Patients and their caretakers should be informed in detail of any potential side effects of an operation, including during the perioperative practices, associations with materials or medications used in the procedure, and effects that could occur during the recovery period. This allows patients to provide informed consent to the procedure, as well as manage their expectations and resources for the complete duration of their procedural timeline.

Resources for Patient/Family Education

One of the medical-surgical nurse's responsibilities is patient and family education. Regulatory bodies such as TJC and CMS clearly identify patient education as a need that must be fulfilled in order to promote optimal patient outcomes. The preoperative nurse is in a unique position of being able to provide education on the immediate next steps (entering the OR suite, monitoring, positioning, induction of anesthesia, emergence from anesthesia, transitioning to post-anesthesia care unit [PACU]) in addition to identifying discharge planning needs. However, discharge planning begins at the time of admission, and much education is based on preparing the patient and family on postoperative care at home.

Resources for education lie in a variety of areas. The medical-surgical nurse can verbalize the preoperative plan of care in addition to providing visual resources, such as written preoperative instructions. The nurse may provide a

192

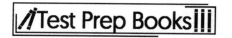
pamphlet or video for the patient and family. Hospital libraries and Internet databases are often good resources for educational materials. Some facilities offer preoperative classes, particularly with joint, spine, and cardiac surgical patients. Human resources such as case managers, disease-specific educators (e.g., diabetes educator, CHF educator), specialty physicians (e.g., endocrinologists, infectious disease physicians), social workers, chaplains, and physical therapists are beneficial to the nurse in providing specialized education to the patient and family.

It is important for the nurse to realize educational barriers and know how to address them. Anxiety is a common barrier to learning, and the patient and family may be overwhelmed by the entire process leading them to the preoperative area. The nurse may need to repeat the education several times for it to be "heard." Considering health literacy, the nurse must present the information in plain, clear language the patient and family can understand. If language barriers are present, the nurse can use an interpreter and material printed in the patient's language to ensure the proper delivery of information. During the educational process, the nurse should verify patient and family understanding of the information. This can be done by asking the patient and/or family to repeat back or paraphrase the information given to them.

Documentation of Perioperative Education

Patient education during the perioperative period is imperative to achieving successful health outcomes. Documentation of the educational activities provides a record regarding the patient's understanding of the teaching and identifies gaps in knowledge. Any deficiencies should be addressed throughout the surgical experience and included in the nursing care plan as potential diagnoses. The educational concepts vary at every perioperative stage.

During the preoperative phase, the nurse performs an admission interview to evaluate the patient's knowledge of the exercises and physical activities that will be required after surgery. For example, the nurse may introduce the use of an incentive spirometer to prevent atelectasis, leg exercises to prevent blood clots, and early mobility to prevent pressure ulcers. The nurse then evaluates the patient's understanding by using a teach-back method, where the patient demonstrates the techniques that they were taught.

Postoperatively, the nurse re-emphasizes preoperative teaching, including early ambulation, pain management, and the need for frequent vital signs. Depending on the type of procedure, the nurse may initiate early teaching on dressing changes, catheter care, and drain management. Education is also provided to the patient's family to ensure continuity of care after discharge.

Documentation should include the concept being taught, demonstration of the activity, and the patient's understanding of the teaching. The nurse also re-evaluates the nursing care plan to ensure knowledge deficits have been addressed.

Health Literacy

Health literacy refers to how capable patients are of understanding their diagnosis, treatment plans, prognosis, and follow-up health instructions. A high degree of health literacy is associated with the ability to make personal health decisions, higher confidence in personal health decisions, and higher compliance with medical instructions.

Teaching Methods

Patient teaching takes place in different settings and formats. The method of choice can be determined by a variety of factors, including learner preference, educator preference, the topic, the setting, and the availability of time and resources. Learning can occur with the help of audio, visual, written, or activity-based methods, and learners tend to fall on a wide spectrum of preference. Typically, individuals require several exposures to new information before it is retained. Additionally, factors such as age, level of education, language barriers, emotional state, desire to learn, pain level, disability, and many others can significantly impact the ability of an individual to take in and retain new

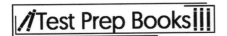
information. Therefore, patient teaching requires individual consideration and benefits from the use of a variety of teaching methods over a span of time.

The following are some of the common methods used to facilitate teaching:

Written materials: Written handouts, brochures, or pamphlets include information about various topics (e.g., disease, procedure, treatment, or medication). These are often accompanied by visual tools to support written information and are often more affordable and convenient for teachers. They can be reviewed repeatedly over time and taken from the care site to the patient's home.

Visual tools: Charts, graphs, pictures, posters, and drawings can provide a visual way to convey a significant amount of information at once and can organize complex ideas. They can be reviewed repeatedly over time and are cost-effective resources. Some visual materials, like brochures, can be taken from the care site, while other materials, like posters, remain at the care site.

Audio and audiovisual materials: Video clips, video programs, recorded interviews, podcasts, or recorded demonstrations can provide learners with opportunities to review information as often as needed and can also be a more interesting method of facilitating patient learning. This can be more costly for organizations to create and is also somewhat limited to individuals who possess the technology required to view the materials; it is also limited by a patient's comfort and desire to use the given media.

Discussion: In-person, virtual, telephonic, email, support group, workshop, or classes provide an opportunity for two-way dialogue between learner and teacher. Discussions can be individual or group-based and can occur in a variety of settings. Teachers have an opportunity to provide learners with a variety of teaching methods to facilitate learning.

Demonstration: Models and training equipment can be utilized in live or recorded sessions to supplement learning through visual representation of a process or procedure. This method is often accompanied by verbal discussion. Live demonstration can provide opportunities for repetition or focus on a specific portion of the demonstration. Patients can also sometimes have the opportunity to handle and practice with training equipment or models in order to increase comfort and decrease anxiety.

Teach Back Method

The "Teach Back" method is an interactive educational technique that fosters rapport, communication, and information sharing between healthcare providers and patients. It encourages the healthcare providers to explain medical diagnoses, prognoses, and plans of care to patients in clear, non-medical terms. Then, patients are asked to explain the medical situation and plan of care to the healthcare professional, utilizing their own understanding. This empowers patients to actively engage in their care plans and understand their health in a new way. It also allows the healthcare provider to determine whether or not the patient has an appropriate understanding of their health situation and how to manage care once they are out of the medical setting. Providers should remain calm, compassionate, and responsive during this process, even if the patient is unable to correctly teach back right away.

Health Promotion

Advanced practice nurses provide various types of counseling to patients. Counseling arises from the need to educate patients on certain risks and conditions that can affect their health decisions. For example, as part of the non-drug therapy for Type 2 diabetes, counseling is necessary to help patients understand the important diet and lifestyle modifications. Patients with Type 2 diabetes should try to decrease their consumption of processed foods, simple carbohydrates and refined sugars, and overall caloric intake, while increasing physical activity. These interventions help to decrease the requirement of antidiabetic medications and prevent long-term diabetes-related complications.

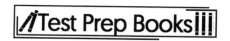
Risk Assessment

After performing a health history, a **genetic risk assessment**, which includes questions about health conditions in their family history, can be obtained. Parents and siblings are considered immediate family. Grandparents, aunts, and uncles are part of the extended family and are important to include in the assessment. Genetic conditions include HTN, cancer, diabetes, high cholesterol, obesity, drug addiction, alcoholism, and mental illness. Bringing awareness to the probability of disease in patients is a method of **health promotion** and risk reduction. Lifestyle risk factors can also contribute to disease and chronic illness. Establishing patterns during the health interview allows for education and counseling. Exercise habits determine a patient's activity level and the potential for the development of sedentary lifestyle–related illnesses, such as obesity and high blood pressure. Patients should be counseled on exercise plans that meet their physical needs. Poor nutrition can lead to heart-related conditions. Nurses should assess their patients' dietary habits and provide counseling on meals that meet their dietary requirements.

Tertiary Prevention

Tertiary prevention focuses on reducing the negative impact that a disease or illness has on a patient who is currently experiencing the issue. Tertiary preventive measures may involve treatment or rehabilitation actions that decrease the impact of deficits associated with acute or chronic disease and maximizing the patient's recovery potential. Effective tertiary prevention limits the negative effects of disease, improves quality of life indicators, and limits disease progression by minimizing potential risk factors and developing a relapse plan for disease progression.

Participation in cardiac rehabilitation, quit smoking programs, and medically managed weight loss programs are examples of tertiary prevention for adults that focus on minimizing the effects of an existing disease or eliminating unsafe behavior. Tertiary prevention can improve surgical outcomes; for example, it can consist of preoperative physical therapy for common orthopedic surgeries such as arthroplasty of the knee or hip or correction of scoliosis. Minimizing the effects of existing diseases becomes more complex and potentially less successful in the elderly, who may have multiple chronic conditions. Tertiary prevention programs may be focused on a population group. For instance, the incidence of Lyme disease is higher in New England than in other regions of the United States. Population-specific treatment plans are in place to minimize the long-term effects of the disease, which can include facial nerve palsy and arthritis.

Resources Available for Patient/Family and Health Information to Meet Patient Needs

Healthcare providers utilize a variety of resources to meet patient and family needs, exchange health information, and promote better health outcomes. In the hospital setting, these resources can begin with specialized counseling services (e.g., lactation consultants, diabetic educators). Hospitals may also collaborate with case management and insurance providers to coordinate the provision of medical equipment (e.g., medical beds, assistive devices, continuous oxygen, etc.) to meet a variety of patients' needs. In the outpatient care setting, providers are increasingly using at-home testing to help identify and treat issues such as cardiac dysrhythmia or sleep apnea.

Smartphone technology has also opened a massive database of potential resources for patients and families. There are applications that allow users to track nutrition intake, which can be used for health promotion activities. Other applications provide access to resources and exercises to help reduce stress and anxiety or offer the ability to track health data, such as weight, blood pressure, or menstrual cycles, for health promotion. Additionally, there are applications which provide a means to track caregiving tasks more effectively. Those patients and family members who do not have access, the desire, or the ability to utilize smartphone apps can also benefit from the use of printed or written materials to track health data.

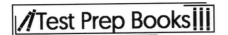

Palliative/End-of-life Care

End of life issues can be complicated from both a logistical and an emotional perspective. For many patients, end of life issues may not have been discussed or resolved with family members; a nurse or other medical staff member may have to step into the role of facilitating this sensitive subject. Even when the situation has been planned for, it can come unexpectedly for both the patient and family members. Most end-of-life situations will require managing the physical and emotional pain of the patient and family members, helping the patient transition in a dignified manner, and dealing with legal paperwork. Many healthcare providers report not feeling emotionally equipped to handle these aspects, do not feel they have time on the job to adequately do so, or feel there is no financial compensation to provide these services. Being aware that job duties may require these uncomfortable tasks can be the first step in being able to provide some level of effective end of life support for the patient and family. Understanding common end of life issues can also help.

More healthcare organizations are beginning to allow family members to be present during end-of-life procedures, including intense procedures that can be harrowing to watch. New research shows this can be beneficial for family members as they cope in the long-term. While remaining present with the patient is often the wish of family members, they may be unaware of the emotional upheaval they may feel when watching a loved one go through resuscitative procedures. Nursing staff should be equipped to be able to continue working even with the presence of distraught family members and be able to provide compassionate and honest support if needed.

In health care, there are two different goals of care: curative and palliative. **Curative care** focuses on restoring the patient back to health after an illness. **Palliative care**, on the other hand, focuses on maximizing quality of life, sometimes when the disease process has reached a point at which a cure is no longer possible. In this case, the goal of care is to comfort the individual and provide pain management, spiritual support, and as high a quality of remaining life as possible. Withholding and withdrawing treatments are a component of palliative care. They are most commonly seen in tragic, traumatic events or in hospice care. These procedures occur when a patient is believed to be terminal, and interventions that were previously being utilized to sustain the patient are gradually ceased in order to let the patient pass comfortably. Withholding and withdrawing treatments are often requested by patients who are aware of their situation and are ready to move on, but they may also be done at the request of family members or a medical proxy if the patient is in a vegetative state.

End of life care refers to guidelines and procedures to comfort terminal patients. Depending on the patient and the condition, this period may last a few days or can last months. During this time, patients may be moved into a hospice facility, receive comfort measures at home, create any legal documents that support their family members in decision-making (such as advance directives or wills), and receive grief counseling with their loved ones.

When caring for the patient who is dying, it is of utmost importance that the health care team respect the wishes of the patient and family. At some point, very difficult decisions regarding care may have to be made by the patient, the family, and the health care team. The nurse should be a comfort and help to the patient and the family during this difficult time. Sensitivity to the emotional and physical needs of the patient and the family will help guide care.

Resources for Patients and Caregivers

Palliative care services focus on the management of symptoms impacting quality of life. Chronic pain management is one of the more common benefits of palliative care. However, palliative care providers can help patients manage many troubling symptoms ranging from fatigue and insomnia to nausea, anorexia, and constipation. Providers utilize traditional therapies as well as **integrative/complementary care** strategies to provide holistic care support. Examples of integrative care include supplements, acupuncture, massage therapy, art and music therapy, spiritual services, and cognitive behavioral therapy. Palliative care strategies can be utilized alongside curative treatments, and they can also be continued once treatment is discontinued.

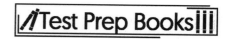

Hospice is one major resource available to patients and caregivers of patients nearing the end of life. Eligibility requirements include patients with a general life expectancy of approximately six months or less who are discontinuing life-prolonging and curative treatments for their illness. Focuses of hospice care include comfort, dignity, and support services for patients and their families. Benefits of this care include extended Medicare coverage for skilled nursing services, medical equipment, and medication, which eases the financial burden. Patients under hospice care are also provided more extensive pharmacological options for pain relief and anxiety. Patients and families have access to education, emotional support services, and bereavement counseling. Additionally, families have access to **respite services**, which provide short-term relief coverage so caregivers can take a break to rest and recover while caring for their dying family member.

Physical Changes and Needs as Death Approaches

As a patient approaches death, the nurse will play an important role in ensuring physical comfort. The patient may have increased pain, skin irritation, decreased control over bowel and bladder, decreased mobility, and decreased consciousness. There are concrete steps that the nurse can take to ensure the patient is as comfortable as possible during the last stage of life.

Monitoring the patient's level of pain is important. Pain medicine as necessary will be used to provide adequate comfort. The nurse should watch for nonverbal signs of pain, such as body tension, moaning, and facial grimacing.

Elimination may become difficult if the patient loses consciousness and mobility. The nurse can make elimination easier for the patient by assisting them to a bedside commode or bed pan, and/or checking for incontinence in order to perform perineal care to keep the patient clean and dry.

The patient's skin may become dry and brittle. Breathing through the mouth can cause the oral cavity to dry out quickly, sometimes called **cotton mouth**. Applying lotions, balms, and moisturizers to skin and lips, as well as making sure the oral cavity is well moisturized, are all steps that can relieve skin discomfort. Mouth sponges or swabs can be dipped in water to wet the mouth. Some patients find these sponges comforting to chew on or take a few drops of water from.

Preventing pressure ulcers or preventing existing pressure ulcers from worsening at the end of life is a consideration for nurses to keep in mind. These can cause additional pain and discomfort that might be avoided. Using pillows to prop and position at-risk areas, such as heels, buttocks, elbows, and the back of the head will help minimize pressure.

The patient will likely have difficulty regulating body temperature, and may experience periods of feeling hot, cold, or both. The patient may not be able to verbalize these needs, but the medical-surgical nurse can watch for nonverbal cues such as shivering or sweating. It is important to keep the patient comfortably warm or cool, using blankets and fans. Electric blankets should not be used, as the patient may not be able to verbalize if it is too hot, risking burn injuries.

Breathing may become difficult for the patient. They will likely develop increased secretions in the airway. The patient will likely be too weak to clear these secretions, resulting in a rattling or gurgling sound. Turning the patient's head to the side, providing a cool-mist humidifier (if available), and using suction equipment are all interventions that can alleviate the patient of these secretions. The patient may be given supplemental oxygen via nasal cannula for comfort. Monitoring to make sure the prongs of the nasal cannula are in place and not causing discomfort to the patient is important.

The patient may not appear to be awake, but still may be able to hear and perceive what is going on around them. Because of this, it is always important for the nurse to identify oneself to the patient when entering the room and tell the patient what they are doing in the room. This courtesy may comfort a patient who is otherwise alone. The

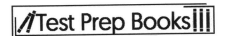
nurse should talk to the patient, provide quiet music, and keep the lighting low and/or natural. These environmental changes can all soothe the patient and should be guided by the patient and the family's wishes. Some patients may prefer a room full of visitors and others may be more private, preferring only a few close relatives and friends.

The nurse needs to be mindful of the family's needs as well. Again, their grief and emotional response in the moment may cause them to forget their own basic needs, such as eating and getting proper rest. It is important to remind them to rest when they need to, offer them drinks and snacks as appropriate, warm blankets, and any other offering available to comfort them during this difficult time.

The end of life need not be a lonely, miserable experience, lacking warmth, thoughtfulness, and care. The medical-surgical nurse can assist the health care team in providing comfort for the patient's physical needs as well as creating a soothing environment around the patient as they approach death.

End of Life Preference

As with other aspects of patient-centered care, end-of-life preferences are individualized and require collaboration of the healthcare team with patients and their families. Preferences may include specific comfort-care requests (e.g., administration of pain and anti-anxiety medications), requests for specific environment preferences (e.g., room layout, temperature, lighting, music, etc.), preferences regarding visitation and communication with healthcare providers (e.g., who may be present, how and when healthcare providers can enter and check in, etc.). They can also include specific rituals, cultural practices, or religious practices (e.g., who provides post-mortem care and how it is performed, how long the family stays with the patient after death, when and how the patient is removed post-mortem, religious ceremonies and prayer, etc.).

Another key end-of-life preference that is discussed with patients and their families is code status. In the absence of known and/or documented preference, patients are assumed to be full code, which means that all life-sustaining and life-saving measures can and will be performed in an emergency. In certain cases, even after careful discussion and after going over the realities of cardiopulmonary resuscitation (CPR) on frail, elderly or fragile patients, the decision may be made to maintain full code status. This can become an ethical dilemma for healthcare providers who may view these extreme measures as harmful. In some cases, hospital ethics committees may need to intervene to determine what is best in a situation, but circumstances are very individualized and sensitive to navigate.

At any time, patients and families can change a patient's code status. Examples of alternative code statuses include Do Not Resuscitate (DNR; no CPR), Do Not Intubate (DNI; no advanced airway), and Comfort Care (DNR-CC; only comfort care measures, no life-sustaining or life-saving measures). These orders can vary based on individual preferences; therefore, careful discussion and clear documentation are critical to this process.

To assess and identify a patient's and family's end-of-life preferences, the nurse should be attentive, assess needs, educate, and always provide respect and empathy when speaking with a patient and their family. It also requires respect for their wishes. Additionally, nurses may act as a mediator, identifying resources and options available for patients and family to promote comfort and fulfillment of end-of-life wishes.

Cultural and religious practice may require specific processes, which can be space and time sensitive. Specific resources, individuals, or religious leaders may be required to complete these rituals. Nurses can support this by providing respect, communicating with family and staff members, and facilitating problem-solving to address requests. Nurses can also assist with ensuring privacy and quiet for the patient and family.

Patient Self-Determination (PSDA)

The **Patient Self-Determination Act (PSDA)** is administrative legislation that requires healthcare facilities to inform patients of their medical rights, requires that facilities note before a scheduled surgical procedure if patients have

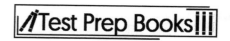

legal documentation relating to advance directives and DNR decisions, and requires that healthcare staff have an understanding of general advance directives and DNR decisions. However, the PSDA is a controversial act. Many critics believe an end-of-life discussion with the attending physician is necessary in order for the patient to make fully informed healthcare decisions; however, this is not part of the PSDA.

Advance Directives and DNR

Advanced directives are legal documents that note how a patient would like to receive or guide medical treatments in the case of terminal cases, cases where the patient is in a vegetative state, or in other end of life contexts. Having this document prepared in advance is extremely helpful for healthcare providers and the patient's family, as the patient's personal decisions are known and can be accounted for. However, many people do not take the time to develop these. Advance directives may only be utilized when a physician has declared the patient to be in an end-of-life state. Other rules may vary by state, so it is useful to be informed of the particular guidelines set forth by the state in which providers are practicing. In emergency cases, support staff do not usually have the legal rights to follow instructions written in an advanced directive until a physician confirms that the patient will not recover. Therefore, support staff must continue to provide comprehensive, life-sustaining care unless otherwise instructed.

Do Not Resuscitate (DNR) instructions are legal instructions provided by a patient, the patient's family, or the patient's power of attorney before serious medical procedures in which heart or lung failure could occur. These instructions guide medical providers to allow a natural death rather than repeated attempts at resuscitating a patient. Elderly and immunocompromised patients often have a slim chance of survival in these contexts, and DNR instructions aim to minimize invasive, potentially ineffective, and costly procedures for patients who may not benefit from them.

Pre-Operative Considerations

Advance directives, such as a living will or durable power of attorney, are forms that state a patient's choices for treatment, including refusal of treatments, life support, and stopping treatments when the patient chooses. **Do not resuscitate (DNR)** status, and its varying types, is also included in advance directives. The preoperative interview should include discussion of advance directives and DNR status. If the patient has advance directives, a copy should be placed in the medical record, and they should be reviewed by the nurse and physician. If the patient has a code status of anything other than full resuscitation, a conversation among the surgeon, anesthesiologist, and patient is necessary to discuss the patient's wishes in detail. Older schools of thinking suggest all patients, regardless of preoperative DNR status, are considered full code while in the operating room; however, this is not true. A patient with DNR status of no intubation and no **cardiopulmonary resuscitation (CPR)** may proceed with the surgical procedure if the surgeon and anesthesiologist have a conversation with the patient and a plan is agreed upon among them.

Consent must be obtained by the patient if there is a change in status or a suspension of the DNR order during surgery. However, if the patient wishes to keep DNR status of no intubation and no CPR during surgery, the surgeon and/or anesthesiologist may deem the patient a nonsurgical candidate. If a patient is entering surgery with a DNR order of anything other than full code, this must be communicated to the entire surgical team and documented in the medical record.

Allow Natural Death (AND)

It may be beneficial for nurses to discuss "**allow natural death**" practices and decisions with patients and their families. "Allow natural death" decisions most commonly take place in instances where a surgery is not successful and the patient experiences an event that leads to full or partial brain or heart failure. These events often lead to patient death or a drastically reduced quality of life (such as prolonged life in a vegetative state). Before surgery, patients and their families can make the decision to allow medical staff to gradually decrease life sustaining measures in order to allow the patient to naturally die in comfort.

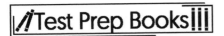

Post-Mortem Care Procedures

After the patient has passed, the first step the nurse can take is to determine the family's needs. This is a time when spiritual and cultural considerations need to be respected. Some families may linger and talk over the body for hours before leaving the room, while others may say a brief goodbye and leave. The health care team should determine if there are any specific burial preparations that need to be done. Funeral and/or burial arrangements, such as cremation or embalmment, will be determined.

Once these considerations are determined, the health care team can prepare the body. Generally, the body will need to be cleaned, as bowel and bladder incontinence happens after death. Having an assistant, usually a nurse, is necessary, as the body will be difficult to move by a single person. Any excess tubes or IVs will need to be removed by the nurse or the nursing assistant, depending on facility policy. The body may need to be placed in a body bag, if in a facility with a morgue. This can be done using the same turning and repositioning techniques used to perform bath care.

The nurse should be aware that there are sights and sounds that one might see in a dead body that might be alarming and unexpected. For example, there may be a release of air from the lungs of the body as the nurse is cleaning or turning that may sound like a gasp or cry. The body may also have muscle twitches and slight movements as the neurological and muscular systems shut down. Both of these are normal. If the nurse and/or doctor have confirmed official death, post-mortem care can proceed.

After the body has been bathed and placed in a body bag, the body will be transferred to a gurney or some sort of transport stretcher. The body is then transported to the morgue. A **morgue** refers to the refrigerated room where deceased bodies are held pending funeral and burial arrangements. The cold temperature drastically slows down the decomposition process in the bodies, preserving them for the funeral presentation.

Some nurses may find post-mortem care to be uncomfortable, disturbing, and even depressing. This is an initial reaction, and many adjust to it with time and experience. Dealing with dead bodies is not something that the general public is used to experiencing. The nurse must keep in mind that post-mortem care is a continuation of respecting and caring for the patient. Everyone dies, and their bodies must be taken care of afterwards. Thinking of it as an act of respect and courtesy is perhaps the best perspective. The deceased must be treated with dignity, even in death. The nurse is in the unique position to provide such dignified care to the individual.

The reason that one enters the health care field should stem from an earnest desire to help others and care for them in their time of need. This extends beyond their life to their death by taking care of their remains appropriately and respectfully.

Organ Donation Process

Organ donation and tissue donation refer to the process of removing healthy, functional organs or tissues from the patient's body after death and transplanting them to another patient in need. This may be a topic that the patient has already considered; for example, many people make this decision when applying for a driver's license and have it notated on their card. Common organs that can be donated include the heart, lungs, liver, and kidneys. Common tissues that can be donated include heart, skin, components of the eyeball, and bone.

When a patient is approaching death or has recently died in the hospital setting, hospitals are required to follow protocols for identifying and managing the organ donation process. Organ donation status may be registered under the patient's state-issued identification or driver's license. Additionally, the patient may have discussed and/or outlined their wish to be an organ donor via their living will and/or designated power of attorney. Family and next of kin may donate a patient's organs and tissues post-mortem; however, family legally cannot deny organ donation if the patient had registered or outlined intent to be an organ donor.

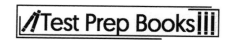

The legality surrounding organ and tissue donation follows a different pathway than the traditional informed consent practices that healthcare providers are accustomed to. Post-mortem organ donation falls under "gift law," which provides a legally binding agreement based on an individual's intent to donate, their agreement to opt into the process, and the designated organ procurement organization (OPO) accepting the donation. Informed consent is not required for this process.

When it becomes known that death is imminent, the hospital is required to contact and report to the OPO. The OPO will confirm if the patient had previously registered to be an organ donor. Review of the patient's medical history through collaboration with family and/or the healthcare organization will determine if the patient has any healthcare conditions that would prevent them from being an organ donor. Some of these conditions include diabetes, cancer, HIV, hepatitis, and uncontrolled high blood pressure.

One important way that healthcare providers can assist in this process is by encouraging patients to discuss their organ donation status with their family. Extreme emotional distress as well as legal and financial implications can occur when family members disagree with and question the patient's donor status. By encouraging patients to make their family aware of their intent, this can help to limit some of the distress involved with the process of organ donation.

Regulatory Requirements for Reporting Death

When a patient dies in certain unusual or sudden circumstances, the hospital is legally required to notify and cooperate with the local coroner's office, who will examine and investigate the deceased patient. These **coroner's cases** are required to be reported in cases when an individual dies suddenly or because of an accident, suicide, homicide, or occupation-related circumstance. Additionally, suspicious deaths or deaths associated with medical treatment and care are legally required to be reported.

After calling to report the death, the hospital must comply with all requests for information made by the coroner's office. HIPAA privacy laws require that hospitals may disclose private health information to coroners and funeral directors without the necessity of consent from family or the patient. Healthcare providers are also required to leave any attached medical devices in place (e.g., IV catheters, endotracheal tubes, etc.) and any medications that were administered around or at the time of death. The coroner's office coordinates collection and transportation of the deceased patient, and an autopsy is performed. The death certificate is required to be signed within 48 hours and is completed by the physician caring for patient at the time of death, the coroner, or the medical examiner, depending on the circumstances of the death.

Practice Quiz

1. Which of the following is the *best* example of a patient-centered health goal statement?
   a. Patient will demonstrate safe and effective self-administration of insulin.
   b. Patient will complete IV antibiotic therapy in two days.
   c. Patient will be able to walk for ten minutes, twice daily, before discharge.
   d. Patient will verbalize pain level of five out of ten or less throughout day shift.

2. Which of the following patients is *least* likely to experience suboptimal patient care related to implicit bias?
   a. A 45-year-old Caucasian male receiving treatment for congestive heart failure
   b. A 23-year-old Hispanic female receiving treatment for pneumonia
   c. A 78-year-old Caucasian male receiving treatment for urinary tract infection
   d. A 50-year-old African American female receiving treatment for breast cancer

3. An elderly patient is receiving teaching about the use of a home blood pressure monitoring device. Which statement made by the nurse would be the *least* effective for assessing patient comprehension?
   a. "Show me how you will measure your blood pressure."
   b. "Where does the cuff go?"
   c. "Tell me which button you will press to see previous results."
   d. "Do you have any questions?"

4. A nurse is caring for a 52-year-old male patient who was admitted for treatment of a bowel obstruction. This patient has a history of stage 3 colon cancer and is currently receiving maintenance chemotherapy treatment. Additional assessment reveals that the patient has a history of chronic pain and nausea. This patient would benefit most from a referral to which specialty?
   a. Hospice
   b. Pain management
   c. Palliative care
   d. Mental health

5. A nurse is caring for a 40-year-old female patient who is actively dying. The hospital reports to the organ procurement organization (OPO), and it is determined that the patient is registered to be an organ donor. The patient had not communicated their wish to be an organ donor, and the family is distraught. The patient's next of kin is present and expresses that they decline consent for organ donation. The nurse knows that which of the following is true:
   a. The next of kin may only deny organ donation if the patient did not sign informed consent.
   b. The family member may not deny organ donation if the patient is registered.
   c. The family member may override the patient's organ donor registration status.
   d. The ethics committee must determine whether the family member may deny organ donation.

See answers on the next page.

Answer Explanations

1. C: "Patient will be able to walk for ten minutes, twice daily, prior to discharge." is the *best* example of a patient-centered goal statement. Effective goal statements can be formulated using the *SMART* goal criteria: specific, measurable, achievable, relevant, and time-bound. Choice *A* is not the best example of a patient-centered goal statement, as the statement could be more specific and is not measurable or time-bound. Choice *B* is also not the best example of a patient-centered goal because this is not patient-driven and is not specific or measurable. Choice *D* is also not the best choice because this goal does not provide a specific means to achieve the pain level of five out of ten or less.

2. A: The patient described in Choice *A* is the least likely to experience suboptimal care relating to implicit bias. Implicit bias is the unconscious stereotypes, beliefs, and values that influence our decisions and behaviors. Females, people of color, and the elderly are all at risk for receiving substandard patient care relating to negative stereotypes. Therefore, Choice *B* is not correct because this patient is a Hispanic female. Choice *C* is incorrect because this patient is elderly. Lastly, Choice *D* is incorrect because this patient is an African American female. Patients with lower socioeconomic status and non-heterosexual orientation are also more at risk for experiencing the adverse effects of implicit bias. Lastly, individuals with disabilities, mental health disorders, history of drug abuse, and obesity are also at increased risk of receiving substandard care related to caregiver bias.

3. D: Choice *D* is the least effective statement to assess for patient comprehension, as this is a closed-statement question that does not require the patient to demonstrate or verbalize proof of comprehension. Choice *A* would be incorrect, as this statement would be the best way to assess a patient's overall understanding of the process. Choice *B* is incorrect because the patient is able to demonstrate whether they understand appropriate blood pressure cuff placement. Choice *C* is also incorrect because the patient is required to verbalize or point to the appropriate button to access previous measurements, which assesses understanding of how to access that feature.

4. C: This patient would most benefit from palliative care referral. Palliative care will be able to address many of the patient's symptoms, including constipation, pain, nausea, and lack of appetite. Choice *A* is not correct because the patient described in the example is not described as being at the end of life, which means that hospice would not be an appropriate referral at this time. Choice *B* is not the correct choice because pain management referral would only address the patient's pain symptom. Choice *D* is not correct because although there are likely to be mental health concerns for a cancer patient, there is no direct mention of mental health being a priority issue for the described patient.

5. B: Choice *B* is the correct answer because family members cannot legally deny organ donation if a patient expressed intent via registration or written end-of-life documentation. Choice *A* is incorrect because organ donation does not follow the same laws as other healthcare procedures and does not require informed consent to be legally binding. Choice *C* is incorrect, as family members cannot override a patient's intent to be an organ donor. Lastly, Choice *D* is incorrect because the hospital ethics committee does not have the authority to grant the family member's request.

Elements of Interprofessional Care

Nursing Process/Clinical Judgment Measurement Model

Nursing Process

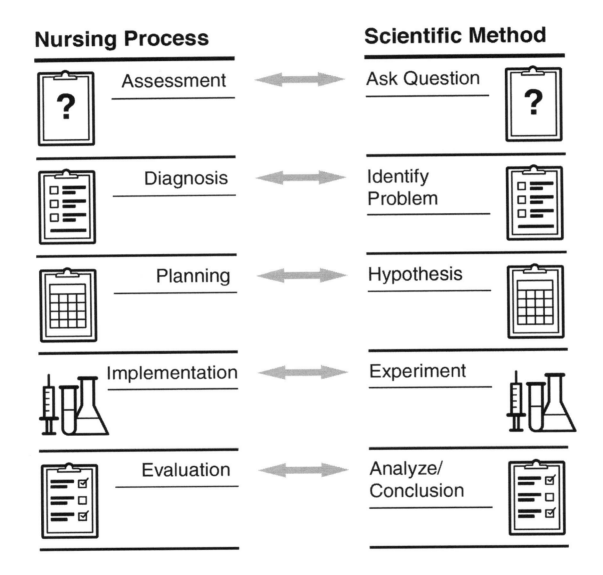

Nursing Process		Scientific Method
Assessment	⟷	Ask Question
Diagnosis	⟷	Identify Problem
Planning	⟷	Hypothesis
Implementation	⟷	Experiment
Evaluation	⟷	Analyze/ Conclusion

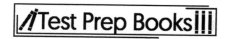
Strategies to Individualize Care

The purpose of providing individualized care is to provide the best medical interventions with the patient's preferences considered. The older healthcare model, which focuses on the concept of "Doctor knows best," does not allow the patient the right to be at the forefront of decision making. While the medical team is responsible for making a care plan for each patient, the goal with individualized patient care is to make the care plan geared toward the specific patient, rather than just the disease process or medical condition.

For example, consider a patient that is being treated for chronic anemia. Under the previous healthcare model, the medical team would have created a care plan that included parameters for a blood transfusion, iron supplementation, and a vitamin regimen. While all of those are appropriate medical interventions, this specific patient is a Jehovah's Witness (a religious group that opposes blood transfusions). Creating a care plan with the patient's considerations and preferences in place can help prevent miscommunications and poor patient care throughout the patient care experience.

The three main aspects of patient individualized care are effective communication, respect, and empathy. Effective communication is a broad concept that is often overlooked due to time constraints, staffing issues, and poor staff training and/or leadership. Not only is open, effective communication important for the nurse-patient relationship, but it is equally important for the nurse-interdisciplinary team relationship. For example, consider a nurse-patient relationship where there is open, effective communication. The patient tells the nurse that he wishes for a priest to visit him on Sundays, as he is Catholic and receives communion every Sunday. The nurse places a note in the documentation system but does not contact the priest. The patient goes two Sundays before a priest visits. While this isn't an error solely for the nurse alone, it is a lapse in interdisciplinary communication that results in a poor outcome for the patient, both spiritually and emotionally.

Respect is another concept that can be overlooked but is critical for individualized care. To respect the patient regarding their own healthcare services, the nurse must place significant weight on their preferences. Respect, in this situation, is understanding that the medical team does not possess the only voice in the care plan. Rather, the team should consider and ultimately respect the patient's cultural, financial, spiritual, emotional, and physical attributes for the patient to receive patient-centered care.

Lastly, empathy is an important aspect of providing individualized patient-focused care. While respect and empathy can often be thrown into the same category, the nurse needs to understand that empathy is what brings personalization to specific patient care. Effective communication and respect can be present, but without empathy, the emotional aspect of nursing cannot be achieved. Empathetic nursing provides an honest, caring relationship where the patient is heard, which results in trust and openness. Healthcare settings can be intimidating, but empathy provides the bridge needed for the patient to see the nurse as a person as well as a healthcare professional.

Interprofessional Collaboration

Role Within the Interdisciplinary Team

Interdisciplinary Teamwork

Nurses, physicians, surgeons, nurse aids, physical and occupational therapists, mental health professionals, and medical assistants are just some of the members who may be collaborating on the care of one patient. Perception of power between various professionals can sometimes create a stressful environment that can also affect patient outcomes. The ability of each one to collaborate with the other is imperative so that patient safety does not become an issue. Collaboration involves joint decision-making activities between all disciplines rather than nurses only following physician orders. Although each role may have a particular focus throughout the assessment and plan

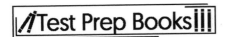

of care activities, they must jointly come together to formulate the best possible treatment plan. Studies show that an attentive communication style between nurses and physicians has the most positive impact on patients.

Communication

One skill that all nurses in all settings must possess is effective communication. Medical-surgical nurses must be able to execute effective listening skills, and they have to use the information provided to decipher what information indicates a significant risk for the patient. Medical-surgical nurses will also have to engage various individuals throughout the different stages of a surgical procedure, including the patient, the patient's family, the surgeon, the anesthetist, and other members of the health care delivery team. Communication may be verbal or written; thus, the medical-surgical nurse should be able to review and process a lot of information as well as identify which pieces of data are most relevant and require further discussion.

Interdisciplinary Rounding

Interdisciplinary rounding can provide an opportunity for team collaboration after a patient's surgery. Much like a clear hand-off process, interdisciplinary rounds reduce patient care errors, decrease mortality rates, and improve patient outcomes. Interdisciplinary rounds are an excellent place to discuss social service needs, nutritional care services, and transportation needs with all teams coordinating care for the patient in a single setting.

The patient's service needs may vary in depth for the inpatient stay and at the time of discharge; however, there should be an evaluation of these needs and a coordination of care for those services in which there is a need. Nurses document the action plan as it relates to services and requirements for the patient and collaborate with members of the interdisciplinary team to see that next steps are executed in a timely fashion. In many instances, rounding may not be possible due to the rapid pace and turnover of the perioperative environment, and thus, clear documentation will be an absolute must to allow for synchronous care coordination.

Care Coordination

Care coordination is an important factor of providing holistic patient care. This concept focuses on the collaboration of the patient's medical team, the patient's family, and the patient themself. The end goal is to treat the patient as a person with physical, social, financial, spiritual, and emotional needs and preferences. The two main concepts that are essential in providing adequate care coordination are **triage** and **transfer**.

First, the nurse must understand that triaging a patient is a more complex concept than just getting the first set of vitals and demographic information. Effective triaging is the responsibility of every nurse. The primary care nurse is responsible for recognizing a patient in the early stages of respiratory distress and referring the patient to the ED. The medical-surgical nurse is responsible for recognizing a patient with altered LOC and hypoxemia and calling for a rapid response team (RRT). The home health nurse is responsible for recognizing worsening lower extremity edema in the congestive heart failure patient and ensuring the patient is either referred to their cardiologist or that the cardiologist is contacted for further orders. These forms of nursing triage are all essential to proper care coordination.

Next, the nurse must understand the importance of transferring a patient—typically referred to as "giving report" or nurse-nurse handoff report. Most nurses will only think of this in regard to in-facility transfer (e.g., ED to ICU, ICU to telemetry, etc.), but facility-to-facility transfers and long-term forms of transfer are just as critical for effective care coordination. For example, a patient in the primary care setting being transferred to the ED would require a detailed report of the patient's presenting symptoms or chief complaint, as well as any medical intervention provided. Similarly, the importance of documentation and effective handoff reports can follow a patient throughout their lifetime. Care coordination is fluid, and the nurse should be prepared for inevitable changes, whether it's from a new medical condition, patient request, or changing healthcare standard.

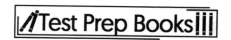

Collaborative Problem Solving

Some of the benefits of collaboration include improved patient outcomes, decreased healthcare costs, decreased length of stay, improved patient and nurse satisfaction, and improved teamwork. Collaboration related to patient care has been widely studied and is considered as both a process and an outcome, which occurs when no single individual is able to solve a patient problem. Collaboration as a process is defined as a synthesis of diverse opinions and skills that is employed to solve complex problems. As an outcome, collaboration is defined as a complex solution to a problem that requires the expertise of more than one individual. This view of collaboration characterizes the process as a series of actions by more than one individual, which creates a solution to a complex problem.

Initially, all members of the collaborative team must identify their own biases and acknowledge the effect of these mental models on the decision-making process. In addition, members must also be aware that the complexity of the problem will be matched by the complexity of the mental models of the collaborative team members, which will influence the decision-making process. It is also essential for team members to recognize the elements of diversity in the group. For instance, while stereotyping is obviously to be avoided, there are gender differences that should be considered.

Research indicates that men tend to be more task oriented, and women tend to be more relationship oriented in the problem-solving process; this means that consideration of both points of view is necessary for genuine collaboration. Another requisite skill of the collaborative team is the development and usage of conflict resolution skills, which are required to counteract this common barrier to effective collaboration. Team members are required to separate the task from the emotions in the discussion. Effective collaboration also requires that members of the team display a cooperative effort that works to create a win/win situation, while recognizing that collaboration is a series of activities that require time and patience for satisfactory completion.

Common barriers to effective collaboration include conflicting professional opinions, ineffective communication related to the conflict, and incomplete assessment of the required elements of the care plan. Research indicates that physicians tend to stress cure-related activities while nurses tend to encourage care-related activities. This means that some resolution of these differences is required for effective communication. Although the Synergy Model defines collaboration as a necessary part of the process that matches the patient needs with the appropriate nursing competencies, it is also possible that the end product may be the best solution for the patient and at the same time be totally unacceptable to the patient. Collaborative team members should also be aware that while successful collaboration improves patient outcomes, research indicates that genuine collaborative efforts are rarely noted in patient care, often because the group is unable to integrate the diverse mental models of the group members.

Care Coordination and Transition Management

Community Resources

After a patient undergoes a surgical procedure, the care that follows focuses on recovery and rehabilitation. The type of discharge resources needed will be dependent on the patient's surgical experience. The nurse will need to collaborate with the interdisciplinary team, such as case managers and social workers, to provide the patient with the necessary community resources to achieve an optimal health status. For example, a patient with a total hip replacement will require physical therapy during the recovery process to ensure full mobility is restored. Depending on the patient's age, additional caregiver services may be required for assistance with activities of daily living.

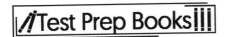

Interdisciplinary Collaboration

For most patients admitted to any health care facility, each provider added to their case is expected to provide the best possible care. While working to ensure that the best care is provided, each practitioner must also be considerate of how their patient will manage once they are discharged from the hospital. In other words, discharge planning begins at admission. Each diagnosis-related group (DRG) generally requires and responds to certain treatments within a specified amount of time. With that basic knowledge, a generalized template on the treatment for each DRG, or clinical pathway can be generated.

A **clinical pathway** is defined as a detailed list of elements, related to the care of the client, that are expected to be completed within a specified period of time. Within the pathway, or care map, is a breakdown of the strategies necessary to achieve the goals outlined in the plan of care. Immediately upon the admission of any patient, discharge planning also begins. Once the patient is stabilized, the care team will be assembled.

Typically, the care team consists of physicians, nurses, physical and occupational therapists, and the psychologist or social worker. The care team will periodically convene, or "round," to discuss the plans for each patient on the unit. The team will collaborate to determine the level of care needed by each patient, the time it will take to accomplish the desired level of functioning, and which disciplines will be active in the care plan. This strategic goal-setting continues daily, adjusting as needed for any unexpected incline or decline in the patient's status. Any provider that becomes aware of the possibility that a treatment deadline may not be met must follow up for feedback. This accountability is meant to provide that the care team is capable of providing consistent, efficient, and cost-effective care. As the patient improves and moves closer to discharge, a discharge plan will be formulated with the assistance of the patient's caregivers and the social worker.

Discharge Planning

Nurses are commonly tasked with discharge planning—the set of procedures that guide patient experiences once they have received written clearance by a physician to leave the medical facility. This transition is a critical one for the patient, who may be physiologically able to leave the inpatient setting but may still require physical and psychological follow-up care in the home. Additionally, some patients may transition to another department, a rehabilitation facility, a hospice home, or somewhere else that is not their primary residence. The patient may also require medical appointments at regular intervals to monitor recovery. Finally, caregivers of the patient may also need counseling on this transition.

Effective discharge planning covers several different areas with the primary goals of ensuring a stress-free transition for the patient and decreasing the chance that the patient will need to be readmitted for any issues related to their current medical case. Discharge planning requires a multidisciplinary approach that may be spearheaded by the medical-surgical nurse. It is important to note that discharge can take place from an inpatient unit or at a facility. For patients recovering from surgery, **discharge planning** for the patient begins with the decision that the patient needs to have a surgical procedure. Patients who have comorbid conditions or are a part of the elderly population are at greater risk for postoperative surgical complications. Discharge planning is a fundamental component of reducing the risk of this complication and readmission.

Discharge planning should begin with noting the health status of the patient, ideally by an interdisciplinary group of healthcare providers. This analysis should be discussed in detail with the patient and any relevant caregivers, with ample opportunity for both the patient and the caregiver(s) to discuss any questions or concerns. Assuming all questions and concerns have been discussed satisfactorily, logistical planning for the transition can begin. This may include determining how and where the patient will be physically moved, what equipment or medical staff may be needed in the next place that the patient will be residing, instructions for caregivers, and instructions for the patients. If extra support or professional support is needed after discharge, the nurse should provide referral information or arrange the referral for the patient. Finally, any follow-up appointments should be scheduled and reminder cards provided.

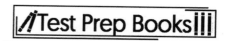

Poor discharge planning that is conducted without reviewing these options or done in a rushed manner can result in poor patient satisfaction, poor patient health outcomes, re-admittance, and/or costly medical errors. Having strict and standardized operating procedures for discharge planning in which all medical staff are cross-trained can help the overall process be comprehensive and beneficial for both the patient and the organization.

Continued collaboration between patients and a representative of their healthcare team promotes positive recovery outcomes. Patients who are contacted regularly after discharge to review their health, medical records, instructions, and satisfaction are less likely to experience poor recovery or be readmitted to the medical facility. Additionally, nurses who collaborate with other health professionals to create patient discharge plans are also associated with improved patient outcomes. This correlation is likely due to input from a variety of medical perspectives that allows the discharge plan to address all potential patient needs.

Functional Mobility Assessment

The physical capacity of a patient determines their functional mobility. Assessing the patient's ability to perform activities of daily living is essential in determining their physical functionality. The Katz Index of Independence in Activities of Daily Living is a tool that assesses the areas of bathing, dressing, toileting, transferring, continence, and feeding. Each category is worth 1 point, and a total score of 6 classifies a patient as independent. Mobility can further be assessed by asking patients about their ability to walk, balance, and perform fine-motor movements, such as opening jars. The patient's ability to prepare meals, shop for groceries, and administer medications are activities that assess independent living. If a patient is unable to perform these instrumental activities, the medical-surgical nurse should consider collaborating with case management for available services and resources.

Functional Assessment in the Presence of Injuries

Once the nature of the injury, required devices, and client needs are determined, an individualized assessment of the patient is also imperative. A typical functional capacity assessment includes an evaluation of an individual's ability to perform basic and job-specific tasks. An interdisciplinary team consisting of physicians, physical therapists (PTs), occupational therapists (OTs), and psychologists collaborate to interview, assess, and diagnose the patient in relation to their ability to perform the duties associated with their current job description and associated activities. The case manager's responsibility is to help locate the appropriate providers, facilitate the necessary appointments, and support the patient through the assessment process. With the use of the necessary assistive devices, the patient's functional threshold is established. Any deficits in functioning are addressed and, if required for the patient to return to work, added to a PT or OT plan of care.

One of the objectives of the functional assessment is to answer several questions in relation to the injury: Can you do your job? Can you do your job in your current work environment? How well can you do your job in your current work environment? Are the assistive devices truly necessary? Are you able to manipulate the assistive devices, or are they too cumbersome? The answers to the aforementioned questions help to build a simulation of the type of work environment, average daily tasks, and associated time frames. Baseline performance levels and endurance of treatment are obtained to be compared with the final assessment. Although maximum effort from the patient is expected, the assessment is not meant to be punitive or severe. The PT or OT will typically plan the activities to build upon themselves, progressing in difficulty as the client's mobility and/or range of motion improves. Barriers to the achievement of the most favorable outcome are identified, and strategies to intervene and correct the problems are developed. Once completed, the inventories will guide further intervention and assist the care team in recommending the individual for a return to work.

The nurse must also assess the patient's needs as the patient themselves perceives them. Do the devices provided aid or support their ability to accomplish the tasks of daily living? Does the patient feel they can perform the necessary tasks with only the devices provided? Has the patient considered an alternate occupation if a return to work is not obtained? How supportive is the patient's home environment? What, if any, emotional or psychological deficits need to be met?

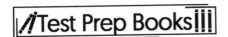

How best can the interdisciplinary team support the patient in working through those concerns? Is the patient willing or able to seek out other sources of emotional support through this process? The answers to these questions are also crucial, as the treatment plan can be adjusted. If the patient's needs have changed during the assessment process, those needs can be addressed and added to the plan of care. Whenever necessary, the team should involve the family and caregivers in the discussion, so that their concerns can also be addressed. Upon the completion of the final report, the case manager will then guide the patient's return to work, with any assistive devices, prostheses or orthotics deemed necessary for the patient to perform at an optimal level of functioning.

Health History Assessment from Multiple Sources

Health history assessments encompass a wide array of medical disciplines with the potential for different informants. The nurse admitting the patient, the medical provider, any specialist providers, and additional nurses providing care over the patient's healthcare experience all have a form of a health history assessment. Add in the documentation from respiratory therapists, occupational therapists, speech therapists, physical therapists, medical social workers, chaplains, and nursing assistants, and there can be a lapse in historical accuracy without effective interdisciplinary communication. Then, factor in the potential for a different perspective with each assessment (e.g., obtaining historical data from the spouse instead of the patient), and the importance of using the healthcare team becomes clear.

While the nurse cannot solve every single lapse in interdisciplinary communication, performing a thorough health history assessment and relaying pertinent information can help in the process of providing consistent care. The phrase "trust, but verify" is a vital nursing tactic in acting as a patient advocate. It is in the best interests of the patient for the nurse to ensure correct documentation so that the care plan can reflect what is needed. If a nurse notices a discrepancy in documentation, or anything that sounds questionable, it is critical for the nurse to follow up. Trusting the medical team and co-workers is a vital aspect of becoming a successful nurse, but verifying information is important for the safety, health, and satisfaction of the patient.

Discharge Procedures

Like the care plan provided during the healthcare experience, the discharge plan is a crucial responsibility of the interdisciplinary team. The goal of discharge planning is for the patient to feel confident in moving forward with their own healthcare once the necessary education, tools, and assistance have been provided. The importance of this is highlighted by federal regulations that closely monitor readmission to the hospital within thirty days of discharge. In some circumstances, readmissions for the same chief complaint can be considered a continuation of services, which lead to penalties related to reimbursement. So, what can the nurse do to provide the patient with a sufficient discharge plan?

First, the nurse must **work closely with all members of the interdisciplinary team**. Some facilities require a meeting of the entire medical team prior to the discharge to ensure the plan is consistent. Some patients may have a relatively simple interdisciplinary team consisting of the medical provider, nurse, nursing assistant, and medical social worker, while other patients may have a complex medical team consisting of ten or more medical professionals.

Next, the nurse must **provide education on the specific disease process** related to the admission. While this should occur routinely throughout the healthcare experience, the nurse needs to closely assess the patient's understanding of the education and provide any resources needed.

Next, the nurse must **perform a detailed medication reconciliation**. A discharge medication reconciliation includes reviewing new medications, changed medications, and discontinued medications, as well as reviewing the specific times to take each medication. The nurse should also provide the patient with education regarding medication side effects.

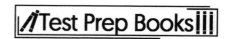
Next, the nurse should **provide the patient with detailed education about any specific complications and whom to contact in the event of complications**. Complications related to the disease process, medications, or medical therapies should be thoroughly reviewed, and the patient should be informed of whom to contact or where to go if they experience these issues.

Lastly, most patients will require assistance with organizing their lives outside of the healthcare setting. The nurse should **ensure referrals are in place for assistance**, typically from the facility case manager or medical social worker. Assistance can include scheduling follow-up appointments, ordering durable medical equipment (DME), and providing community resources.

Pain Management Counseling

Pain management is a vital component of discharge care. Not only does the patient need to be comfortable, but it is also important that they receive correct medication, dosing, and follow safe guidelines for any therapeutic recommendations. Patients may not be able to effectively manage their pain if they fail to follow dosing instructions of prescription medications. They may inadvertently engage in unsafe behavior if they do not follow limitations of certain prescription medications. For example, opioids are highly addictive and make routine behaviors, such as driving a vehicle, dangerous. Therefore, it is crucial that pain management counseling is provided as a part of discharge services. Following up with patients who have documented pain and management techniques may also mitigate risks. This practice can additionally allow nurses to review and modify pain management plans as patient needs change over time, while also noticing if there are any early causes for concern.

Patient/Family Centered Care

Patient-centered care is a healthcare concept in which the patient is at the center of all healthcare decisions. While the concepts of patient care seem simple, they are complex to put into practice within the fast-paced healthcare environment. The steps to provide patient centered care include the following:

- Showing respect to the patient and family about healthcare decisions and personal preferences or cultural and religious practices

- Ensuring the patient is provided the medically appropriate services requested (e.g., having a chaplain visit after the family requests or having the dietary staff bring only kosher foods after the patient requests)

- Providing the patient with holistic care, treating all aspects of the patient and not solely focusing on the chief complaint or primary diagnosis

- Ensuring the patient has access to support systems (i.e., family and friends) as much as possible within any medical constraints

- Guiding the patient through the healthcare process to empower them in making confident healthcare decisions

Care Coordination and Transition

Transitioning care refers to any context in which the patient's care level and/or specific caregiver changes. This could be as simple as a nursing shift change, where the nurse attending to a particular patient changes, or as complex as moving the patient from a healthcare facility to their place of residence when the patient requires in-home medical staff and equipment. Any time there is a change in care level, there is an opportunity for the quality of care to decline. This can be due to a lack of communication between healthcare providers, a lack of

211

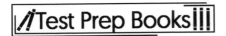
communication between healthcare providers and the patient, a lack of education provided to the patient about their care, a paperwork mix-up, or some other type of unintentional error. Therefore, standardizing transition procedures and documentation can be a critical and valuable component to quality patient care.

Initial patient boarding is an important moment of data collection. Whether it is the patient's first admission into the healthcare system or a transition into a new system, documenting as much information as possible about the patient's personal history, medical history, the condition that brought the patient into the facility, any documentation of advanced directives or medical proxies, and initial health assessments can be valuable as the patient's time in care progresses. A standardized electronic medical record that can be continuously accessed and updated by all healthcare providers who play a role in the patient's care can prevent complications that arise from lack of communication. Otherwise, comprehensive intake forms at each transition can help minimize the chance of the patient receiving inadequate or improper care.

Post-Operative Transfer

Once a patient is ready for transfer to the **post-anesthesia care unit (PACU)**, the perioperative nurse will complete handoff documentation and a report. The toolkits, policies, and procedures that the unit implements and uses should be those that a multidisciplinary team has come together to create. Various members of the interdisciplinary team must take an active role in identifying the structure and process for transferring a patient. Members of this team may include the following:

- Nurses (e.g., medical-surgical, perianesthesia, perioperative, or critical care)
- Physicians (e.g., resident or surgeon)
- Allied professional team (e.g., radiology or certified surgical tech)
- Other licensed professionals (e.g., social worker or physician's assistant)
- Support staff (e.g., patient care assistant or unit clerk)

This multidisciplinary team can help ensure that various perspectives are integrated into any standard or guideline put into place for the unit.

Shift Change Transfer

While each facility will have a specific protocol regarding hand-off reports from shift-to-shift, some basic data points are important to ensure consistency of care in any healthcare setting. Basic demographics and past medical history are important points of preview to ensure the chief complaint/primary medical condition is discussed in further detail. Next, any medical intervention provided over the shift should be discussed (including new provider orders, therapies, PRN medications, and so on). Any patient changes, such as flagged lab results or worsening pain, should be discussed with consideration to the patient's baseline. While these are all important topics of discussion regarding shift change reporting, the nurse should also consider the physical location of the handoff report. Performing the handoff report at the bedside can be beneficial for both the nursing staff and the patient, as well as the patient's family. Not only can the bedside handoff report lead to improved patient-centered care by including the patient/patient's family, but it can also improve continuity from nurse to nurse. Trust can be established from shift to shift, and any errors noted by the patient can be discussed.

Level of Care Transfer

Level-of-care transfers are simply that—a change in patient acuity that results in a change of care (e.g., from telemetry unit to ICU, from ED to med-surg, from PACU to step-down unit). Like shift change transfers, each facility will have a specific protocol for level of care transfer. The main points will be similar to that of a shift change transfer, but will require a detailed review of what necessitated the change in level of care. For example, a medical-surgical nurse giving the transfer report to an ICU nurse would need to include why the patient now requires intensive care.

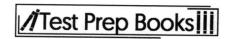

Interprofessional Roles and Responsibilities

The difficult part of coordinating care and ensuring consistency is the number of interprofessional roles and responsibilities within the healthcare team. Each individual healthcare professional working toward the goals stated in the patient's care plan introduces the possibility of unintended overlap and miscommunication. The nurse's role in preventing these discrepancies is to understand who does what and why. That may sound generic, but understanding the dynamics of the healthcare team can help prevent lapses in patient care as well as provide the patient with a better healthcare experience:

Doctors:

- Consists of medical doctors (MDs) and doctors of osteopathic medicine (DOs) Both MDs and DOs receive the same amount of training, but DOs specifically train with additional holistic models of care.

- Roles and responsibilities include diagnosing the patient, formulating treatment plans with additional diagnostics/therapies/medications, providing preventative healthcare, and providing information regarding healthcare decisions.

Advanced Practice Providers:

- Consists of nurse practitioners (NPs) and physician assistants (PAs)
- Advanced practice providers can function with the same roles and responsibilities as the doctors, but may require oversight depending on the state's scope of practice.
- Advanced practice providers receive less schooling and clinical training than a doctor.

Nurses:

- Consists of registered nurses (RNs) and licensed practical nurses (LPNs, also sometimes referred to as licensed vocational nurses [LVNs])
- Roles and responsibilities of the nurse include performing routine patient assessments, administering orders from doctors or advanced practice providers, being a patient advocate, providing patient education, and coordinating care.
- The difference between RNs and LPNs is the level of education and treatments provided. The RN is able to perform more complex medical therapies, while the LPN provides more direct patient care.

Nursing Assistants:

- Roles and responsibilities include duties assigned by the doctor/advanced practice provider or nurse that are within the state's scope of practice (e.g., bathing, feeding, and toileting).

Medical Social Workers:

- Roles and responsibilities include providing counseling, providing referrals for community resources, being a patient advocate, and using tools to assess the patient's well-being.

Additional Interdisciplinary Team Members:

- Can consist of physical therapists, speech therapists, occupational therapists, respiratory therapists, dieticians, spiritual counselors/chaplains, healthcare specialists, or mental health counselors

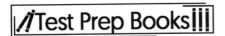

Continuum of Care

Continuum of care refers to the healthcare team's ability to provide consistent services throughout the process of the patient's healthcare experiences. The healthcare team should be able to follow the patient throughout transfers of care and patient changes while providing the services needed over the patient's lifetime. There are multiple effective continuum-of-care models, but the main aspects include prevention, treatment, and maintenance.

Preventative healthcare can take the form of wellness checks, routine dental visits, and scheduled vaccinations, but the concept is evolving. It can mean education regarding heart health or weight management as well. Essentially, preventative healthcare is the attempt to prevent the need for further healthcare intervention.

This aspect of treatment is present in any healthcare environment, but it's most often found in EDs, urgent cares, specialty offices, and primary care provider offices. Treatment can take the form of medications, surgical interventions, therapies, or procedures.

The aspect of maintenance has the main goal of reducing the progression or symptoms of the disease process. Maintenance can include rehabilitation, therapies, medications, lifestyle changes, and education regarding compliance.

Patients at Risk for Readmissions

One of the healthcare team's primary goals is to prevent the need for patient readmission and to recognize those patients that are at a higher risk of readmission. Readmission is defined as the readmission of a patient to an acute care facility with the same chief complaint within thirty days of discharge. While not all readmissions can be avoided, there are some steps the healthcare team can take to recognize risk factors and provide the necessary resources.

Certain Disease Processes

Disease processes with complexities (especially progressive diseases) increase the need for readmissions, even with adequate treatment and education. These disease processes can include CKD, heart failure, COPD, sepsis, CVA, and MI.

Patient Demographics

Patient demographics that increase the likelihood of a readmission include advanced age, male gender, and lower-income individuals. The patient's education level can also be an issue regarding comprehension of medical treatment.

Inadequate Healthcare

Inadequate healthcare refers to gaps in interdisciplinary communication and poor discharge instructions. If the patient is discharged without proper follow-up, extensive discharge information, and a clear understanding of the path forward, the likelihood of readmission is high.

Noncompliance

Lastly, patient noncompliance with the medical treatment plan increases the likelihood of readmission. The nurse can assist in the prevention of noncompliance by thoroughly reviewing the importance of each aspect of the treatment plan (e.g., taking furosemide as ordered to prevent another heart failure exacerbation).

Social Determinants of Health

Social determinants of health can be an overwhelmingly complex concept for the nurse who cares for a diverse patient population. Each nurse should understand the general social determinants of health, representing the

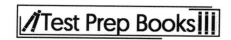
nonmedical factors that directly or indirectly affect the patient's healthcare experience. Several general talking points fall under social determinants of health: economic stability, level of education, access to quality healthcare, community resources, and environmental status—essentially, each patient's socioeconomic status.

Economic stability refers to the patient's level of consistent income. Poor economic stability can affect the foods a patient eats, the medications the patient can take, the resources the patient can utilize, and access to certain forms of healthcare. Level of education includes the highest level of education achieved, along with general access to education. Access to healthcare relates to the patient's ability to physically get to anything healthcare related (e.g., a patient without a car in a rural area would have a harder time getting to routine doctor's appointments) as well as the quality of healthcare provided. Lastly, the community factor includes the safety of the neighborhood/housing as well as community resources available. Considering that all these points are related and each one can impact the others (e.g., economic stability could affect the level of education), social determinants of health will vary from patient to patient and will require the nurse to closely assess for gaps in healthcare needs.

Regarding the nurse's understanding of social determinants of health, the main goal is to ensure safe, consistent patient care with appropriate referrals in place. Low-income patients with a low level of education are at a higher risk of poor care coordination, noncompliance, and gaps in healthcare. The nurse can provide patient-appropriate education (i.e., education resources that are appropriate for the patient's education and understanding level), ensure follow-up appointments, and assist in referrals to community resources.

Quality Patient Outcome Measures

Medical-surgical nurses should understand that the patient outcomes rely on a complex combination of the patient's individual biological pharmacotherapeutic profile, degree of adherence with the plan, socioeconomic factors, and existing comorbidities. Much of the research on patient adherence focuses on economic factors, while many providers believe that the patient outcomes should be the top priority. Quality improvement activities at the administration level can address many of these issues by standardizing the provider approach to the development of the therapeutic plan. Some of the issues addressed can include methods of education, monitoring procedures for drugs with known or high-risk for the development of adverse drug reactions, and examination of hospital readmissions following the administration of the target drug.

Nurses promote best patient outcomes by providing education to patients and families by utilizing best practice guidelines and using these in the nursing process. Ultimately, the purpose of education, care bundles, core measures, and guidelines is to promote the best possible **patient outcomes**. Patient outcomes are identified as high priority by nurses, physicians, patients, families, professional organizations, and governing bodies. One of the quality objectives of the **Affordable Care Act (ACA)**, enacted in 2010, is fewer avoidable hospital readmissions. Avoidable hospital readmissions are considered negative outcomes for all parties involved, but especially for the patients. The **Institute for Healthcare Improvement (IHI)** is a worldwide driver of health care improvement and best patient outcomes. The IHI's work focuses on improvement capability, person- and family-centered care; patient safety; and quality, cost, and value. These focus groups are all aimed to improve patient outcomes.

The **Centers for Medicare and Medicaid Services (CMS)** was formed in 1977. CMS provides value-based incentives to providers and institutions by tying reimbursement to better patient outcomes. Conversely, CMS withholds reimbursement to institutions and providers if a patient is readmitted to the hospital within thirty days of discharge if the readmission is related to the same problem causing the initial hospitalization. For instance, a patient is admitted to the hospital with CHF exacerbation, treated, and released. Two weeks later, the patient is readmitted with CHF exacerbation. Neither the hospital nor the physician is reimbursed for care related to the readmission.

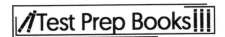

TJC created the Surgical Care Improvement Project (SCIP) with the goal of substantially reducing negative patient outcomes (surgical mortality and morbidity), specifically **surgical site infection (SSI)** and venous thromboembolism (VTE).

Systems Thinking

Systems thinking is defined as a link between individuals and their environment. For nurses, this refers to their ability to understand the influence of the healthcare environment on patient outcomes. Systems thinking is identified as the goal of all of the Quality and Safety Education for Nurses (QESN) competencies, which are acquired by nurses on a continuum that ranges from the care of the individual patient to the care of the entire patient population. The QESN competencies were originally identified to improve patient outcomes in response to extensive research that identified a significant difference between the care of patients and the improvement in patient outcomes resulting from that care. The nursing competencies include patient-centered care, evidence-based practice, teamwork and collaboration, safety, quality and improvement, and informatics. Successful interventions associated with each of these criteria for professional nursing practice require the ability to apply the systems thinking approach to care.

Competency related to systems thinking requires appropriate education and clinical experience, and is also identified as one of the nursing competencies in the Synergy Model. In that model, novice nurses view the patient and family as isolated in the nursing unit rather than being influenced by the healthcare system, while experienced nurses are able to integrate all of the resources in the healthcare system to improve patient outcomes. Several of the learning activities designed to improve nurses' ability to acquire systems thinking include creation of a grid that identifies the nursing competencies across the continuum from isolated, individual care to the level of care associated with systems thinking. There are assessment models that apply this exercise to specialty care units such as emergency care, long-term care, and outpatient care, which identify specific systems needs for these areas. Other exercises include tracking unit statistics for the QESN competencies followed by the creation, implementation, and evaluation of a plan that applies systems thinking to address that competency. All of these activities help nurses integrate patient needs with all available resources in order to improve outcomes.

The Iceberg

A Tool for Guiding Systematic Thinking

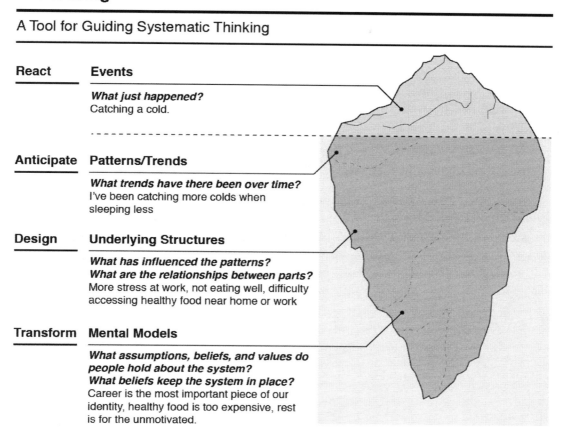

React   **Events**

What just happened?
Catching a cold.

Anticipate   **Patterns/Trends**

What trends have there been over time?
I've been catching more colds when
sleeping less

Design   **Underlying Structures**

What has influenced the patterns?
What are the relationships between parts?
More stress at work, not eating well, difficulty
accessing healthy food near home or work

Transform   **Mental Models**

What assumptions, beliefs, and values do
people hold about the system?
What beliefs keep the system in place?
Career is the most important piece of our
identity, healthy food is too expensive, rest
is for the unmotivated.

Documentation

Documentation

The final step of assessment is the documentation of the findings. The medical-surgical nurse is aware that safe patient care relies on accurate documentation that may or may not be shared in a larger provider network. Documentation is also required to meet reimbursement schedules for Medicaid, Medicare, and other private insurers. The assessment details, the subsequent interventions, and the patient's response to the interventions must be clearly evident and must be recorded in the appropriate EHR format.

A patient's chart is a legal record of observations about the patient and any care given for the patient. Most facilities use an electronic health record, which the nurse will generally be trained to use as a part of new employee orientation. Documentation may include time of observation, time task was performed, what was done, how it was done, and reaction to intervention. There are various charting systems used to document patient data by patient care facilities. Documentation requirements will be dictated by facility policy and regulatory guidelines. Two methods—charting by exception and comprehensive charting—are used.

Charting by exception means that besides recording of vital signs, only abnormal findings are documented. This charting method is somewhat controversial as so much information about the patient is usually left out. It is

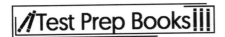

sometimes argued that this is the safer way to chart, as only what is deviant from normal is noted, and thus, there is less room for documentation errors. The normal is assumed, unless otherwise noted. This method also saves time, as less information needs to be documented, leaving more time for patient care.

Some facilities prefer a **comprehensive method** of documentation, charting everything about the patient—normal and abnormal—in a very thorough manner. This way, when the patient's chart must be reviewed, especially in the case of a safety incident (e.g., a pressure sore develops or a patient falls), all details surrounding the event should be present in the medical record. This method works as long as everything is actually documented, although it can be quite time-consuming and take away from patient care time.

Documentation provides a defense for health care workers and patients in the case of patient incidents to show what was done for the patient. There is an adage that says, "If it wasn't charted, it didn't happen." The nurse needs to be mindful that the medical record is a legal document—a complete, thorough, and accurate documentation of care, according to facility policy.

Perioperative Documentation
Clinical documentation of each phase of the perioperative spectrum serves as a baseline of care coordination and communication while providing for patient safety. It provides a historical snapshot of care given to the patient and the patient's response to each intervention by various members of the health care team.

While most documentation is done electronically, nurses should also be familiar with the policies and procedures for paper documentation in the event of computer system downtime.

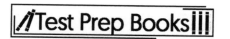
In an effort to adhere to federal and state regulations and accreditation protocol, many facilities maintain documentation of invasive or operative procedures. An intraoperative report is a permanent part of the patient's record, and it can provide insight into the patient's status postoperatively.

Pre-operative Record

Pre-operative

Patient Name .... Surgeon .... Date ....

Procedure ....

Arrival .... **ID** ☐ Verbal ☐ Nameband **Pt Verbalizes** ☐ Procedure Site ☐ Surgeon **NPO** Since............................

Allergies: ☐ NDA ☐ Latex ☐ Other............................ ☐ Drugs ....

Lab Data: ☐ CBC Reports: Consents: Blood Products - # of units

☐ Urinalysis ☐ EKG ☐ Surgical in OR ....

☐ Chemistry ☐ Chest ☐ Blood Blood Bank .... ☐ Autologous ....

☐ Coag Studies ☐ H & P ☐ Anaesthesia ☐ Type and Screen .... ☐ Directed ....

.... ☐ Pregnancy Test ☐ Other ☐ Type and Cross .... ☐ Homologous ....

Equipment: ☐ IV's ☐ Foley ☐ Ventilator ☐ Cardiac Monitor ☐ IABP ☐ Other ....

Prosthesis: ☐ None ☐ Ophthalmic ☐ Optic ☐ Dental ☐ Jewelry Disposition of Prosthesis ....

Orientation: ☐ Awake ☐ Oriented ☐ Sedated ☐ Confused ☐ Agitated ☐ Crying

Implants / Other Comments: ....

.... RN SIGNATURE ....

Intra-operative

Identification: ☐ Verbal ☐ Nameband Scrub Nurse: ☐ Sees Permits ☐ Aware of Allergies

Skin Condition: ☐ Intact ☐ Presence of Lesions - Type/Location ....

Skin Prep: ☐ Betadine ☐ Hibiclens ☐ Other ....

Position: ☐ Supine ☐ Prone ☐ Lithotomy ☐ Lateral ☐ Jackknife ☐ Fracture Table

☐ Other .... Positioned by ....

Equipment Codes: Supports:

= - Safety Strap applied by .... ☐ Kidney Rest ....

X - Grounding Pad applied by .... ☐ Stirrups ....

T - Tourniquet applied by .... ☐ Arms @ Side ....

- Pressure Pads applied by .... ☐ Arms on Armboard ....

S - Sandbag applied by .... ☐ Action Pads ....

R - Roll applied by .... ☐ Black Leg Positioner ....

A - Action Donut applied by .... ☐ Bean Bag ....

Z - Zoll Defib Pad applied by ....

Tourniquet Unit #............................ mm/Hg .... Inflated .... Deflated ....

Warming Blanket Unit #............................ Temp .... On .... Off ....

Electrocautery Unit #............................ Coag @ .... Cut @ ....

Pad # .... Exp. Date .... ESU Pad Skin Site ....

Defibrillator # .... Time / Joules ....

BiPolar Unit # .... Setting .... Other Equipment ....

Comments............................

.... RN SIGNATURE ....

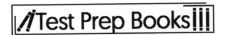

Narcotic Medication Management

Narcotic medication management has its own set of guidelines, including distribution and documentation of narcotic usage. The potential for narcotic abuse guides strict documentation of narcotic chain of custody. Most institutions use a central form of medication dispensing, such as a Pyxis system. Pyxis is managed by the institutional pharmacy and is stocked by pharmacists and pharmacy technicians. Access to Pyxis is granted to those approved to remove and use the medications; generally, nurses and anesthesiologists.

When a narcotic is removed from this system, the narcotic count is verified by the person removing the narcotic, and the narcotic is then removed and administered to the patient. If the person initiating narcotic removal discovers an incorrect narcotic count, the Pyxis system shows the last transaction involving the medication, including the name of the person who removed it and the prior narcotic count. The discrepancy must be resolved at that point, or the issue is turned over to pharmacy and/or hospital security. If a narcotic is removed from the system and the full dose is not administered to the patient, the narcotic must be wasted with another licensed person (such as nurse or anesthesiologist) witnessing the waste. This is documented either on paper or in the Pyxis system.

Electronic Health Records

One way of improving patient outcomes is with the use of **electronic health records (EHRs)**. EHRs help health care providers to access complete and accurate health information in a timely fashion. EHRs have also been shown to reduce (and even prevent) medical errors due to misinterpretation of handwriting. EHRs also allow built-in systems designed to prevent treatment errors. All documentation is typically added to an electronic health record (EHR), due to the need to maintain patient privacy and confidentiality. Anyone who accesses this information will be tracked and monitored. Most institutions will conduct routine audits to see who has been accessing which records and if they were authorized to do so. The use of paper records continues, but due to the sheer volume of information collected and the need to ensure the security of this record, this practice will soon be phased out. Basic standards of care require the EHR contains all pertinent information and that it is updated frequently as the plan of care changes. Basic demographic information, along with treatment protocols and correspondence, is readily available to be accessed by the necessary practitioners associated with the case. Further, the meaningful use of file sharing is expected. Meaning, one of the main stipulations of the use of the EHR is that the client and provider benefit from the use of the EHR in quantifiable and qualitative ways. For this reason, it is imperative that all health care providers periodically document in the EHR, addressing the client's progress throughout the treatment plan.

Downtime Procedures

Downtime procedures can vary from facility to facility, but the nurse should be prepared for both planned and unplanned downtime. First, what is downtime? Considering healthcare predominantly uses electronic health records, downtime is any time that an aspect of the electronic health record system is not working. Downtime can be a planned situation during which staff is informed of a certain time frame where the system will be down for updates, repairs, or a reset. It can also be unplanned in the event of an IT malfunction, cybersecurity issue, or loss of power.

During downtime, the greatest concern is patient safety, as the safeguards in place through the electronic health record are no longer accessible. The nurse's role in downtime procedures, both planned and unplanned, is to be prepared to access paper health records, understand the policy for paper documentation, and ensure no lapses in communication related to downtime. There will be minor setbacks with downtime procedures, but the goal of the nurse is to continue to provide safe, effective care to each patient.

Coaching for Documentation Performance Improvement

The nurse should become familiar with the phrase "if it wasn't documented, it didn't happen." While this may seem dramatic, it is unfortunately true in the world of the patient experience. The nurse can provide extensive care with

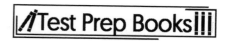

timely intervention and implementation of all provider orders, but if that care isn't documented, the medical team will not be aware of it. Not only will the medical team be out of the loop in terms of patient care provided, so will the insurance companies, as well as the legal team in the event of a lawsuit. Proper documentation is not only the chance for the nurse to record all care provided to the patient, but also the opportunity to improve the continuum of care and quality of care.

Coaching to help improve nursing documentation should demonstrate the following:

Document everything as soon as possible. An interval of time that is too long can lead to forgetting important details or mixing up patients.

Follow facility protocol on times to document and any abbreviations allowed.

Do not assume in documentation. The nurse should not say the patient "seems" a certain way—they should record only objective data or reporting from the patient.

Be detailed enough to "paint the picture" or "tell the story."

Follow up in a timely manner when a medical intervention is provided.

Technology

Technology, Equipment Use, and Troubleshooting

While it is easy to assume technology in healthcare revolves around electronic health records, the nurse will be able to use other types of technology including complex equipment. The nurse should be prepared to use and troubleshoot the equipment in their field of practice, including but not limited to IV pumps, mechanical ventilators, bladder scanners, and/or smart beds. To review, listed below are a few of the more common types of equipment the nurse should feel comfortable using and troubleshooting.

IV Pump

IV pumps are seen in the critical care, med-surg, outpatient, and home health population. Every manufacturer provides a slightly different set of instructions, but there are a few basic steps in using any IV pump. The IV pump is in place to help the nurse provide a consistent administration of ordered medication or fluids, but it is the nurse's responsibility to ensure the correct flow rate, medication, and compatibility with other medications (if applicable). IV pumps need to be inspected routinely for accuracy, but there are still some alarms that the nurse will need to troubleshoot. The two alarms that the nurse should be prepared to troubleshoot are the presence of air in the tubing and a distal occlusion. In the event of air in the IV line, the pump should be stopped, and the air should be removed from the line prior to administration of any further infusions. Regarding a distal occlusion, the catheter is either in a place that allows the patient's movement to affect flow (e.g., flow can be obstructed by bending an elbow with an AC catheter) or there is a kink in the IV line.

Bedside ECG Monitor

Depending on the clinical setting, the patient may be set up on a continuous bedside monitor or telemetry. For these monitoring tools to be effective, the nurse must be prepared to recognize arrhythmias and respond accordingly. Common issues with the use of continuous bedside monitoring include misplacement of electrodes, not replacing electrodes routinely, and faulty wiring or a faulty monitor that requires maintenance or new batteries.

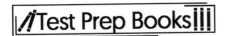
Feeding Tube Pump

Like IV pump alarms, enteral feeding pumps sound an alarm in the event of a blockage or air present in the tubing. A blockage can be the result of a few things and will require the nurse to use nursing judgement. The blockage could be the result of administering a medication that was not intended to be crushed or was not adequately crushed, not flushing the line after administering medications and food, or a kink in the tubing. Nursing interventions include removing any formula present in the tubing and attempting to flush with warm water. Using a feeding tube syringe, a pull-push method can be used gently to try and clear the tubing. Air in the tubing may alarm as "NO FOOD," as the device does not detect the enteral formula, but detects the air bubble instead. Adequately priming the tubing and removing air bubbles will resolve this issue.

Mechanical Ventilator

Mechanical ventilators are seen in the critical care environment and in the home health environment for long-term usage. The nurse should be prepared to recognize and respond to vent alarms, as a ventilator is a life-sustaining piece of equipment. The main alarms the nurse must be prepared to respond to are high-pressure alarms and low-pressure alarms. High-pressure alarms sound in response to high amounts of pressure fighting back on the ventilator. The causes can include the patient coughing, the patient fighting the vent, the presence of a mucus plug or thick secretions, or a kink in the tubing. Low-pressure alarms sound when there is not enough pressure detected and are most often the result of the patient not receiving adequate amounts of ventilation. The causes include disconnected tubing, a dislodged trach tube or ET tube, or an air leak in a cuffed ET tube. For both ventilator alarms, the nurse's first step is to assess whether the patient is in any distress. Interventions can be provided when the airway is patent and respirations are being provided.

Technology Trends in Healthcare

Nurses will need to stay current with IT trends and engage in ongoing education and exposure to technology. Continuing education and training can be accomplished through independent reading, e-learning, and live classroom instruction.

Nurses may encounter a broad range of technologies in the following areas:

- Robots
- Medication delivery devices
- Instruments
- Biotechnology and nanotechnology
- Digital tracking
- Mobile and wireless devices
- Nursing informatics

Radio frequency identification (RFID) provides support for real-time surgery scheduling. This technology has been shown to drastically enhance the structure and functions within medical software. RFID functions on wireless networks and helps to "tag" items and track the movement of the items as they remain on or leave a particular unit. This may be especially important when tracking equipment or supplies that are used to care for the patient or during a surgical procedure.

Nurses may assist in the development of standards for EHR (electronic health record) or other clinically based IT systems that nurses utilize for their sphere of health care. In today's landscape, many nursing applications fall into a variety of categories including the following:

- Internet-based patient education systems
- EHR

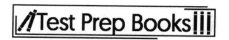

- Telemedicine and telenursing

These systems have the capacity to exchange information and enable the decision-making process to progress along the continuum.

Some nurses possess a master's degree in informatics and also work in a variety of roles to assist with development of clinical systems designed to support nurse activities including the following:

- Business or clinical analyst
- Project management
- Software developer

These systems are designed to accommodate patient education resources, nursing procedures, and critical pathways, to name a few.

Nurses may also serve in the role of perioperative robotics nurse specialist. As robotic surgery utilization continues to evolve into standard practice, the robotics nurse specialist supports a variety of tasks ranging from scheduling maintenance to assisting during surgery.

Health Care Informatics and Technology

Information technology (IT) is a field of nursing that continues to evolve with the rest of health care. Nurses must not only understand the science that is associated with nursing, but they must also be able to navigate various forms of technology. While there are nurses still in the workplace who can recall what it was like to physically fill out forms and track vitals on paper, there are also nurses who have no concept of having documented their activities in these systems. All nurses must be able to function within today's technologically advanced world.

IT is important for many reasons including the following:

- Cost savings/reduction of costs
- Need to decrease or eliminate medication errors
- Improving documentation efficiency by removing paper charting
- Enhancing accessibility to quality health care

Medical technology needs to be fully integrated with a larger system within an institution to support the continuum of patient care. This connection provides information sharing throughout each stage of the treatment period and eventually allows for the collection of statistical data at a later date.

Next, medical technology has to support the user's ability to navigate without difficulty. The goal here is to not slow down the pace of the medical environment but allow for increasing efficiency so that technology is seamless. These qualities then allow for real-time data and real-time decision-making capabilities while reducing the risk of errors or redundancy.

There are a few gaps that remain on the IT front of the medical environment that have their roots in the computerized physician order entry (CPOE) arena. In some instances, CPOE software is not able to meet the needs of various interdisciplinary roles in the OR. The reason for this is that it tends to favor the inpatient setting.

Health care IT, or HIT, has characteristics that are steeped in supporting broad processes or functions.

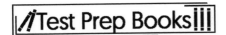

HIT is software that can perform operations associated with the following:

- Admissions
- Scheduling
- Clinical documentation
- Pharmacy
- Laboratory
- Clinical Information Technology

Clinical IT (CIT) concentrates on a particular set of clinical tasks, instruments, equipment, and imaging.

Practice Quiz

1. A patient's ankle/brachial index is 0.39. Which of the following is an expected finding associated with this report?
   a. Chronic edema
   b. Increased pigmentation of the feet
   c. Lower extremity pain at rest
   d. Medial malleolus ulceration

2. Studies have shown that which of the following practices has the most positive impact on patients?
   a. Personalized comfort measures in their post-operation room, such as a favorite snack or book
   b. Internet and television access during their clinical stay
   c. An attentive communication style between their nurses and physicians
   d. Visible operation and safety checklists that staff members regularly check and notate

3. A natural disaster, internet outage, software glitch, and mass casualty event can all result in which of the following?
   a. Improved patient access
   b. Triage
   c. Downtime
   d. An increase in tetanus vaccinations

4. Which statement best describes the evaluation phase of the nursing process?
   a. Subjective, objective, and psychosocial data are gathered in this phase.
   b. Nursing diagnoses are formulated during the evaluation phase.
   c. Evaluation happens across the continuum of the nursing process.
   d. This phase often begins with educating the patient on expected outcomes.

5. What should take place during a postoperative follow-up call by perioperative staff?
   a. Assess for any changes in health status, address patient and family concerns, validate medication regimen, and provide additional education.
   b. Conduct patient satisfaction surveys.
   c. Assess for changes in health status, but avoid excessive reinforcement education activities.
   d. Focus on positive postoperative outcomes instead of highlighting discrepancies in the patient's recovery.

Answer Explanations

1. C: An ankle/brachial index of 0.39 indicates severe peripheral arterial disease, which is commonly associated with lower extremity pain at rest because the amount of oxygen supplied to the tissues is insufficient to meet the metabolic demands of the tissues. The remaining choices are associated with chronic venous insufficiency that is associated with venous congestion that is responsible for the manifestations. Therefore, Choices *A*, *B*, and *D* are incorrect.

2. C: Patients respond favorably to positive intrapersonal communication between their attending nurses and physicians. The other options may be nice for patients, but studies indicate that nurse and physician relationships have the most impact on a patient's overall experience.

3. C: In healthcare, downtime refers to periods when the electronic medical record/electronic health record and/or other clinical software critical for clinical and administrative operations stop working or are inaccessible. This can occur due to technology issues such as internet outages, software problems, or hardware concerns; they can also result from natural disasters and mass casualty events when patient volume becomes too high for electronic systems to be used efficiently. For example, in mass casualty events, patients often end up being seen in in makeshift areas where computers and lab equipment are not available. During downtime periods, patient access to care is often compromised. For example, providers may not be able to use their normal systems to order labs or other medical interventions, and patients typically cannot access their own medical records and documents. Therefore, Choice *A* can be eliminated. While triage may be used during times of natural disaster, mass casualty events, or other instances of overcapacity, this process is typically not implemented due to internet outages and software glitches, so Choice *B* can be eliminated. An increase in tetanus vaccinations is not directly linked to any of the listed causes, so Choice *D* is incorrect.

4. C: The final phase of the nursing process is evaluation; however, evaluation happens across the continuum of the nursing process, not just at the end. The nurse frequently evaluates the effectiveness of care plans, adjusts as necessary, and reevaluates. Data is collected during the assessment phase. Nursing diagnoses are formulated in the diagnosis phase. The implementation phase often begins with educating the patient on expected outcomes.

5. A: Postoperative follow-up calls are an opportunity for perioperative staff to assess recovery of the patient, address questions, provide reinforcement education, and identify any discrepancies that could have a negative impact on the patient's postoperative period. Patient satisfaction calls are not typically conducted by the perioperative staff.

Professional Concepts

Communication

Chain of Command

In any workplace environment, an established chain of command is vital to streamlining communication and improving efficiency. In healthcare, the chain of command can get confusing with so many disciplines and titles and with the frequency of changes. Each individual nurse will need to become familiar with their specific employer's nursing chain of command, but there are general guidelines that the nurse in any clinical setting should recognize:

Chief Nursing Officer (CNO):

- Top tier of nursing leadership, working aside the CEO of the healthcare facility/agency
- Oversees all aspects of nursing care within the healthcare facility/agency

Director of Nursing (DON):

- Administrative nursing with a more hands-on leadership role
- Reports directly to CNO

Advanced Practice Registered Nurse (APRN):

- Includes nurse practitioners (CRNPs), nurse specialists (CNSes), nurse anesthetists (CRNAs), and nurse midwives (CNMs)
- Provides direct patient care in coordination with MDs and/or DOs

Nurse Manager/Unit Manager:

- Manages the nursing staff within an entire unit/department (e.g., nursing manager for all nursing shifts within the Medical ICU)

Charge Nurse:

- Manages the nursing staff within a nursing shift (e.g., charge nurse for the day shift at the Medical ICU)
- Provides direct patient care with assigned patients

Registered Nurse (RN):

- Associate's or Bachelor's degree in nursing
- Provides direct patient care with varying complexities

Licensed Practical Nurse (LPN):

- Diploma/certificate in practical nursing
- Provides basic nursing care in communication with the RN

Nursing Assistant:

- Provides assistance with appropriate ADLs
- Obtains vital signs within scope of practice

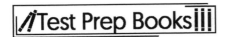

Communication Skills

Similar to the chain of command, effective communication skills are crucial in any workplace but especially in healthcare. While some industries are focused on a product, healthcare is focused on the patient—specifically safe, efficient, and effective patient care. The nurse can provide this level of care through the following elements:

- Practicing active listening
- Utilizing effective verbal and non-verbal communication
- Utilizing effective written communication
- Practicing mediation techniques

Active Listening

The nurse is responsible for being a patient advocate. The best way to truly advocate for a patient is not just to listen but to fully comprehend what the patient wants. To do this, the nurse must practice active listening. This form of listening requires the nurse to receive information by listening to the words, watching the body language, and gauging the feelings of the patient; process the information; and respond accordingly. Active listening not only improves the healthcare practice of patient-centered care but also helps to establish a trusting relationship.

Verbal Communication vs. Non-Verbal Communication

Effective verbal communication is not just simply speaking out loud, but also speaking clearly in the language and form that the patient best understands. The nurse can speak clearly and concisely, but if the patient cannot understand the jargon the nurse used, the verbal communication is not effective.

Nonverbal communication encompasses body language, facial gestures, eye contact, and posture. The patient would not feel as comfortable sharing sensitive information with a nurse that is visibly disconnected with her arms crossed and poor eye contact. Nonverbal communication is the way that the nurse can physically show the patient that they are listening.

Written Communication

Written communication is important throughout the entire healthcare journey, but it becomes especially important with discharge information and medication education, both of which are prominent nursing responsibilities. Providing detailed education or education on multiple topics to the patient can become overwhelming. The patient may only remember bits and pieces of the information and could leave the interaction confused. Providing the patient with written communication can allow the patient to follow up on the information in their own time.

Therapeutic Communication

Overcoming barriers to communication requires practicing therapeutic communication. Therapeutic communication is a type of communication that assists the patient in the healing process rather than hindering it. There are a number of useful communication techniques the nurse can employ to aid in therapeutic communication:

- Sometimes, silence is the best way to get clarification from a patient, or simply asking them to clarify when one does not understand.

- Nurses may offer themselves to support the patient without providing personal details, by sympathizing and saying, "Yes, I have been through something similar."

- The nurse may ask the patient to summarize their thoughts or identify a theme when stories go on at length. This helps redirect communication in a positive direction.

- Asking the patient how certain events made them feel is a way to investigate the patient's emotional status.

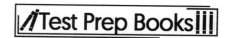

- The nurse may give information about their role and make observations, such as "I noticed you seem tense," to open the door to more fluent conversation.

- Giving the patient praise and recognition without overt flattery is a way to show support, such as complimenting a noticeable effort during a physical therapy session.

- The nurse may want to determine the chronological order of events, which can be helpful for reporting information.

Employing therapeutic communication aids smooth collaboration and cooperation between members of the health care team. Incorporating smart, simple, therapeutic communication techniques and overcoming barriers to communication are important parts of achieving this goal.

Conflict with Patients or Family Members

Nurses sometimes must contend with aggressive and violent behavior from patients or their family members who may be distressed. An aggressive or violent patient can be characterized by the exhibition of any nonverbal behaviors or verbal communication that intend to cause conflict, harm, pain, or injury. An aggressive or violent patient may invade personal space, make verbal threats or obscene gestures, mimic or follow through with physical threats, speak unnecessarily loudly or in a hostile manner, or be generally abusive in some other verbal or physical way. The causes motivating these behaviors are variable. Patients may show aggressive or violent behavior due to a psychiatric or physiological issue, such as drug abuse, delusions, head injuries, and infections of the brain. However, aggressive or violent behavior can also be a result of the patient's personal background and history, such as family upbringing, socioeconomic status, and current personal stressors.

While mediators are available for complex situations, the nurse will need to be prepared to practice basic mediation techniques. It is important for the nurse to remain consistent, not allowing varying emotions to dictate the care they provide. Effective mediation practices include the following:

- Discussing conflicts in detail to verify understanding
- Identifying root issues
- Establishing goals for conflict resolution
- Context reframing

Nurses should assess each patient for potential aggressive or violent behavior. This can include looking for known risk factors on intake forms (e.g., medical and psychological history, documented history of violence or substance use, history of detention or imprisonment, or personal stressors such as unemployment). This can also include assessing the patient directly and taking note of appearance, mental and physical state, pupil size, level of perspiration, mood, tone of speaking, and any comments made by the patient that could indicate current feelings of hostility or anger.

Nurses should be knowledgeable of their health care setting's policies and local laws as they relate to managing or sedating aggressive or violent patients. To protect the safety of medical personnel, the patient, and other patients in the vicinity, if a patient becomes visibly aggressive or violent, physical restraint may need to be provided by a dynamic team from the facility. In some cases, it may be necessary to administer antipsychotic medication or sedation.

Nurses should keep the following principles in mind when handling conflict or communicating with family members:

- Recognize that the family is the constant in the patient's life while the service systems and personnel within those systems fluctuate.

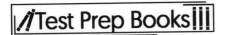
- Be aware of family strengths and individuality and having respect for different methods of coping.

- Encourage and facilitating family-to-family support and networking.

- Share complete and unbiased information about the patient's care with family members on a continuing basis in a supportive manner.

- Design accessible healthcare delivery systems that are flexible, culturally competent, and responsive to family needs.

Information Sharing

Information sharing can be overwhelming for even the most experienced healthcare workers. With a high caseload of patients, varying acuity levels, and only so much time in the day, gaps in communication can easily occur. This is why using communication tactics for sharing pertinent information is so important. The nurse should be prepared to practice both informal and formal types of information sharing.

Standardized Communication Tool

A standardized communication tool sets the same parameters for requested information each time an instance communication occurs. By asking for specific answers to the same set of questions, regardless of who is sending information and who is receiving it, standardized communication tools aim to reduce variability in communication, incomplete or partial communication, and irrelevant communication. In the medical setting, standardized communication tools are associated with improved quality of care, improved patient outcomes, and improved patient satisfaction. Electronic medical records, the SBAR hand-off technique, and safety checklists are examples of standardized communication tools.

Standardized Communication Plan

Standardized communication plans are a component of National Patient Safety Goals. Clear verbal, non-verbal, and written communication between healthcare providers is essential for patients to receive high quality care. Communication is especially crucial during patient transitions, such as nursing shift changes, as these periods are when patients are most likely to experience adverse outcomes. The Joint Commission recommends the SBAR communication technique when one healthcare provider is sharing information about the patient to any other provider. SBAR stands for Situation (why the communication is taking place), Background (the status and medical history of the patient), Assessment (the speaker's perspective of the problem), and Recommendation (what action the speaker believes would be most beneficial to the patient).

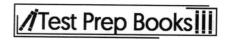
Closed-Loop Communication

Closed-loop communication is commonly seen in the surgical setting, where the surgical team will frequently reiterate instructions given and ensure follow-up to prevent surgical errors, retention of surgical instruments, and postoperative infections. While this is a vital practice in the surgical setting, the healthcare team should also utilize this type of information sharing in routine practice. See the figure below for a visual of how this cyclical communication tool works in practice. It is important for the nurse to practice the check-back communication to "close the loop" and verify that the information obtained is consistent with both parties.

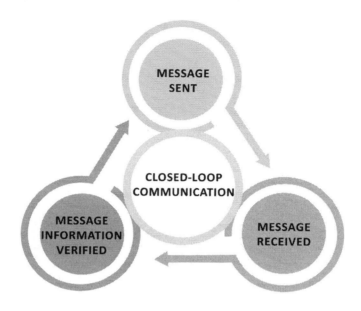

Huddle

Nursing huddles are short, scheduled meetings that occur routinely (such as daily or weekly) to review issues, patient safety data, and any new information (e.g., policy changes). Not only is this a good time to promote teamwork and open communication, it is also a good time for the frontline staff to voice any concerns (e.g., a new supply not working as well as the previous one used).

Bedside Report

Giving the change-of-shift report at the bedside is a practice that every nurse should adopt for the improvement of patient-centered care. Not only can this form of report save time by including the patient/family in all handoff information, it also reduces the risk for medical errors. Performing a bedside report can also allow both nurses to be hands-on with relaying assessment information.

Interdisciplinary Team/Group (IDT/IDG)

Interdisciplinary communication ensures patient safety. Although documentation in the EMR provides quick access to the patient's clinical history, any immediate concerns should be verbally communicated to the appropriate provider. The interdisciplinary team is composed of professionals within various disciplines and specialties. The nurse must be knowledgeable of the roles and responsibilities of each health care team member to ensure purposeful communication.

Interdisciplinary meetings can be formal or informal but will require structure to be effective. Some healthcare facilities like to do bedside IDT meetings, while others prefer a more formal structure such as using a meeting room. The importance of this type of information sharing cannot be overstated. Every aspect of the patient's care—

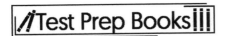

physical, emotional, spiritual, financial, mental, and social—will be discussed in this setting of information sharing. Changes in the patient's level of care, medications, and therapies will be discussed, along with pertinent discharge planning, social/community resources, and any spiritual or cultural concerns/needs.

SBAR

The **SBAR technique** is a highly favored method that nurses utilize for hand-offs. SBAR stands for Situation, Background, Assessment, and Recommendation. The advantages of using SBAR include the following:

- Enhancement of situational awareness

- Promotion and utilization of critical-thinking skills

- Predictable and reliable communication

- Provision of a framework that reduces bias commonly seen with organizational hierarchy and experience

- Expansion of collaborative interactions between nurses and physicians

- Advancement of collaborative discussions in nurse-to-nurse exchanges

Situation

For the situation, the nurse identifies what is happening with the patient. The overview should be concise. It is a succinct statement of the problem. Examples of situation details include the following:

- Demographics (patient and surgeon names, other physicians, age, admission date, surgery date)
- Problem
- Patient stability

Background

In reviewing the background, the nurse provides information about the patient's clinical background that is applicable and relevant to the patient's current situation. He or she is answering the question, "What got us to this point?" Examples of background information details include the presentation history.

Assessment

For the assessment component, nurses should describe findings and provide an analysis of possible options and considerations. Examples of assessment details include the following:

- Procedure-specific assessment
- Vital signs
- Temperature (route of temperature)
- Blood pressure (e.g., cuff or arterial line)
- Monitoring
- Hemodynamic pressure
- Pulse (e.g., apical or peripheral)
- Respiratory status
- Breath sounds
- Oxygen saturation
- Mechanical ventilator settings
- End-tidal carbon dioxide

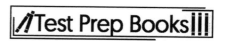
- Monitoring
- Lab results
- Neurological function (e.g., level of consciousness)
- Intake and output (e.g., intravenous [IV] fluids)
- Location(s) of IV access
- Pain
- Pain rating
- Sedation level
- Dressings and drains
- Condition of the skin
- Drainage (type, color, amount)
- Scores
- Scores associated with the procedure itself
- Monitors and readings (including cardiac monitor)

Recommendation

Finally, the recommendation aspect of the hand-off report should serve as a discussion among professionals about what should happen next. This discussion focuses on next steps and concerns. It is an excellent opportunity to identify if there is a need to update the plan of care or notify the surgeon or physician of any findings, medication adjustments, and pending laboratory data.

Read-Back/Repeat

Some organizations incorporate an additional R, which is known as the read-back or repeat. This extra step is where staff can read back orders to ensure that there is a mutual understanding of the need.

It is a sequential process that challenges individuals only to include pertinent and relevant data. The recipient of the information validates their understanding of the information. This clarification period gives the communicator an opportunity to clarify details if necessary or to take any essential action.

The SBAR method allows nurses to spend less time writing. This effect, in turn, increases the amount of time they can focus on patient care. Studies demonstrate that use of the SBAR technique reduces the risk of adverse events, including death, and increases communication among nursing staff. It has become an industry best practice according to The Joint Commission, and as a result, organizations use electronic tools that reflect the SBAR framework to comply with The Joint Commission on Accreditation of Healthcare Organizations' National Patient Safety Goals.

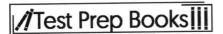

S Situation

I am calling about ....

The patient's Code status is ....

The problem I am calling about is ....

e.g. I am concerned the patient is going to arrest

I have just assessed the patient personally:

Vital signs are: Blood Pressure   .... / ....   Pulse ....

Respiration ....   Temperature ....

I am concerned about the:

Blood pressure because it is	**over 200** or	**less than 100** or	**30 mmHg below usual**
Pulse because it is	**over 130** or	**less than 40 and symptomatic**	
Respiration because it is	**less than 8** or	**over 30**	
Temperature because it is	**less than 96** or	**over 104**	
Urine output because it is	**less than 25 ml/hr** or	**200 ml/8hrs**	
O₂ because it is	**less than 88% on 6/liters**	**nasal cannula**	

Other ....

B Background

The patient's mental status is:

Alert and oriented to person, place, and time

Confused and   cooperative or   non-cooperative

Agitated or   combative

Lethargic but conversant and able to swallow

Stuporous and not talking clearly and possibly not able to swallow

Comatose   Eyes closed   Not responding to stimulation

The skin is:

Warm and dry   Pale   Mottled

Diaphoretic   Extremities are cold   Extremities are warm

The patient   is not or   **is on oxygen**

The patient has been on .... (l/min) or (5) oxygen for .... minutes (hours)

The oximeter is reading .... %

The oximeter does not detect a good pulse and is giving erratic readings.

A Assessment

This is what I think the problem is ....

"Say what you think the problem is"

The problem seems to be   cardiac   infection   neurologic   respiratory

I am not sure what the problem is but the patient is deteriorating

The patient seems to be unstable and may get worse, we need to do something

R Recommendation

From Physician ....

Transfer the patient to Critical Care   Come to see the patient at this time

Talk to the patient or family about Code status   Ask a consultant to see patient now

Are any tests needed:

Do you need any test like   CXR   ABG   EKG   CBC   BMP

Others ....

If a change in treatment is ordered then ask:

How often do you want vital signs?

How long do you expect this problem will last?

If the patient does not get better when would you want us to call again?

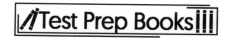

Transfer of Care

When possible, a face-to-face discussion will take place between the team transferring the patient and the staff receiving the patient. A patient qualifies for transfer to a different unit once their health status stabilizes and transfer of care does not create a safety risk. Nurses must document all transfers of care within the patient's medical record.

Here is an example of an SBAR intraoperative hand-off to the PACU:

Components of an Intraoperative SBAR Hand-Off to PACU	
Situation	<ul><li>Patient name</li><li>Surgical Procedure (including site)</li><li>Anesthetist provider name</li><li>Surgeon name</li></ul>
Background	<ul><li>Anesthesia administration</li><li>Medications and dosage (including antibiotics)</li><li>IV fluids/sites</li><li>Blood type/products</li><li>Specimens (type, location, quantity, tests requested)</li><li>Estimated blood loss</li><li>Urine output</li><li>Surgical sites</li><li>Dressings, tubes, drainage (including location)</li><li>Unexpected or adverse events in the OR</li></ul>
Assessment	<ul><li>Hemodynamic stability</li><li>Respiratory/airway/oxygenation status</li><li>Pain status and pain management</li><li>Body temperature (i.e., hyperthermia or hypothermia)</li><li>Neuro status</li><li>Monitoring (e.g., equipment, lines)</li><li>Special needs (e.g., autism, disabilities)</li><li>Safety risks</li></ul>
Recommendations	<ul><li>Implement postoperative orders</li><li>Allow for time to answer questions of PACU staff before, during, and after transfer of patient</li><li>Actively support patient transfer activities (including lines, equipment, and patient)</li><li>Address any known family concerns</li><li>Discharge from the PACU once stable</li></ul>

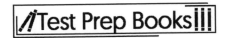

Handoff Report

As one shift ends and another begins, there is a **handoff report** that is given from the off-going team to the oncoming team. The medical-surgical nurse who has completed the shift will tell the nurse beginning the next shift all pertinent information related to each individual patient.

The communication experience during the hand-off process should be a work of art that demonstrates all of the characteristics of a clean exchange of information among professionals. **Hand-offs** not only allow for the dissemination of information from one profession to another but serve as an opportunity for the receiving professional to ask questions and identify concerns. They act as a means to protect the patient from harm and enable professionals to provide a high level of continuity of care.

Patients are most susceptible to an adverse event during the hand-off time frame, as with most transitions in care during the perioperative period. The reasons for the enhanced risk are closely related to organizational behavior and patterns during the perioperative process that may influence the hand-off process. Common distractions that arise include patient volume in the receiving unit, the need to maintain a rapid and "efficient" pace during the turnover phase, and reduction of abrasion with surgeons.

The hectic pace of the perioperative environment increases the risk for mistakes and inexplicable communication errors. According to one study, sentinel events occur as a result of poor communication practices that take place during the hand-off process. Nurses can become complacent in this exercise because it is very much part of their routine activities. Organizations must follow a standardized method for hand-off communications to reduce the danger of any impact to patient safety. This standardized approach is a requirement of The Joint Commission.

The requirement dictates that professionals must allow adequate time to exchange information and ask questions and to allow for responses. The benefit of following a standard practice helps to reduce errors and potentially avoid exclusion of pertinent data. Nurses can follow a consistent method for the following:

- Documentation practices
- Review and discussion of critical information
- Adequate preparation and delivery of patient care

A standardized shift handoff procedure can provide a seamless transition between two different medical staff members who may be providing care for the same patient. It can provide detailed and crucial information about the patient and the case; equally important, it can serve as a tool that indicates that official responsibility has moved from one provider to another. This provides a clear mechanism for providing accountability for the individual who is overseeing specific tasks between staff members.

Internal handoffs occur within the same healthcare facility, including, but not limited to, shift handoffs and inter-department handoffs (e.g., a physical therapist is working with a patient in the orthopedic surgery ward). All established healthcare facilities will have their own internal handoff protocols. This can include procedures such as formal handoff training for new staff, continuing training for established staff, verbal handoff protocols, written handoff forms, and stringent repercussions for staff members who fail to meet handoff standards.

External handoffs occur between two separate healthcare entities or during a transition of care. Unless the two systems involved have similar procedures, external handoffs can be compromising situations for the patients and prone to errors.

Errors in handoffs can occur when procedures are not standardized—that is, they do not occur in the exact same manner and convey the exact same information each time a handoff occurs. Developing formal, written standard operating procedures can eliminate the occurrence of various human errors. Standardizing a process may include (but is not limited to) a written checklist, a process flowchart, a meaningful acronym, or an audit tool for staff

236

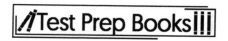

members to follow. Additionally, errors in handoffs can occur when established standard operating procedures are ignored, written poorly, or are too broad for the scope of the procedure. Errors in handoffs can also occur if medical staff are rushed, are unsure of the team members they are working with, or receive incorrect information anywhere along the duration of a patient's stay.

Read-Back for Verbal Orders

Read-back occurs when staff reads back orders to ensure that there is a mutual understanding of the need. It is a sequential process that challenges individuals to include only pertinent and relevant data. The recipient of the information validates their understanding of the information. This clarification period gives the communicator an opportunity to clarify details if necessary or to take any essential action.

Ideally, verbal orders should only occur when the provider is physically unable to write out the orders due to an emergency or other extenuating circumstances. Verbal orders must be carefully read back to the provider to ensure accuracy. The verbal order process includes receiving, reading back, documenting, and executing the order. During the read-back, the nurse must repeat the order that was given as it is interpreted. The provider must then confirm the read-back with the nurse.

After the verbal order has been given, the nurse must document the date and time of the order as well as the provider's name. After the emergency situation has passed, the provider must review the verbal order for accuracy and sign the order, including the date and time. Verbal orders must be physically signed by the provider within 24 hours of being given to the nurse.

Perioperative Interdisciplinary Communication

During the preoperative stage, the nurse performs a health history assessment on the patient. Information such as the patient's allergies, medications, acute and chronic illnesses, past surgeries, and overall health status must be obtained. Relevant history must be communicated to the appropriate heath care provider. The relevancy depends on the procedure.

For example, a patient with a fractured tibia will undergo internal fixation with implanted hardware. The procedure will require intraoperative imaging studies with the use of contrast media. The patient reports an allergy to shellfish during the health history assessment. The nurse must document this information in the patient's medical record and inform the surgical team prior to the procedure. The patient also reports adverse effects to general anesthesia during a past surgery. The nurse would communicate this concern to the anesthesiologist. Additionally, the patient's latest laboratory results indicate a potassium level of 6.8 mmol/L. The nurse identifies this result as a critical value. Hyperkalemia can result in cardiac arrest and must be corrected prior to surgery. Postoperatively, the nurse must continue to communicate the patient's health status with the interdisciplinary team. For example, after surgery, the patient has episodes of hypotension and verbalizes dizziness when sitting upright. A consult to physical therapy has been ordered. Before the physical therapist can assess the patient, the nurse must communicate the patient's hypotensive episodes and weight bearing status.

Communication with the interdisciplinary team must be relevant and succinct. The use of SBAR (situation-background-assessment-recommendation) can guide nurses to communicate concerns effectively. *Situation* provides a brief statement of the current problem. *Background* should include pertinent information that relates to the current situation. *Assessment* can include physical findings, lab results, and objective and subjective data. *Recommendation* is a request for resources, medications, or further guidance. For example, a patient who had abdominal surgery has end stage renal disease and is being managed by a hospitalist, nephrologist, and general surgeon. Postoperatively, the patient develops fluid volume overload. The nurse would contact the patient's nephrologist to communicate the patient's condition. Following the SBAR technique, the nurse would include the following information: "The patient recently had abdominal surgery and has developed symptoms of fluid overload.

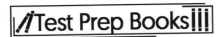
The patient has history of end stage renal disease and currently has +3 edema to the extremities and crackles upon auscultation. Should a diuretic be anticipated?"

Communication Barriers

Prior to providing effective communication, the nurse will need to assess any communication barriers present. It is easy to just associate language with communication barriers, but the nurse will need to assess for more than that to ensure communication is both received and comprehended by the patient/family. Communication barriers can present in the form of a language barrier, cultural barrier, cognitive impairments or limitations, and physical impairments.

Language/Cultural Barriers

Language barriers can vary from completely different languages to mild accent differences. The nurse will need to become familiar with the facility/agency translation services. Each healthcare facility/agency will have an approved translation procedure to use. Using an approved interpreter can not only improve communication but can also provide cultural sensitivity/phrasing. Language barriers can also present with the use of slang or complex medical jargon.

Cultural barriers can present without a language gap. The nurse will need to be prepared to care for patients with varying cultural backgrounds without judgment. For example, some Asian cultures highly value stoicism when experiencing pain. If the patient states a verbal pain score of 10/10 and remains expressionless, the nurse will be responsible for communicating with the patient and treating the patient accordingly, as this is a cultural difference in reception and expression of pain.

Cognitive Impairments/Limitations

Cognitive impairments or limitations can occur due to neurological damage (e.g., CVA, TBI), a congenital disorder, or just the standard progression of childhood understanding. Cognitive impairments or limitations will require the nurse to establish the appropriate form and level of communication. For example, educating a five-year-old patient on an upcoming procedure will require the nurse to recognize the cognitive limitations present. The attention span, memory, and comprehension are not that of an adult, so the nurse will need to provide age-appropriate teachings.

Physical Impairments

Physical impairments include anything that would physically hinder the patient from speaking or hearing effectively. A common example is a hearing deficit that would require the nurse to speak clearly and slowly, without shouting at the patient.

De-escalation Techniques

De-escalation in healthcare can be a complicated balancing act between empathizing with the individual and establishing boundaries of mutual respect. There are a few techniques that the nurse should feel comfortable practicing in the event that a patient, family member, or even coworker needs to be de-escalated.

First, the situation should be taken to a private area with a safe exit for the nurse at all times. Not only can the stimuli from a public environment worsen agitation, it can also create a situation in which an altercation is more likely to occur.

Next, the nurse needs to focus on maintaining a calm demeanor. Regardless of the individual's level of anger, the nurse should always maintain a non-threatening posture and calm voice. Using active listening and empathy, the nurse can attempt to de-escalate the individual.

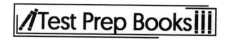
Lastly, the nurse needs to ensure that firm boundaries are in place. The concept of respect will need to go both ways, and it is appropriate for the nurse to calmly reiterate the consequences to certain actions.

Critical Thinking

Time Management and Prioritization of Care

The ability to establish priorities is one of the nurse's most important skills. The nurse must be able to look at their patient load for the day, assess the needs of each patient, organize tasks in chronological order, and prioritize each task based on its importance and necessity.

When prioritizing the tasks for the day, the nurse must first employ their knowledge of the body, how it works, and what it needs to function. The nurse starts with ABC: airway, breathing, and circulation. Are any patients compromised in these respects? If so, they are immediately placed at the top of the list of priorities. If the patient cannot breathe, they are hemorrhaging, or their heart has stopped beating, they require the nurse's immediate assistance. The ABCs are considered the first priority of patient needs:

- A: Airway
- B: Breathing
- C: Circulation
- D: Disability
- E: Examine
- F: Fahrenheit
- G: Get Vitals
- H: Head to Toe Assessment
- I: Intervention

After the ABC patient needs are taken care of, the nurse can move down the scale to the next priority. A helpful acronym to remember is M-A-A-U-A-R. These are considered second-priority needs:

- M is for mental status changes and alterations

- A is for acute pain

- A is for acute urinary elimination concerns

- U is for unaddressed and untreated problems requiring immediate attention

- A is for abnormal laboratory/diagnostic data outside of normal limits

- R is for risks that include those involving a healthcare problem such as safety, skin integrity, infection, and other medical conditions

Along with the ABC-MAAUAR methods of prioritization, the nurse may also utilize Maslow's hierarchy of needs. Maslow argues that physiological needs such as hunger, thirst, and breathing are among the first that have to be met. The same goes for patients. For example, a patient in pain needs to be addressed before a patient who needs education on a procedure that is to happen tomorrow.

After the basic physiological needs have been met, the nurse knows that on the next level of the pyramid are safety and psychological needs. Mental health fits on this tier of the hierarchy and is a crucial step toward wellness. Love and belonging follow; for this part of care the nurse can enlist the help of social services and family members. The

239

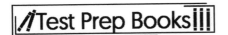

next level of Maslow's hierarchy is "self-esteem and esteem by others." In nursing terms, this level represents the patient's need to feel they are a respected and esteemed member of the care team. The final level of Maslow's hierarchy is self-actualization, in which a person reaches their fullest potential and highest level of ability. The nurse does everything they can to help the client reach this level, pushing them to do their best and be their best at all points in the care journey.

Recognizing the patient's needs and establishing priorities based on Maslow's hierarchy, the nurse can then move on to the next step of the process. After goal-setting and client care delivery comes the evaluation stage. In fact, evaluation does not happen only at the end. The nurse must be continually evaluating the plan of care for each patient. The plan may need tweaking and revision throughout the day, based on how the patient responds to interventions. Quality evaluation of interventions ensures needs are being met and proper care is being delivered.

Sound nursing judgment will guide the nurse as they endeavor to prioritize and adequately meet the needs of their patients in a timely manner.

In the event of a medical emergency, there are specific steps to take depending on the situation. There will be written policies for these types of emergencies in the workplace that are used for patients, staff, and/or visitors.

Crisis Situations and Resources

While not every nurse will work in an emergency care or critical care environment, every nurse needs to be prepared to manage the initial stages of a crisis situation, as well as be aware of readily available resources. Nurses in home health, med-surg, outpatient, step-down, and primary care (just to name a few) will need to recognize, assess, and promptly respond to warning signs of a crisis. So what are the warning signs of a pending crisis? While most healthcare facilities will have an Early Warning System (EWS) in place, the nurse will need to know the specific parameters and when it is time to increase the level of care. Generally, EWSes look at the following assessments to determine if there is a pending crisis:

- Temperature
- Heart rate
- Blood pressure
- Respiratory rate
- LOC
- UO

In the event that one of these assessment readings falls either above or below the set parameters, further assessment is required. An EWS has a scoring system based on the severity and the accumulated score of all assessments, with a key in place to give information on the total score. With that being said, the nurse will need to be prepared to apply nursing judgment. For example, if a medical-surgical nurse is caring for a patient who was extubated 12 hours prior and has a respiratory rate of 35 (shallow) with audible stridor, the nurse will need to immediately enact the emergency protocol—in this case, the rapid response team (RRT). The nurse should quickly recognize that this could be post-extubation laryngeal edema that would require immediate assessment and intervention.

For outpatient crisis referrals, the nurse will need to instruct the patient to go to the emergency department for the appropriate level of care. But for the inpatient nurse, the RRT becomes a vital resource in the event of early crisis intervention. The RRT is a multi-disciplinary team of critical care clinicians that can provide preliminary care to stabilize the patient while the appropriate level of care is established. The nurse outside of the critical care environment should use this resource in the event of any acute deterioration in a patient's health.

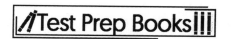

Crisis Management

While discussing a crisis, the immediate thought in healthcare is a physical crisis (e.g., cardiac arrest, hemorrhage, collapsed airway, etc.). But the nurse will need to be prepared to provide crisis management for various types of events. A crisis can be caused by life-changing events like birth, death, marriage, and divorce, as well as by accidents, illnesses, natural disasters, or social issues like violence and war. A crisis can also vary significantly from person to person, depending on their ability to cope with stressors.

While there are different stages of crisis, there are also different levels of nursing intervention. In the earlier stages of a crisis, the individual will have notable anxiety but can still somewhat cope with the stressor. The nurse in this situation must practice active listening, empathize with the individual, and demonstrate respect, without demonstrating any threatening body language or non-verbal gestures. Crisis resolution is the goal in all stages of crisis management but can be easier to attain in the early stages.

Later stages of crisis include severe levels of uncontrolled anxiety. The individual may become combative and lose the ability to reason. The important elements for the nurse and individual in these stages are de-escalation and safety. The individual may be a threat to themselves or others in the later stages. The patient may not be receptive to assistance and could even grow argumentative, but it is important for the nurse to not argue or engage with the patient. Establishing boundaries and getting assistance when needed is key for the nurse caring for an individual in an advanced stage of crisis.

Critical Thinking

Critical thinking is a skill that comes from experience (both successes and failures). The nurse-to-be can be the smartest person in the classroom, making perfect scores on every test, but will not be able to provide quality care without using critical thinking. Common practices for using critical thinking in nursing include the following:

- Using self-regulation
- Practicing problem-solving
- Analyzing and interpreting information
- Making appropriate inferences
- Using the nursing process

Self-Regulation

Self-regulation is a responsibility of every nurse. To self-regulate, the nurse must first fully understand their individual scope of practice (federal, state, and agency regulations). Practicing within the established scope of practice, the nurse's goal is to provide effective, safe, and ethical care practices.

Problem Solving

Problem-solving skills are essential in the practice of critical thinking. Using critical thinking to recognize the problem is important, but the nurse must also cultivate the mindset of finding potential solutions. Problem solving can be seen formally in care plans, but the nurse will need to understand the importance of putting this into practice.

For example, say a patient is prescribed digoxin, and the nurse is due to administer the medication. The nurse with critical thinking skills will check the heart rate prior to administering the medication. Upon further assessment, the heart rate is 40 bpm. The nurse with problem-solving skills will recognize that this medication should not be administered, and the medical provider should be contacted for further orders.

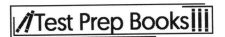

Analysis, Interpretation, and Making Inferences

Additional key practices in critical thinking include analyzing data, interpreting results, and making inferences based on that interpretation. Why is the patient's heart rate 40 bpm? That would be the question the nurse needs to analyze, and they could find that information by looking through past vital sign trends, medications, comorbidities, and procedures. It is important for the healthcare team not to stop at just recognizing the problem and solving it, as that does not likely prevent the problem from happening again. Analyzing the data gives the nurse the information to interpret and then allows them to make clinical inferences based on the results.

For example, if the previously mentioned patient was also taking ivabradine, an HCN channel blocker for progressing heart failure, the nurse could infer that the combination of ivabradine and digoxin is the culprit of the patient's bradycardia. The following is a breakdown of the critical-thinking process in this scenario:

- **Analyzing** the medication administration record
- Interpreting the results
- **Inferring** that the synergistic effect of the medications can cause the problem

This process of critical thinking allows the medical team to either closely monitor the patient on both medications or make a medication change to acknowledge the problem.

The Nursing Process

While the nursing process is an accumulation of the previously discussed components of critical thinking, the nurse will need to understand the cycle of the nursing process. Below is a visual to demonstrate the steps of the nursing process.

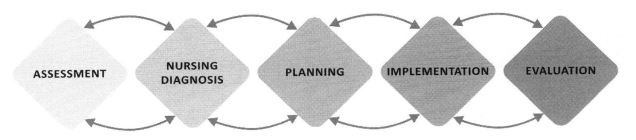

It is important to note that the cycle of the nursing process does not just move in one direction, and it may take multiple steps back to get to the solution. If the nursing diagnosis is no longer applicable, the nurse will need to go back to the assessment phase. Using this method of critical thinking gives the nurse an overview of the procedural process while also allowing for the flexibility needed in healthcare.

Perioperative

The perioperative experience can result in multiple patient complications. Invasive procedures carry risks ranging from infection, hemorrhage, accidental injury, hemodynamic instability, and prolonged recovery periods. At every stage, the nurse must use critical thinking skills to maintain the patient's health and safety. Critical thinking skills are acquired through years of bedside experience and knowledge gained from training programs and continuing education. Nurses must use a variety of problem solving and intuitive skills to ensure patient care issues are prevented or addressed in a timely manner.

In the preoperative stage, nurses must use critical thinking skills to determine if a patient is stable enough to undergo an invasive procedure. Although the determination is made collaboratively with other members of the healthcare team, nurses oversee the entire patient experience. It is crucial to perform interventions such as conducting a physical assessment, reviewing laboratory results, and assessing a patient's physical and mental well-

242

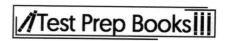
being before the procedure. Any concerns must immediately be reported to the healthcare provider. For example, if a patient will be sedated for a prolonged period of time, a respiratory assessment is a priority. Should the nurse auscultate crackles in the lungs or note any respiratory abnormality, the patient may need further screening to determine the stability of their health status. Anticipating potential problems and promptly reporting abnormal results is an essential critical thinking skill that can prevent intraoperative complications.

Postoperatively, the nurse must assess the patient's ability to recover. Interventions in the immediate postoperative period include monitoring vital signs, maintaining fluids, controlling pain, and assessing the surgical site. Any abnormalities that can hinder recovery should be reported immediately. For example, if the nurse notices decreased capillary refill and discoloration to an extremity that underwent a wound debridement, these findings may indicate a potential problem with wound healing and recovery. Before the nurse receives orders from the healthcare provider, interventions to maintain circulation would be implemented (i.e., maintaining a stable blood pressure, ensuring adequate hydration, and preventing immobility).

Ethical Dilemmas

Healthcare providers routinely face situations with patients where they must analyze various moral and ethical considerations. In the medical-surgical unit, where quick judgment and action can be necessary to care and where patients are often not fully sound in body or mind, ethical dilemmas can arise without much time to process resolutions.

Above all else, nurses have the responsibility to do no harm while advocating for, promoting good health outcomes for, minimizing injury to, and protecting the overall health and functioning of their patients. It is important to consider the patient holistically when applying these values, such as considering what the patient may view as a good quality of life, what family values the patient holds, other family members that may be affected (such as a spouse or children), legal considerations, and logistical considerations (such as how much time and medical resources are available). When patients are unable to make decisions autonomously, or even to indicate consent to treatment (as can be common in emergency cases), nurses should act from these responsibilities to make wise and compassionate decisions on the patients' behalf.

Dilemmas that can arise for nursing staff include situations where the patient may have cultural or personal beliefs that prevent lifesaving treatment. For example, a female patient may not want to be treated by any male staff, or a patient that needs a blood transfusion may not accept this procedure due to religious beliefs. In cases where the patient is able to directly communicate their wishes, the nurse may need to defer to the patient's wishes in order to preserve the patient's autonomy. This may mean providing alternative means of care (such as finding available female medical providers to assist with the female patient that does not want to be treated by male staff).

It may mean withholding treatment that the patient refuses. If the patient's life is in question and rapid medical action is necessary to save the patient's life, nursing staff may need to intervene even if it is against the patient's wishes. Ethical considerations like these will vary by case and patient and will depend on the severity of the case, the medical and personal history of the patient, and the judgment of the nurse in question. In all cases, it is ideal if the nurse and patient are able to communicate openly with each other about the case and potential medical options, and hope that the resolution is able to be for the greatest good.

Healthy Practice Environment

Workplace Safety

Personal Protective Equipment

Personal protective equipment (PPE) refers to any equipment used to protect the wearer from hazardous materials such as bodily fluids, chemicals, radiation, noxious gases, blunt objects, or other items that could cause personal

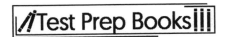

injury upon contact, consumption, or inhalation. OSHA requires that employers train all workers in the safety precautions that pertain to their industry and job role. Healthcare providers often work with PPE that protect them from infectious patients. These commonly include items like gloves, surgical masks, surgery gowns and booties, and protective eyewear. Healthcare providers also require PPE that protect them from hazardous material that is not biological in nature, such as medicinal compounds or disinfecting agents, especially if they regularly work in a laboratory setting.

Hands-Free Zone

Hands-free zones are used to minimize risks from sharps handling. Research shows that most sharps injuries occur when healthcare providers are passing them to one another. Hands-free techniques recommend that only one healthcare provider holds a sharp at a time, therefore eliminating passing sharps between two people. Instead, healthcare providers should place a sharp down in a designated area, known as the neutral zone, where the next person can retrieve it. Most healthcare facilities use designated areas in which only a single sharp can be placed and a standardized verbal hand-off technique to pass the sharp. In addition, some healthcare facilities take hands-free handling one step further by using tools such as forceps to handle any sharp, even to place it in the neutral zone. This practice aims to ensure that a healthcare provider does not ever make actual hand contact with a sharp.

MSDS

A material safety data sheet (MSDS) was regularly found in healthcare facilities, laboratories, and other settings where chemicals are used. It provided information about relevant chemicals, how to store and use them, potential risks, and how to manage hazards that may occur. After 2012, the United States adopted the safety data sheet (SDS) information system, which stems from the Globally Harmonized System of Classification and Labelling of Chemicals. This system is an international standard for chemical safety. It covers 16 comprehensive sections relating to chemical mixtures, identifying hazards, ingredient information, first aid responses to potential hazards, action required in the event of accidental spills, handling and storage, exposure, toxicology, ecological considerations, proper waste management, transportation considerations, and regulatory information as set forth by the country of location.

Safe Handling of Chemotherapeutic Agents

Medical-surgical nurses may care for patients with cancer at some point in their treatment. They are not generally required to administer IV chemotherapy because this is a function typically managed by a physician or oncology nurse. The surgeon may administer chemotherapy in the OR during a surgical procedure, or this may take place following the procedure in another location. However, medical-surgical nurses may have to handle these chemotherapeutic agents.

Chemotherapeutic Agent	Medication Class	Route of Administration
Biodegradable Polymers	Alkylating agent	Intracranial, intracavity
Methotrexate	Antimetabolite	Intrathecal
Mitomycin	Antineoplastic antibiotic	Intravesical instillation, topical ophthalmic
Cytarabine	Antimetabolite	Intrathecal
Pegaspargase	Enzyme	Intramuscular injection

These agents can be a hazard to nurses who are handling them due to the antineoplastic agents, which are toxic compounds. Therefore, these agents require special handling and disposal. They have the label of being on the "P-list" or "U-list." These lists help to identify which commercial chemical products are "hazardous." There are three items or sets of criteria that must be met for an agent to receive the designation of P or U:

- The formulation has to contain a chemical on the P- or U-list.

244

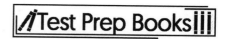

- The chemical in the waste must be unused.
- The chemical in the waste has to be the only active ingredient.

Evidence-based practices for safe handling of chemotherapeutic agents are imperative for the safety of staff:

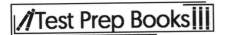

Process	Description
Appropriate Use of PPE	Nurses and physicians should don appropriate PPE during chemotherapy procedures. Proper practices should include: • Double gloving • Wearing a mask • Eye protection • Impervious gown
Transportation and Disposal Procedures	Tips for transportation and disposal procedures include: Chemotherapeutic agent should be verified between pharmacist and registered nurse. Disposable instruments and equipment should be used with chemotherapeutic agents to reduce the need of processing instruments that have been exposed to chemotherapeutic agents. Containers must have a chemotherapy label and should be sent to the sterile processing department. Chemotherapeutic agents should be transported using a puncture-resistant container before and after the surgical procedure. Staff must change gloves after chemotherapeutic agent administration and before proceeding with the surgery.
Sterile Processing	Sterile processing department personnel have to wear PPE and must also double-glove when handling and processing chemotherapy contaminated instruments and equipment.
Documentation Protocol for Chemotherapy	The nurse documents: Names of the chemotherapeutic agent, medication, dose, route of administration, date, and time of administration Name of the physician administering the agent Name of the nurse checking the agent prior to administration
Medication Safety and Chemotherapy Time-Out	Nurses must monitor patient safety at all times and know what medication and orders the physician has created for the patient. Route of medication administration is especially important in the OR setting.
Acceptable Environment	A designated area should be used for the preparation of chemotherapeutic agents.
Physician Orders	Verbal orders are not acceptable for chemotherapy administration. Orders should be written on a designated chemotherapy order form.

Processes and procedures should address items such as the following:

- Appropriate use of PPE
- Transportation and disposal procedures
- Sterile processing

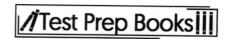

- Documentation protocol for chemotherapy
- Acceptable environment preparation of chemotherapeutic agents
- Physician orders
- Medication safety and chemotherapy time-out

Proper Body Mechanics

Ergonomics is the science of matching the physical requirements of a job to the physical abilities of the worker. Musculoskeletal injuries can occur if physical demands are greater than the individual's physical capabilities. Body mechanics refers to how the body moves during activities of daily living.

The hospital environment can present potential hazards that increase risk of injury to the nurse. Proper body mechanics should be consistently followed to prevent injury. There are three foundational principles of proper body mechanics that should be followed by nurses. First, bending at the hips and knees instead of at the waist uses the large muscle groups of the legs instead of the back muscles and helps to prevent back injury. Second, standing with feet at about shoulder-width apart helps to reduce risk of injury by providing foundational support. Finally, the nurse should keep the back, neck, pelvis, and feet aligned when turning or moving. Twisting and bending at the neck and waist can increase risk of injury.

As a standard of care, many healthcare institutions have mandated use of **safe patient mobilization (SPM)** equipment in an effort to reduce injuries as well as to promote patient safety. SPM equipment can be used during patient transfers and positioning.

Slide sheets are often used in patient transfers. These sheets are placed underneath the patient prior to lateral or vertical transfer. They decrease the surface tension, making transfers easier. However, since the slide sheets do decrease surface tension, they must be removed after use, so that the patient is not at risk of sliding off the bed.

Inflatable blankets can be placed under the patient to assist in lateral transfers, as well. When engaged, the forced air blanket helps to support the weight of the patient, making lateral transfers easier. The mattress should be deflated after completion of transfer.

Another type of SPM equipment is lift equipment. Lift equipment works by placing a sling under the patient's limb or underneath the entire patient, connecting the sling to the lift machine, and programming the machine to lift the body to the desired height. The weight limits of these machines vary, so the medical-surgical nurse must ensure the patient's weight does not exceed the weight limit set by the manufacturer.

Hazardous Waste Management

According to the Institute of Hazardous Materials Management (IHMM), a **hazardous material** is defined as "any item that has the potential to cause harm to humans, animals, or the environment, either by itself or through interaction with other factors." A hazardous item may be biological, chemical, radiological, and/or physical in nature. Agencies such as the United States Environmental Protection Agency (EPA) and the Occupational Safety and Health Administration (OSHA) provide regulation and guidelines as to how hazardous materials are handled.

Hazardous materials in the medical environment can include biological, chemical, radiological, and physical hazards. Biological hazardous materials are commonly referred to as **biohazards**. These are materials that present a threat to the health of living things, primarily humans. Biohazards are typically introduced into the medical environment in the form of patient body fluids and excreta. Examples of biohazardous materials are blood, body fluids, viruses, and bacteria. Items in the medical environment that have been exposed to biohazardous materials are considered to be biohazardous, as well, until the decontamination process is completed. For example, used surgical instruments are considered biohazardous until they have been cleaned of bioburden and sterilized.

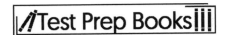

Chemical hazardous materials in the medical environment include solid, liquid, or gas materials that pose a threat to health. Primarily, solid and liquid chemical hazards include materials used to clean, disinfect, and sanitize the medical environment. They may also include cytotoxic and chemotherapy medications. Gas chemicals are primarily anesthetic gases. Containers for chemical hazards are labeled with symbols representing the type of potential hazard, along with instructions for steps to take in the event of exposure.

Radiological hazards found in the medical environment are seen in the forms of thermal, radioactive isotopes and electromagnetic radiation. The most common thermal radiological hazard is in the form of lasers. The use of lasers exposes the patient and the health care team to risk of eye damage, as well as increasing the risk of fire in the operating room. Laser operators must be trained on the correct usage of the laser, along with indicated safety precautions. Radioactive isotopes are used in brachytherapy. **Brachytherapy** is a form of cancer treatment where radioactive beads are inserted near or inside a cancerous tumor in order to deliver a high dose of radiation to the tumor while sparing the surrounding healthy tissue. Electromagnetic radiation is seen in the form of x-ray and ultraviolet radiation. During a procedure where electromagnetic radiation is used, the patient is protected by shields and/or drapes specifically designed to minimize exposure to the radiation. The perioperative team utilizes shields, gowns, and eyewear to minimize radiation exposure.

Physical hazards also exist in the medical area. **Autoclaves** are used to steam sterilize surgical instruments, and this steam can potentially cause burns. Removing surgical instruments straight from the autoclave can cause burns to the hands if the proper gloves are not used. Liquid on the floor can cause someone to slip or fall, causing injury. Handling carbon dioxide tanks or cryogenic material can cause severe burns to the hands if gloves are not worn.

The types of hazards should be discussed at the beginning of employment in the medical environment. This should include identifying the potential hazards and known hazards, steps to minimize exposure to them, and discussing the necessary steps to take in case of exposure. Healthcare facilities are required to provide material safety data sheets (MSDS) and keep them in a central area. For most healthcare facilities, education on hazardous materials management is done on an annual basis.

Infectious Waste

Infectious waste refers to waste that occurs during medical examination, treatment, autopsy, or some other procedure relating to human or animal tissues, bodily fluids, or bone. Infectious waste includes items such as blood, plasma, fecal or urine matter, bacterial or viral cultures, materials used in surgery or recovery, pharmaceuticals, syringes, and so on. This type of waste must be handled differently from traditional waste due to its infectious and pathogenic nature. In the medical setting, it must be collected separately from other types of waste and marked as such. Infectious waste is then removed from the building and sterilized at an external facility before it is landfilled or recycled.

Emotional Workplace Safety

A nurse is guaranteed to experience heightened emotions in one form or another throughout their professional career. Between the tasks, the patients, the environment, the administration, and so much more, the nurse will be subject to a wide range of emotional situations. Feeling overwhelmed from being new on the unit, frustrated by inadequate staffing, or sad because of a patient dying are all realistic feelings in the field of nursing. So how can the nurse manage these emotions effectively to actually improve patient care?

The key element in managing emotions for the betterment of patient care is the culture of the healthcare facility/agency. A culture with harsh reprimands and the silencing of issues can create an emotionally toxic workplace where staff members don't feel comfortable discussing issues, reporting errors, or even working as a team (out of fear and lack of trust). The nurse needs to ensure that the culture allows growth through asking questions, stating concerns, and promoting teamwork. Honesty, trust, and open communication are necessities in the workplace to ensure emotional workplace safety.

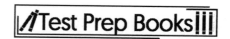

Workplace Violence

Workplace violence in nursing refers to threats or actual incidents of violence, aggression, intimidation, harassment, or force. Workplace violence can occur by former or current colleagues, by someone from the nurse's personal life, or by individuals who have no relationship to the nurse or workplace. Statistically, nurses experience a higher rate of workplace violence, most often from patients they are treating or from someone associated with the patient. Nurses are most likely to report experiencing physical assault (e.g., kicking, hitting, pushing, hair-pulling), being screamed at, being spit on, and needing to restrain patients. This is perhaps due to the fact that they are regularly dealing with mentally unwell populations or patients that are heavily medicated from procedures; in fact, psychiatric nurses experience the most incidents of workplace violence among all nursing specialties. Additionally, healthcare settings may cause extreme feelings of stress and fear in patients, their friends, and their family, especially if they are worried about the patient's prognosis or financial issues. They may be unable to healthily express or cope with such extreme feelings; therefore, they become hostile.

Workplace violence in specific healthcare settings has been associated with high turnover and staff shortages. Additionally, nurses who experience workplace violence often have to take one or more days off from work to recuperate. Not only are these experiences taxing and scarring for affected healthcare professionals, but they are also extremely costly for the healthcare facility. Hiring, training, firing, providing severance, and other human resources tasks are expensive for the organization.

Nurses may also feel uncomfortable about reporting incidents, as they may believe that doing so goes against their nursing oath to protect the patient or fear that it could jeopardize their job security. Such situations can have long-lasting negative health effects on nurses; they may fear going to work or experience stress disorders after a violent situation occurs. Healthcare workers who experience workplace stress are more likely to experience job-related fatigue, burnout, medical errors, and poor patient outcomes. Some healthcare systems have begun to make administrative changes to address workplace violence, including the presence of metal detectors, security escorts, alarm systems that nurses can activate when needed, and system-wide surveillance and monitoring of patients. Additionally, more hospital staff members are receiving training on de-escalation techniques.

Personal Limitations and Seeking Assistance

Working in the hospital environment can be stressful, overwhelming, and physically demanding. The day-to-day activities involve more physical activity than in other care areas. Staff members are frequently on call and working overtime. The medical-surgical nurse is only able to provide the best patient care when they have also taken care of themselves. It is important to remain aware of physical, mental, and emotional health. The nurse should be aware of personal limitations, physically and mentally, and be cognizant of responsibilities that may put the nurse at risk. Whenever needed, the nurse should seek assistance.

Nurse Resiliency and Well-Being

Nurse resiliency is a key characteristic in the prevention of burnout. The emotional toll and working conditions can become stressors for the nurse, especially in healthcare settings with high-acuity patients or high turnover. Nurse resiliency is essentially the nurse's ability to overcome or adapt to adversities in the healthcare setting.

Nurse resiliency and well-being can be closely connected with the concept of emotional workplace safety. An important component of nurse resiliency is communication and positivity. If the workplace culture does not promote open communication, the nurse is less likely to report the feeling of pending burnout, resulting in worsening burnout and a likely decline in positivity.

How can the nurse promote their own resiliency and well-being? First, the nurse must recognize their own present or potential stressors. One nurse may feel overwhelmed with multiple patients but be flexible with their schedule,

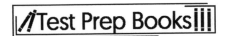

while another nurse may feel comfortable with multiple patients but be uncomfortable working back-to-back twelve-hour shifts. While these stressors may not always be resolvable, the nurse recognizing them is an important step in developing resiliency. Taking action to recognize and reduce stressors for physical, mental, emotional, spiritual, and social well-being is the most important form of nursing self-care. Common examples include regular exercise, getting adequate sleep, practicing relaxation techniques, and setting goals and boundaries.

Next, the nurse must feel comfortable utilizing any agency/facility resources present for combating burnout, promoting open communication, and furthering education. Nurse resiliency and well-being is a responsibility of both the individual nurse and the healthcare agency/facility.

Unintended Consequences

Healthcare providers, like other service-oriented professions, are at a higher risk of experiencing burnout, compassion fatigue, post-traumatic stress disorder (PTSD), and other stress related health issues. The incident rate of stress-related disorders in healthcare professionals, especially nurses, increased significantly due to the COVID-19 pandemic. Burnout is a type of overload and comprehensive exhaustion that occurs directly from work-related tasks. It is not considered a formal diagnosis like other mental health disorders. Symptoms include loss of interest in work, unhappiness at work, physical ailments, and symptoms that overlap with depression. Nurses may experience burnout from staff shortages, long work hours with no breaks, highly repetitive and taxing cases, administrative challenges, or limited professional and personal support.

Compassion fatigue, or secondary traumatic stress, occurs when people are constantly exposed to other people's traumas during the course of their workday. Symptoms are similar to that of burnout, depression, and anxiety, but they also include numbness and inability to empathize. Nurses experiencing compassion fatigue may find it difficult to sympathize with patients' suffering; they may outwardly show irritation and apathy, or they may blame the patient for their condition.

PTSD is a mental health disorder that occurs directly as a result of experiencing a highly stressful, scary, or otherwise traumatic event. Symptoms include recurrent, difficult thoughts; detachment; anger; and flashbacks of the traumatic event. Nurses may experience PTSD after difficult cases in which a patient does not survive or after interacting with violent and aggressive patients. These situations are highly taxing on their own, but chronic stress can lead to physical health problems such as hypertension, insomnia, and musculoskeletal pain.

Seeking professional counseling can be an important way to cope with stress, as counselors can tailor interventions to their clients' unique stressors. Caregiving professionals are accustomed to taking care of others during their workdays and may need to take care of their own families and dependents during their time away from work. Therefore, sustainable self-care is a crucial part of stress management for nurses. Nurses should seek out lifestyle behaviors that will nourish their well-being in the long run, such as getting adequate sleep, exercising, eating nutritious foods, drinking enough water, resting, participating in leisurely activities that are not related to work or caretaking, and spending time with supportive friends and family.

Moral Distress and Moral Injury

Prominent causes of burnout in the nursing profession are moral distress and moral injury. The nurse feels moral distress when their moral code does not align with what is or is not happening. Moral injury occurs when the nurse can no longer cope with the moral distresses, leading to impaired psychological functioning.

For example, if the nurse is caring for a geriatric patient with a terminal illness, but the family is making the patient a full code, the nurse may have moral distress. Knowing the consequences of resuscitation on a patient, especially a geriatric patient that is actively dying, the nurse could feel morally torn between what is required and what they feel is ethical. The nurse may also feel distress when there is a staffing issue leading the nurse to not perform the level of care that they think is necessary.

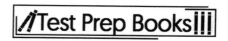

Another example of an ethical dilemma is the practice of disaster triaging. With a mass casualty, patients are tagged based on their acuity level. While the nurse knows that it is necessary for the greater good by preserving time and resources, placing a black tag on a patient can be a devastating moral injury for the nurse. The best practice for the nurse experiencing moral distress is to first recognize it and then use available resources to work through the emotional turmoil.

Resource Allocation

Resource allocation in healthcare is a complex topic without a clear-cut solution. There are some key points for understanding the nurse's role in resource allocation, and the bulk of it revolves around being a patient advocate. Adequate staffing, reducing staff turnover, and ensuring equipment safety (both in availability of equipment and in proper usage and storage) are all important aspects of resource allocation. Adequate staffing and reducing staff turnover can go hand in hand. If the nurse feels comfortable with the patient caseload and that there are adequate resources available, there is a lower likelihood of turnover. Reduced staff turnover also results in effective cost management, improved patient satisfaction, and safer patient care.

Peer Accountability

As a nurse, it can become difficult to balance the day-to-day responsibilities like nursing procedures, documentation, interdisciplinary communication, and providing education. While these short-term responsibilities are of vital importance, the nurse must not forget the importance of their own ethical responsibilities.

Peer accountability is one of those ethical nursing responsibilities, as the main goal is providing safe and effective patient care. Peer accountability often gets misconstrued as tattling or whistleblowing, when in reality it is simply a chance for continuing education and improved patient safety. The goal is not to get someone in trouble but to fix the issue at hand. For example, if a nurse witnessed another nurse not using proper aseptic technique when inserting an indwelling urinary catheter, further education would need to be provided for the nurse to provide safe catheter care.

Scope of Practice and Ethics

Scope of Practice and Code of Ethics for Nurses Per Local and Regional Nursing Bodies

Scope of Practice

Another responsibility of the nurse is to work within their own scope of practice. So the main questions become: what is the nursing scope of practice, and how does the nurse stay up to date on changes?

Nursing scope of practice simply means what the nurse can legally and ethically practice based on competency through active licensure and any testing required. Federal regulations are geared towards the general practice of safe patient care and advancements in practice, while each state will have a specific set of laws that will be defined in the Nursing Practice Act (NPA). Standards of nursing practice will be thoroughly defined in this document to give the nurse in each state a specific scope of practice. Each facility will also have a set of regulations that the nurse should know.

For example, federal regulations and certain state laws approve of an LPN initiating a peripheral IV as long as competency tasks have been completed. With that being said, if the specific agency does not approve of LPNs initiating a peripheral IV, the scope of practice of the LPN within that agency will be to not initiate peripheral IVs. For this reason, the nurse will need to ensure the use of federal, state, and agency resources to ensure appropriate and ethical nursing practice. Following nursing regulatory bodies (NRBs), the state board of nursing (BON), and agency policies and procedures can help the nurse know, and practice within, the approved scope.

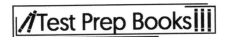

Code of Ethics

Similar to the scope of practice, the nursing code of ethics can slightly vary between healthcare agencies. With that being said, there are certain ethical practices that are consistent for all practicing nurses. The Code of Ethics for Nurses with Interpretive Statements gives the nurse a list of ethical practices to utilize for all patient care. The Code, created by the American Nurses Association (ANA), includes the following practices:

- Practicing with compassion and respect
- Providing care with the patient being the primary responsibility
- Providing care being a patient advocate
- Keeping up to date with nursing scope of practice to provide safe patient care
- Ensuring self-care to prevent burnout and provide safe, efficient patient care
- Working towards any advancements or improvements in safe patient care
- Working towards furthering education
- Ensuring effective interdisciplinary collaboration for improvement of patient care
- Promoting social justice and nursing integrity/values

Similar to the Code of Ethics for Nurses with Interpretive Statements, the Academy of Medical-Surgical Nurses (AMSN) Scope and Standards gives the nurse a frame of practice for providing ethical care. Standard V of the AMSN Scope and Standards includes the ethical framework of medical-surgical nursing, including the following:

- Maintaining a professional relationship with the patient
- Maintaining patient confidentiality and establishing professional boundaries
- Reporting any discrepancies in ethical nursing practice
- Assisting in resource allocation to ensure safe patient care
- Supporting differing values, practices, and decisions
- Maintaining a nonjudgmental and nondiscriminatory attitude towards all patients

Just as it is the responsibility of the nurse to practice within their approved scope, it is the ethical responsibility of the nurse to stay up to date on the ethical practices of nursing.

Patients' Rights and Responsibilities

Patients have rights and responsibilities when it comes to their health care. Generally, these are communicated to the patient in a Patient's Bill of Rights document at the entry point of care. Safety is an inherent patient right and expectation. Patients have the right to be informed on their disease process, treatment plan, and alternatives to treatment. When developing outcomes and interventions, the nurse and healthcare providers must discuss the care plan with the patient. The patient has the right to be involved in decisions involving their care. The patient has a right to agree or disagree with the proposed plan of care. Nurses must also be cognizant of the patient's ability to provide informed consent for an invasive procedure. The nurse may need to refer the plan of care to the next of kin or to the patient's medical power of attorney. The nurse must work collaboratively with the patient and the interdisciplinary team to ensure all parties are in agreement with the care being provided and the expectations of the patient's involvement in their care. In all cases, the nurse must remain an advocate for the patient and implement a plan of care that acts in the patient's best interest.

A patient may access their medical record upon request by following the process set by the health care facility. HIPAA protects patient rights around confidentiality, release of medical information, and privacy.

All patients have the right to affordable, quality care based upon best practices regardless of ability to pay. Patients should be cared for in a respectful, nondiscriminatory fashion. Patients have the right to comfort measures, as well as pharmacological pain management (if ordered by a physician) provided in a manner that is safe. Patients who are

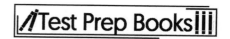

hospitalized have the right to visitors during times allowed by the facility. Evidence-based practice supports open family visitation hours, even in critical care units. Several facilities have adopted policies supporting this practice.

Each patient has certain rights that must be respected. When patients are admitted to a facility, they are put in a position of vulnerability. This special position of power held by the health care provider should never be abused to violate the rights of the patient. Caring for a patient is an honor, and certain rules of conduct should be followed.

The patient has the right to have health information kept private and only shared with those who are given permission to view it. The Health Insurance Portability and Accountability Act (HIPAA) was passed by Congress in 1996 to protect health information. The term HIPAA is often used to reference patient privacy. There are many different ways a patient's personal health information can be shared: verbally, digitally, over the phone or fax, or through written messages.

The nurse plays an important role in keeping a patient's health information private. Sharing personal details—such as a patient's name, condition, and medical history—in an inappropriate way violates the person's right to privacy. For example, telling a friend who does not work in the facility that the nurse took care of the friend's aunt, without the aunt's consent or knowledge, is considered a violation of privacy. Another way a nurse could violate a patient's privacy is to access the medical record when they are not actually caring for that particular patient. For example, if a celebrity has been admitted to a different unit, and the nurse—curious to find out the details—accesses the celebrity's electronic health record, then they are in violation of HIPAA. Those who violate HIPAA and are caught could lose their jobs, among other punitive actions.

Along with protecting the patient's health information, the nurse must be respectful of the patient's privacy in general. Knocking on the patient's door before entering the room, keeping the door shut to the busy corridor outside the room, and not asking unnecessary personal questions are all ways the nurse can extend common courtesy to the patient. The nature of the nurse's relationship with the patient is already quite personal in nature (e.g., the nurse is giving the patient baths, helping him or her go to the bathroom, etc.), so there is no need to exploit that relationship.

Each patient has the right to fair treatment. This means that no patient should be treated any better or worse than another patient for any reason, such as a racial bias or unfair prejudice based on the nurse's personal opinions and beliefs. Giving one patient preferential treatment over another is a violation of the patient's rights, and the nurse will be subject to disciplinary action if they are discovered to be treating patients poorly.

No patient should ever be abused or neglected. This should go without saying, but it is a patient right that is perhaps the most important. Abuse can be physical, emotional, sexual, mental, or financial. Neglect is when the patient's needs are being ignored, usually resulting in patient harm.

The patient has the *right of self-determination*, which means that he or she has the right to make decisions regarding their own health care. Patients are members of the health care team along with the doctors and nurses. What the nurse may think is the right course of action for a patient may not align with what the patient thinks is right, and that is to be respected. The health care team forms the plan of care and educates the patient as to what a plan entails, but it is the patient who makes the final decision to accept or reject a plan. If the patient is not capable of making their own decisions, the *power of attorney*—usually a close family member such as a wife, husband, or adult child—has the power to make health care decisions for the patient.

Along with self-determination, the patients also have the freedom to express themselves and their opinions. Simply being admitted to a facility does not take away their freedom of speech. Patients may have opinions about all aspects of their care, and they have every right to express these feelings. The nurse needs to be respectful, listen, and try to help when there is a problem that can be solved. Issues voiced by patients can always be escalated by the nurse, using the appropriate chain of command.

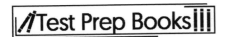

Consent to Treat

Ideally, patients should always provide written consent for treatment. This should also include discussion between the healthcare provider and the patient about what treatment will entail, what the end goal is of treatment, the risks and benefits of the treatment, and the opportunity for the patient to voice any questions and concerns. Patient consent decreases liability for the healthcare provider and increases patient reports of empowerment. Patients also have the right to revoke previously given consent at any time.

However, problems with patient consent do exist. In many healthcare facilities, the consent process can be a rushed one; often, patients receive a large packet of paperwork in which the consent form is included. Many patients sign without reading or do not understand what they are signing but complete the form out of fear, pressure, or to appear informed when they actually do not feel that way. Often, verbal exchange about the form or treatment does not occur. Legally, healthcare providers do not have to provide an explanation of information that is accepted as common knowledge. However, medical topics are often not part of the average person's body of knowledge, and this gap can be complicated to bridge without thorough communication. Healthcare providers can attempt to resolve these problems by taking the time to discuss the consent form with the patient, simplifying consent forms, and providing additional media (such as literature or video links) to patients, especially in the event of more complex procedures.

Informed Consent

An important part of the patient's bill of rights is **informed consent**. This means the patient has been adequately informed about their health care plan, whether that involves new medications, vaccinations, procedures, diagnostic screenings, and so on. The patient is granting their permission to go ahead with the care plan. It is up to the health care team to obtain this informed consent. This usually takes the form of a patient-signed document that goes in the permanent health care record.

Implied Consent

Implied consent does not involve the patient signing a document or even verbally granting permission, but rather it is assumed that any reasonable person would consent to the health care interventions being performed. The most common use of implied consent is in emergency situations in which lifesaving interventions are necessary and there is not enough time to perform informed consent with the patient, such as cardiopulmonary resuscitation (CPR) after cardiac arrest.

Expressed Consent

This type of consent entails that the patient consent to a medical intervention either verbally, nonverbally through a gesture such as a nod, or in writing. This type of consent differs from informed consent in that there is not necessarily an education process that precedes it. This type of consent generally requires a witness.

Patient Incompetence

A patient who is unable to make their own informed decisions about their health care plan is termed **incompetent**. In the case of an incompetent patient, it may be necessary to use a proxy, such as a power of attorney, to make health care decisions for them.

Emancipated Minor

If a minor is legally **emancipated**, it means they are freed from having parental consent to certain things. The legal age for emancipation is generally sixteen. A patient may be medically emancipated if they become pregnant, thus freeing them to give consent with associated medical procedures and maintaining confidentiality of their records at that point.

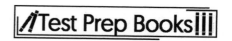

Mature Minor

The **mature minor** concept applies to unemancipated minors and says that if a patient is deemed mature enough and the medical intervention is not especially serious, they may make their own decisions and give their own consent without parental consent.

Responsibilities

As previously stated, the patient has the right to respectful treatment; however, the patient is responsible for being respectful to caregivers. The patient should have a clear understanding of their rights, and health care providers are bound to do everything possible to uphold these. With that being said, the patient should be clearly informed of their responsibilities and be compliant with them.

It is important for the patient to keep scheduled appointments and arrive in a timely manner. If the patient's demographic information changes, the health provider's office should be updated in order to keep the lines of communication open. The patient is responsible for copays, deductibles, and any other fees that align with the health insurance or benefit plan. If the patient is unable to pay, they are responsible for negotiating a payment plan or deferral. If an advance directive exists, the patient must communicate this and provide a copy for health providers. The patient should actively participate in care, asking questions when necessary. To ensure appropriate care is provided, the patient must provide accurate and complete health information to providers; this includes disclosing all medications that are currently being taken. If the patient is prescribed medications, the patient is responsible for keeping medications to self only, not allowing others access to them. When the patient and health provider(s) create a plan of care, the patient should verbalize understanding of it and accept any consequences of decisions made. The patient must also be responsible for following up on instructions as directed.

Professional Reporting and Resources

A discussion in ethical nursing must also include the practice of professional reporting and appropriate resources. Medication errors, procedural errors, abuse, unsafe conditions, and medication diversion are just a few of the reportable incidents the nurse may face in practice.

Reporting will differ in each situation based on the type of incident and the facility/agency guidelines (in compliance with state/federal regulatory bodies). The following points review the typical response to a reportable incident and the subsequent resources to utilize:

Medication administration errors and procedural errors:

- Each facility/agency will have an incident reporting system
- Sentinel events are mandatory to report in certain states

Abuse:

- Nurses are mandatory reporters of any form of patient abuse
- State and facility/agency guidelines will be specific to the patient population (e.g., the elderly, children, etc.) and the reporting agency

Unsafe conditions:

- Unsafe staffing and work conditions are to be reported to the specific state board of nursing

Medication diversion:

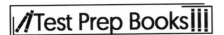

- Reporting diversion of controlled substances will vary based on where or by whom the diversion occurs (e.g., coworker, patient's family member/friend)
- Reporting to facility/agency reporting system in both circumstances with potential for involvement with DEA, state board of nursing, state pharmacy board, and potentially law enforcement

Reporting patient information and work issues in a timely manner and using the correct route on the chain of command are a legal obligation of nurse. Not reporting important information could result in serious ramifications and punitive action for the nurse, up to loss of employment and/or revocation of certification. When important information goes unreported, it can result in patient harm or unresolved conflicts that turn into bigger problems to deal with later on. Addressing patient issues and resolving conflicts all start with accurate and timely reporting. A basic definition of a **report** is the relaying of information that one has observed or heard. When this report is given to an authority figure who can intervene, it will contain different elements, such as patient name, situation, time of event, and circumstances surrounding the event.

Policies; Procedures; Standards of Practice; and State, Federal, and Local Laws

Each healthcare facility/agency will be responsible for following the regulations set forth by local, state, and federal laws and guidelines. The healthcare facility will follow these laws through the implementation of policies and procedures. For any nursing skill or practice, each healthcare facility will have a specific policy/procedure to follow, of which the nurse will likely be assessed for understanding and competency. Policies and procedures are created, reviewed, and revised by the healthcare facility's quality assurance/improvement team. Below are the common healthcare regulatory and accreditation agencies:

Healthcare Facility/Agencies:

- Quality Assurance Team: Includes compliance specialists, administrators, and QA healthcare personnel

Local Agencies:

- Varying local agencies responsible for public health measures and emergency response planning

State Agencies:

- State Board of Nursing **(BON)**

Federal Agencies:

- Occupational Safety and Health Administration **(OSHA)**
- National Institute for Occupational Safety and Health **(NIOSH)**
- Environmental Protection Agency **(EPA)**
- Department of Health and Human Services **(HHS)**:
  - Centers for Medicare and Medicaid Services **(CMS)**
  - Center for Disease Control and Prevention **(CDC)**
  - Food and Drug Administration **(FDA)**
  - National Institutes of Health **(NIH)**

Accreditation Agencies:

- Assurance (NCQA)
- Commission on Accreditation of Rehabilitation Facilities (CARF)
- Council on Accreditation (COA)

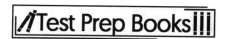

Regulatory Guidelines

The nurse must uphold and answer to certain legal rights and responsibilities within their profession. From simple things like managing a patient's property to more complicated issues such as reporting abuse and neglect, the nurse has a legal responsibility to act or their license could be in danger.

Nurses need a knowledge of the common legal terminology in their practice. The following is a list of terms the nurse should know:

- Common law: Common law is based on legal precedents or previously decided cases in courts of law.

- Statutory law: These are laws based on a state's legislative actions or any other legislative body's actions.

- Constitutional law: Laws based on the content of the Constitution of the United States of America are referred to as constitutional law.

- Administrative law: For a nurse, this is a type of law passed down from a ruling body such as a state nursing association. For example, each state's nursing board passes down regulations on continuing education requirements for licensed nurses.

- Criminal law: This type of law involves the arrest, prosecution, and incarceration of those who have broken the law. Such offenses as felonies and misdemeanors are covered under criminal law.

- Liability: Nurses are liable for their actions while practicing. Thorough documentation and patient charting are important. If an act is not charted, it was not done, so to speak. Nurses must protect themselves legally to maintain their practice.

- Tort: In a nursing context, this legal term refers to nursing practice violations such as malpractice, negligence, and patient confidentiality violations.

- Unintentional tort: Negligence and malpractice may be unintentional forms of tort.

- Intentional tort: On the other hand, torts may be proven to be intentional, including such violations as false imprisonment, privacy breaches, slander, libel, battery, and assault. A nurse using a physical restraint without meeting protocol or getting a physician's order is guilty of false imprisonment. Slander is a form of defamation in which the person makes false statements that are verbal, and libel is written defamation.

Legal Obligations of Nurses

A nurse is legally responsible for maintaining an active licensure according to their state's regulatory board's laws. Failure to maintain licensure requirements such as continuing education credits will result in disciplinary action. Nursing licenses may be revoked or suspended because of disciplinary actions.

Nurses must report abuse, neglect, gunshot wounds, dog bites, and communicable diseases. Nurses are also legally mandated to report other health care providers whom they suspect may be abusing drugs or alcohol while practicing, because they are putting patients and themselves at risk.

Nurses have a legal obligation to accept the patient assignments given to them, if they believe they are appropriate and it is within their scope of practice to perform duties related to these patients. However, if they are assigned tasks that they are not prepared to perform, they must notify their supervisors and seek assistance.

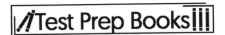

Laws at the national, state, and local level must be complied with by practicing nurses. Such laws include those in relation to the Centers for Medicare and Medicaid services. Another example would be adhering to local laws regarding the disposal of biohazardous waste.

Board of Nursing

Each state and territory in the United States has a Nurse Practice Act, under which a **board of nursing** must be established. This board regulates nursing standards, credentials, education requirements, best practices, and licensure within the state or territory. Each area's board of nursing ensures that once standards for licensure are met, they are meticulously maintained throughout one's nursing career in order to uphold high safety and quality standards. If a nurse fails to maintain standards established by their area's board of nursing, they may lose licensure or undergo other disciplinary and corrective actions. If nurses choose to move jurisdictions, they may need to pass requirements for the new jurisdiction. Nurse practice acts and boards of nursing are in place in order to ensure that all forms of nursing, which can take place in a range of settings and with a wide demographic of patients, exhibit competence, skill, quality, and care in all contexts.

Quality Management

Evidence-Based Guidelines

Nursing guidelines are developed in order to provide decision-making advice as it relates to clinical cases. Their goal is to standardize care by utilizing evidence-based practice, provide documented accountability standards for nursing professionals, and generally guide nursing care. Nursing guidelines may be developed nationally, regionally, or within a specific organization. Guidelines are typically developed by reviewing appropriate and relevant scholarly literature, proposing guidelines based on research and the input of key stakeholders, and testing proposed guidelines in clinical settings to determine what aspects work well and consistently and what aspects need further development. Finally, once guidelines are accepted, they should be continuously reviewed and revised as needed in order to maintain high safety, quality, and efficiency standards while incorporating advances in technology or shifts in the healthcare culture.

Quality Standards and Policies

Similar to the scope of practice and laws/regulations for nursing, the quality standards are established by multiple healthcare organizations. Looking towards organizations such as the American Nursing Association (ANA) and the Joint Commission (TJC) can give the nurse up-to-date quality standards and policies/procedural practices. The quality assurance team within the specific healthcare facility/agency will regularly assess these organizations for creation and revision of policies, procedures, and protocols.

For example, TJC released a standard practice for placing a hard stop date on a medication order that is only ordered for a specific amount of time. Medical providers write in the order to take a medication for a certain number of days (e.g., Bactrim 500 mg BID for ten days), but the TJC standard would require the medication to be removed from the medication administration record at the ten-day mark (upon the completion of the medication). Evidence-based protocols are established to ensure safe, competent healthcare for all patients.

Surgical Care Improvement Project (SCIP)

The **Surgical Care Improvement Project (SCIP)** took place between 2005 and 2010. It was a quality-driven, nation-wide initiative aimed at reducing surgical complications and improving patient outcomes by establishing standardized guidelines for perioperative, operative, and postoperative patient care. These guidelines included directives such as strictly timed antibiotic administration, glucose monitoring, stringent patient preparation requirements, and practices to minimize the risk of postoperative infections. The project produced best practices

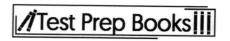
and core measures that were compiled into a specifications manual; this serves as a benchmarking tool used by The Joint Commission to ensure sustained quality in the surgical setting.

Continuous Quality and Process Improvement

Performance Improvement

Performance improvement is a mechanism to continuously review and improve processes in a system to ensure that work is completed in the most cost-effective manner while producing the best possible outcomes. Healthcare facilities are constantly hoping to drive down cost and increase reimbursements while delivering the highest quality of healthcare and utilizing analytical methods to achieve this. These analyses and implementations may be done by top administrative employees at the organization and be executed across the healthcare system or within a particular department. Leadership support is always crucial for positive change to occur and sustain itself.

All processes should be regularly monitored for opportunities for improvement. Common opportunities include areas of reported patient dissatisfaction; federal, state, or internal benchmarks that are not being met; areas of financial loss; and common complaints among staff. While multiple opportunities for improvement may exist, focusing on one at a time usually produces the greatest outcome. When choosing a process to improve, it is important to select a process that can actually be changed by the members involved (e.g., medical staff often do not have control over external funding sources). Processes that can produce positive end results with the use of minimal resources for change are also preferable to costlier improvements. Once the process has been selected, a group of stakeholders that are regularly involved in the process should map out each step of the process while noting areas of wasted resource or process variation. From here, stakeholders can develop a change to test.

PDCA

The PDCA cycle provides a framework for implementing tests of change. *Plan*, the first step, involves planning the change. This will include accounting for all workflow changes, the staff members involved, and logistics of implementation. It should also include baseline data relating to the problem. *Do*, the second step, involves implementing the change. During this step, data collection is crucial. For example, if a department believes that implementing mobile work stations will decrease nurses' wait time between patients, the department should keep a detailed record of the time spent with and between each patient. *Check*, the third step, involves checking data relating to the change with the baseline data and determining if the change improved the process. *Act*, the final step, involves making the change permanent and monitoring it for sustainability.

Quality Improvement Activities

The nursing team should participate in, and initiate, quality improvement activities in an effort to improve patient care and the overall profession. There are constant opportunities for practice improvement, and ideally, the team should foster an environment that is open to exploring these opportunities.

One of the best opportunities to learn about quality improvement activities is at trade shows and poster presentations. It is very beneficial to review what other institutions have researched or implemented in order to improve patient safety and patient care. These projects can range from changes to workflow and process to introducing tools to improve the hand-off of care in between care areas. After learning about these projects, the team can determine if implementing a similar project may be beneficial at their own facility while ensuring there are not overwhelming changes that may be a distraction to the team.

With the adoption of electronic medical records and electronic documentation, another great opportunity for research and improvement is using analytic tools to analyze and interpret the data at the facility. There are many examples of nursing teams using their own data for initiatives such as decreasing postoperative nausea and vomiting (PONV) using premedication or decreasing unnecessary overtime.

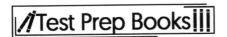

Audit

An **audit** is an inspection of a specific aspect of an organization. Audits can be conducted on procedures, finances, incentives, product counts, or any other area of the business that can be monitored. Audits may be conducted internally or by an external, independent body; most effective organizations perform both types regularly. Audit activities may include checklists of certain processes that must be in place, benchmark score comparisons, and evaluation practices. Internal audits allow organizations to be prepared for external audits. Non-compliance of standards found by an external auditing body, especially if it is a regulatory agency, may result in fines, disciplinary action, intensive monitoring, or a shutdown of the organization.

Best Practice

Best practices refer to a set of procedures that are generally accepted to be the most effective method of accomplishing a specific goal. These are shaped by evidence-based practice, professional expertise, and patient or client input. Organizations should follow established best practices in an industry in order to maintain high-quality standards. If an organization is underperforming in an area, researching established best practices for that area and implementing change to reflect best practices is likely to result in improved quality.

Quality Measures

Quality measures are used to determine how effective a quality process is. These can be classified into three categories: structural, process, and outcome measures. Structural measures refer to tools available within an organization that support high-quality processes, such as software or highly credentialed personnel. Process measures refer to the assessment of actual steps in a procedure, such as determining if nurses are verifying identity before administering a medical procedure. Outcome measures refer to whether structures or processes in place make a difference, such as the number of patients with bedsores in inpatient settings.

Quality Assurance

Quality assurance refers to an established system within an organization that has the function of ensuring that processes and outcomes are free of error. Quality assurance practices use administrative and process controls to ensure that variation from the start of the process to the end of the process are limited, therefore creating relatively standardized inputs that lead to an expected output. These factors are associated with efficiency, cost and resource reduction, and reduced product and service defects. Examples of quality assurance practices in the healthcare setting include electronic medical records, which reduce documentation error within and between different healthcare facilities, sanitation checklists, standardized training protocols for staff, and identity verification before medical procedures.

Quality Improvement

Quality improvement is a framework that analyzes performance on a continuous basis to ensure all steps are as efficient and effective as possible. This concept came from manufacturing, where industries focused on reducing defects in product, reducing cost and waste, and worker safety. From a healthcare perspective, quality improvement focuses on patient safety and satisfaction, decreased mortality and medical complications, and personnel job satisfaction. Effective quality improvement in healthcare requires meaningful data, clean and relevant data collection, managing processes of care rather than micromanaging people, and empowering clinicians to take responsibility for quality factors.

Nursing Professional Practice Model

The nursing professional practice model is a cultural framework for nursing care defined by most healthcare facilities/agencies. The model is put in place within the specific facility/agency to give the nursing staff professional guidelines for communication, care, and collaboration with the facility/agency's values in the forefront. While each healthcare facility/agency will have a different set of values, the general framework for a successful nursing

260

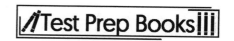

professional practice model is typically the same. The five general subtopics of a nursing professional practice model include the following:

- Core professional values
- Professional relationships
- Professional recognition and compensation
- Care delivery system
- Management/administration

The keys for a successful professional practice model require the following:

Nursing involvement in the creation, review, and revision process

Evidence-based research and literature

A graphic or visual to depict the model

Routine evaluation to evolve with the changes within the organization and general healthcare environment

A nursing professional practice model not only provides the nursing staff with a framework of good nursing practice, but also an opportunity to buy in to the culture. In a large healthcare facility, cultural practices have to be routinely assessed and reinforced.

For example, the administration within a hospice inpatient facility highly values the nurse frequently spending time with the patient (e.g., giving emotional support, conversing with the patient and family). This facility also has a nurse-to-patient ratio of 1:5 with controlled substances being administered frequently. In this situation, there may be a gap in the priority values and the reality in the clinical setting. The administration may value quality time, but the clinical staff may be unable to provide that level of care with the current workload. In this situation, the nurses may state that the nurse-to-patient ratio will need to change to allow more quality of time with each patient.

Adverse Event Reporting

Adverse event reporting can be commonly associated with legal formalities and repercussions, but it serves as a prominent resource for quality improvement measures when used correctly.

First, the nurse must understand what defines an adverse event. An adverse event is a situation where an undesirable clinical outcome occurs related to the care provided, while not being related to the underlying disease process or condition. Types of adverse events in healthcare include medication errors, falls, equipment errors, and nosocomial infections.

Next, the event must be properly reported, not only for the benefit of the patient affected by the adverse event, but also for future patient safety measures. For example, if a fall occurs related to an equipment error, reporting this adverse event can result in quality improvement measures such as in-services on equipment usage and fall prevention.

Never Event
"**Never events**" refer to errors in care that should never occur during a medical procedure, due to the catastrophic effects on patient safety and outcomes that the event could have. Additionally, these events can be costly for the healthcare facility. "Never events" include instances like performing an incorrect procedure on a patient, performing a procedure on the wrong patient, failing to take into account patient history such as allergies, the development of pressure ulcers on patients in care, and other situations that cause adverse outcomes, including

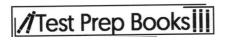

death, to the patient. Associated costs with "never events" include time, labor, and money spent to correct medical errors, lawsuits, and future reimbursements lost due to tarnished reputation.

Patient Customer Experience

Patient experience is essentially the patient's cumulative exposure to the healthcare system. From primary care offices and clinics, to hospitals and acute care facilities, to telehealth and home health services, the patient's healthcare experience can become very disjointed without the assistance of a devoted healthcare team. To improve the patient experience, the nurse should remember the five Cs (consistency, coordination, continuity, caring, and correction):

- Consistency: Consistent patient care is consistency across the entire healthcare experience. From varying nurses to varying shifts, there is vast potential for a lapse in consistency. Effective communication and routine training are key to a consistent nursing practice.

- Coordination: Coordination is the teamwork and communication of the interdisciplinary team. An example of poor coordination would be the nurse educating the patient on a medication that the medical provider just discontinued. Effective communication is essential for coordination of the patient's healthcare experience.

- Continuity: While similar to consistency, continuity of care is the smooth transition of care. Continuity of care can be seen in the nursing shift change. The patient would experience continuity of care if there were no lapse in quality of care during the change of staff at regular shift changes.

- Caring: Caring in nursing can drastically affect the patient experience. Empathy, respect, and the practice of active listening are all key practices involved in being a caring nurse.

- Correction: Lastly, correction can improve an issue a patient experiences in the course of their care. Human error is inevitable, but the patient experience can be improved with the recognition of the issue and measures put into place for resolving the issue or preventing a recurrence.

Service Recovery

As previously discussed, the skill of recognizing an issue and working towards correction is crucial for the nurse. With a lapse in care quality, trust can be compromised, and the patient may lose confidence in the ability of the healthcare team to provide care. The goal with service recovery is restoring trust and restoring confidence in the healthcare team.

Restoring Trust
Restoring trust will require the nurse to acknowledge the issue with honesty. Allowing the patient time to ask questions while maintaining an apologetic attitude can restore respect, which can be an initial step to restoring trust. Making any amends necessary/appropriate can also assist in restoring trust.

Restoring Confidence
Simply put, restoring confidence will include resolving the issue. Fix the issue, follow up, and follow through:

- Fix the issue with the assistance of the entire interdisciplinary team to ensure adequate coordination.

- Follow up by checking with the patient after the issue has been fixed, both to ensure that the issue is in fact fixed and that the patient does not require additional assistance.

- Follow through by ensuring that any promises or plans made are effectively in place.

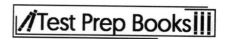
Project Development

While the making of policies and procedures is typically left to the quality assurance/improvement team, understanding project development is good for any nurse. While this business model may seem too formal for the bedside nurse with very little say-so in quality management, the process of project development can be extremely practical and beneficial for the hands-on nurse:

Initiation:

- Understanding the root issue
- Defining measurable goals and outcomes
- Recognizing any limitations or restrictions
- Example: The root issue is a poor documentation system. The goal is to implement a new electronic documentation system. Limitations include potential lapses in documentation during the shift of documentation systems and barriers with technology among staff

Planning:

- Establishing the "how" of obtaining the measurable goals and outcomes
  - Once defined, educating staff on the steps/procedures in place to obtain the goals/outcomes
- Establish all equipment, supplies, manpower, and education needed for the next phase
- Example: The project management team will need to plan for potential downtime for documentation, an expert documentation team, and education in-services on the new electronic documentation system

Execution:

- Implementing the plan
- Example: The new electronic documentation system will be implemented with the planned resources in place

Monitoring/Controlling:

- Closely monitoring the implementation
- Measuring the actual outcome with the planned goals and outcomes
- Monitoring will occur continuously or at regular intervals
- Example: The project management team will monitor documentation standards and staff understanding/compliance

Closing:

- Closing out the process once the implementation process is sustainable
- Example: The project management team will close the project when the documentation system is successfully in use with the routine quality assurance checks in place for documentation standards

Evidence-Based Practice and Research

Legislative and Licensure Requirements

Similar to the procedural scope of practice for nurses, there are legislative and licensure requirements for the use of evidence-based practice (EBP) and research. As with the procedural scope of practice, each state board of nursing

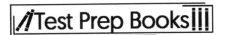

will have specific guidelines for EBP and research practices. The nurse must understand the similarities and differences between EBP and clinical research. While both serve as pivotal tools in the improvement of safe, effective patient care, the actual processes and end results are different.

Evidence-based practice looks towards evidence seen in clinical practice to make informed decisions on patient care. Evidence-based practice puts the gathered information into practice. Research focuses more on validating the current nursing practice and gathering information that is already in practice.

Evidence-Based Practice

Evidence-based practice (EBP) is a research-driven and facts-based methodology that allows healthcare providers to make scientifically supported, reliable, and validated decisions in delivering care. EBP takes into account rigorously tested, peer-reviewed, and published research relating to the case; the knowledge and experience of the healthcare provider; and clinical guidelines established by reputable governing bodies. This framework allows healthcare providers to reach case resolutions that result in positive patient outcomes in the most efficient manner. This, in turn, allows the organization to provide the best care using the least resources.

There are seven steps to successfully utilizing EBP as a methodology in the nursing field. First, the work culture should be one of a "spirit of inquiry." This culture allows staff to ask questions to promote continuous improvement and positive process change to workflow, clinical routines, and non-clinical duties. Second, the PICOT framework should be utilized when searching for an effective intervention, or working with a specific interest, in a case. The PICOT framework encourages nurses to develop a specific, measurable, goal-oriented research question that accounts for the patient population and demographics (P) involved in the case, the proposed intervention or issue of interest (I), a relevant comparison (C) group in which a defined outcome (O) has been positive, and the amount of time (T) needed to implement the intervention or address the issue. Once this question has been developed, staff can move on to the third step, which is to research. In this step, staff will explore reputable sources of literature (such as peer-reviewed scholarly journals, interviews with subject matter experts, or widely accepted textbooks) to find studies and narratives with evidence that supports a resolution for their question.

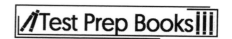

Once all research has been compiled, it must be thoroughly analyzed. This is the fourth step. This step ensures that the staff is using unbiased research with stringent methodology, statistically significant outcomes, reliable and valid research designs, and that all information collected is actually applicable to their patient. (For example, if a certain treatment worked with statistical significance in a longitudinal study of pediatric patients with a large sample size, and all other influencing variables were controlled for, this treatment may not necessarily work in a middle-aged adult. Therefore, though the research collected is scientifically backed and evidence-based for a pediatric population, it does not support EBP for an older population.) The fifth step is to integrate the evidence to create a treatment or intervention plan for the patient. The sixth step is to monitor the implementation of the treatment or intervention and evaluate whether it was associated with positive health outcomes in the patient. Finally, practitioners have a moral obligation to share the results with colleagues at the organization and across the field, so that it may be best utilized (or not) for other patients.

Evidence-Based Practice Flowchart

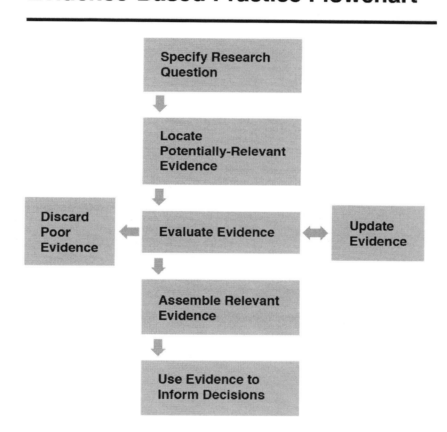

Research Process

The research process in nursing is similar to the research process in any workplace, with the goal of finding and accumulating information in attempts to further knowledge. The importance of routine research within healthcare cannot be overstated. With evolving technology and improvements in care processes, protocols are almost constantly changing. For the nurse to stay up to date in the constantly evolving healthcare system, using the proper form of research is essential. Just as important as the concept of research itself, is the correct practice and use of

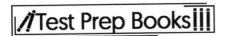

the research. Credibility is of utmost importance in clinical research. The following is a review of the procedural process of nursing research:

1. Select the specific topic: While this step sounds relatively straightforward, the research team will need to understand the importance of selecting an appropriate topic. While there are plenty of issues that warrant discussion, not all issues are appropriate for a research topic. The research team needs to be sure that the topic selected has an attainable solution or outcome. The topic will also need to be specific enough to be measurable.

2. Find additional background information on the specific topic and formulate hypotheses: This stage can be known as the pre-planning phase, as the research team will be looking for general background information to formulate hypotheses. The point of this phase is to further assess the quality of the topic selected for a research project.

3. Design framework for research: This stage can be known as the planning phase. The research team will focus on finding the appropriate forms of data collection and establishing specific roles for the extraction of the data. The goal is to find data specific enough to answer the research topic/question while maintaining practical and ethical values.

4. Utilize approved resources for detailed data collection: Data collection is the meat and potatoes of the research process. It is the unrefined collection of data that is related to the research topic. The importance of data collection is to obtain unbiased information from credible sources. Most facilities/agencies will have a resource library that can be freely used, but access to multiple credible sources is the best research practice.

5. Organize data collected and evaluate findings: Separating the data into quantitative and qualitative sections can help with the organization and evaluation of data. Using visuals for the quantitative data (based on numbers/measurable) and using direct quotes for the qualitative data (interpretive/subjective) can help the research team organize the information to closely assess the general findings.

6. Analyze and interpret data collected: Analyzing the data and interpreting the results is rarely the form of closure to the research topic. This stage usually brings clarity on the need for further research on the topic, research on an additional topic, or revision of the entire research plan. This stage allows the research team to review the interpreted data with the hypotheses.

7. Properly cite any sources: Properly citing sources is not only giving credit to the original author but also avoiding plagiarism. Giving credit to the original source—whether it's a demonstration of the research or written literature—also allows the audience to follow the research.

Clinical Inquiry

Clinical inquiry is an ongoing process that evaluates and challenges clinical practice in order to propose the needed change. Clinical inquiry has several components or attributes, including critical thinking, clinical reasoning, clinical judgment, critical reasoning and judgment, and creative thinking. The process is viewed as the critical structure for the establishment of evidenced based practice and quality improvement efforts. In the Synergy Model, professional nurses employ clinical inquiry to innovate and facilitate interventions that are appropriate to patient care needs. Clinical inquiry is a rigorous process that requires attention to the rules of nursing research, such as attention to sample size, and a correct match among the data, the study design, and the statistical measures.

When used to implement evidenced based practice, clinical inquiry can result in replacing an outdated, even counter-productive nursing intervention with an intervention that effectively addresses the needs of the patient. Nurses who are involved in this form of clinical inquiry are viewed as evaluators and innovators in the Synergy

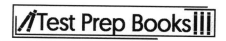

Model. Matching patient needs with nursing competencies means that professional nurses are responsible for challenging all nursing interventions to be sure that they represent current best practice standards. As innovators, nurses are in the best position to research, implement, and evaluate alternative care practices.

Nurses acquire clinical inquiry skills on a continuum that is based on education and clinical experience. As is the case with the other nursing competencies included in the Synergy Model, this progressive development is consistent with Benner's novice to expert model that views the development of nursing expertise as a progressive process that requires ongoing education and clinical experience. Novice nurses are able to implement clinical innovations developed by others, to identify their own learning needs, and to enlist the aid of other nurses to identify critical needs of the patient. Experienced nurses are able to question the adequacy of interventions and to begin to challenge the "we have always done it this way" philosophy that is the most common rationale for many nursing interventions. They are also able to assess the utility of alternative interventions. The Synergy Model views the practice of expert nurses as the point at which clinical inquiry and clinical reasoning become inseparable elements of clinical practice. Expert nurses are able to predict changes in the patient's condition that require revision of the plan of care, and they are also able to develop and implement alternative approaches to address those changes.

Public funds are the most common source of research funding, which means that researchers are obligated to design studies that provide valid results that are applicable to some form of patient care and to disseminate the results appropriately. Common barriers to nursing research efforts include inadequate funding, limited access to appropriate patient populations, and lack of institutional support for research initiatives. The rapid expansion of new knowledge from multiple sources can also inhibit the assimilation and application of new care interventions by expert nurses.

In addition, the final step of the clinical inquiry process, knowledge translation or dissemination, may be the most important step. Knowledge translation refers to the complex process of synthesizing the research findings, disseminating those findings to others, and integrating the findings into clinical practice. Barriers to this process include lack of rigor in the original research design with respect to sample size, data interpretation, and the applicability of the research findings. The failure of nursing researchers to access all possible modes of the dissemination of study results has also been identified as a significant barrier to the application of new interventions. All of these system-wide and individual barriers potentially limit the use of innovative patient care interventions.

Practice Quiz

1. Which of the following is NOT a benefit of using SBAR?
   a. Perioperative nurses spend an excessive amount of time writing, but they are able to draw attention to adverse events using this process.
   b. Perioperative nurses are able to focus on patient care.
   c. The SBAR process increases communication among members of the perioperative staff.
   d. SBAR eliminates the need for face-to-face communication.

2. Which of the following details are necessary in order for checklists to be effective standardization tools?
   a. Checklists need to be aesthetically pleasing to the practitioner's eye, so that he or she is more likely to use it.
   b. Interdisciplinary team members must commit to using the checklist, and all members must use the checklist in the same context.
   c. Checklists need to be varied enough so that a diverse group of staff members has appropriate tasks (pertaining to their job role) to check off.
   d. A checklist must have a global presence in order to be considered a standardization tool.

3. How does each state board of nursing set the standards a nurse is expected to maintain in practice?
   a. Through its Nursing Practice Act
   b. By mandating a minimum number of continuing education units (CEUs) by nurses in all fifty states
   c. By defaulting to each institution's policies and procedures
   d. Individual states do not set these standards; federal guidelines govern these standards.

4. Which of the following is a characteristic of high-quality research evidence?
   a. Results obtained from observational studies
   b. Variable estimates of effect size
   c. RCT study design
   d. Case controlled analytics

5. The nurse is delegating the task of getting a set of vital signs to the certified nursing assistant (CNA). The nurse tells the CNA the task to complete, the CNA repeats the task instructions back to the nurse, and the nurse verifies that the message is correct. This is an example of what kind of communication?
   a. Closed-loop communication
   b. Call-out communication
   c. Feedback communication
   d. Open-loop communication

See answers on the next page.

Answer Explanations

1. D: The SBAR technique is a best practice that allows nurses to focus on providing patient care because it decreases the amount of time they spend writing. Also, the design of this process promotes open communication among the perioperative nursing team. SBAR can be used face-to-face or by telephone, and it should always be a verbal conversation.

2. B: A checklist can only be useful if all active members work together to use it at the same time; otherwise, it cannot produce standardized results. Aesthetically pleasing checklists can be nice but aren't necessary. Checklist tasks should always be repeatable and reliable; therefore, diverse tasks would make a poor checklist. A checklist doesn't need a global presence to be a reliable tool; it simply needs to be accepted by the organization and staff where it's being used as a quality tool.

3. A: Each state board of nursing has a Nursing Practice Act that sets the standards of care a nurse is expected to maintain in practice. All fifty states do not require nurses to maintain a minimum number of CEUs. Policies and procedures vary from institutions within each state. Nursing Practice Acts are regulated by states, not federally.

4. C: The randomized controlled trial (RCT) is regarded as the research design that best controls researcher bias. RCTs tend to be expensive and large-scale; however, the number of subjects often corresponds with the quality of the results. The level of confidence in observational studies is proportional to the control of bias in the specific design, but the evidence is generally considered to be of low quality; therefore, Choice A is incorrect. Variable or imprecise estimates of effect size that require additional investigation before the results of the research can be directly applicable are considered as only moderate-quality evidence; therefore, Choice B is incorrect. Case controlled analytics are also considered to be moderate-quality evidence; therefore, Choice D is incorrect.

5. A: The communication style in which someone sends a message or instruction, someone receives the message, the receiver repeats the message back, and then the initial sender verifies the message is called closed-loop communication. Closed-loop communication is important in the healthcare setting and when delegating tasks to ensure that the instructions are clear and received accurately. Choices B and C are incorrect because they are each only one step of the closed-loop communication style. Choice D is incorrect because in open-loop communication there is no feedback step and the person receiving the instruction does not repeat it back and get the message verified by the sender of the message. This communication style is quicker but allows more room for error.

Nursing Teamwork and Collaboration

Delegation and Supervision

Delegation and Supervision

Nursing staff take on many responsibilities that can be delegated to other clinical and non-clinical colleagues. However, learning how to delegate tasks effectively and safely, while still making patients feel cared for, is a skill that can take time to develop. It requires knowing not only what the needs of the patient are, but also the strengths and weaknesses of assistive personnel and how to best communicate professional needs with them. It also requires personal development in becoming comfortable with outsourcing responsibilities, as the nurse who delegates still remains accountable for the patient.

Assistive personnel may be supervised by nurses, but clinical assistive staff can provide basic medical assistance such as monitoring patients' vital signs, assisting with caretaking duties, monitoring any abnormalities or changes in the patient, maintaining a sterile and safe environment, and any other request made directly by nursing staff. Non-clinical assistive personnel, such as front desk staff, can assist with patient communication (such as wait times), managing paperwork and ensuring it is complete, and performing any other administrative task that may support the nursing staff's cases.

When nursing staff choose to delegate tasks, they may feel worried about risking their own accountability or work ethic. However, relating with assistive personnel, understanding their strengths and weaknesses, understanding their interests, and remaining transparent about the needs that are present in the department can ensure that delegated tasks are a good fit for the person who is taking the responsibility. In this regard, nursing staff take on a leadership and managerial role that requires developing their problem-solving, time management, and interpersonal skills. Some effective tools for delegation can include standardized checklists that cover the procedure that is being delegated, formal and informal meetings about assistive personnel's comfort levels and interests in performing certain tasks, and matching professional needs with individual qualifications. When delegation is effective, it can help the entire department work in a more efficient manner. Additionally, both nursing staff and assistive personnel are more likely to feel like part of a cohesive team and less likely to feel overworked or undervalued.

After the nurse has successfully and effectively delegated a task, the nurse then takes on the role of supervisor of the person to whom they delegated the task. Delegation requires supervision to ensure the task is done appropriately and to protect the nurse's own licensure.

The key to supervision is the follow-up. After the task is delegated, the nurse must then make a note to investigate whether the task was done, whether it was done in a timely manner, and whether it was done correctly. Asking the person who was supposed to perform the task to report back is appropriate. All conversations and interactions must be performed professionally and with respect for both the inferior and superior party.

Many nurses were once certified nursing assistants (CNAs) and understand the role and responsibility of the person they now delegate to. If the two nurses were former co-workers and one has risen to the role of nurse from CNA, tensions may arise. Tensions that arise between nursing staff and those they delegate to may be resolved through careful interactions in which each party is respected and an effort is made by both parties that shows they are both working hard together with the best interest of the patient at the forefront of their minds.

At times, it may be necessary for the nurse to coach and support the staff member, giving tips for better performance where appropriate. Again, this interaction must be done with professionalism and respect. It is

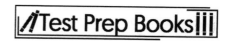
important as an employee in any field to be receptive to constructive criticism as well as being able to offer it when appropriate and allowing plenty of discussion on the point.

The nurse must ensure that the task delegated, such as taking vital signs or cleaning up an incontinent patient, has been appropriately documented. Documentation is necessary for legal reasons, to show that proper care was given to the patient. If the person to whom the task was delegated did not document the task, it is necessary for the nurse to confront them directly and confirm that it was done.

Client Care Assignments

Every day when the nurse reports to duty, a team of patients will be assigned to them. A caseload of patients will vary in size based on the acuity of the patients' illnesses and the policies of the unit that the nurse belongs to.

Acuity refers to the severity of the patient's illness. Some patients are high acuity, meaning a lot of time and resources are put into their daily routine due to the severity of their illness. Others are low acuity and do not require much oversight from the nurse to get through the day. High-acuity patients are a major sore point for many nurses because their care can often take away from the care of others. A team full of high-acuity patients, then, can be a great burden for a nurse to bear.

When patient assignments become too burdensome for nurses, those nursing-sensitive indicators are the first signs that there is a problem. When the nurse is busy with a team of high-acuity patients, it is difficult to perform all the tasks of the day, let alone perform them carefully and thoughtfully. It is then in the best interest of those making team assignments for nurses to weigh carefully the patient load and ensure equitable and fair decisions are made.

Dividing up teams of patients is often the task of the charge nurse. To fairly assign patient teams to nurses, the charge nurse must bear in mind each patient's acuity. Conflict arises when nurses feel that there is inequity in the assignment of patients and they are unduly burdened with an unfair patient load compared to other teams or units.

Nurse satisfaction directly correlates with patient care. If nurses do not feel their patient assignments are fair and the burden is too great, their performance suffers as well as their job satisfaction. Nursing performance can be linked to the following nurse-sensitive indicators: how well patient pain is managed; the presence and treatment of pressure ulcers, patient falls, and medication errors; patient satisfaction; and nosocomial or hospital-acquired infections.

Scope of Practice

Scope of practice refers to the tasks and skills that a person is able to perform within a role. The scope of practice for a particular role may vary depending on the location (i.e., state, facility, department), the situation, and the timing of the situation. For example, in some states, it is within the scope of the emergency medical technicians (EMTs) to start intravenous catheters on patients, while in other states this is only within the scope of the nurse or paramedic. Additionally, scope within certain roles (or titles) may be different across a facility depending on department and training. For example, in one facility, a nurse may be able to perform conscious sedations in interventional radiology, but a nurse on an inpatient floor may not have this scope. Finally, those who are licensed versus unlicensed may be able to perform different tasks. An unlicensed individual may not be able to perform medical tasks and will be less liable or responsible for the patient's safety than the licensed individual. When performing tasks and delegating, it is important to have an understanding of what is within one's own scope of practice and what falls within the scope of practice of ancillary staff.

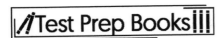

Prioritization Skills

Prioritization skills refer to the ability to decide which task must be performed first. There can be many factors in determining the order in which tasks should be performed. Within nursing, safety is generally considered the highest priority. For example, if the nurse has a patient who is actively falling out of bed, the nurse may prioritize lowering the patient to the ground without injury over leaving to perform another task. Another example of this would be a nurse choosing to administer a time-sensitive medication to a patient in a life-threatening situation before continuing on to administer chronic medications that may not be as time-sensitive. Prioritization is key when it comes to certain disease processes. Understanding which patient to see first based on presentation and assessments is a vital part of a busy medical-surgical nurse's day. However, when there is not necessarily a matter of safety concerns or life-saving measures required, prioritization may become more complicated and less straightforward. Prioritization requires flexibility and critical thinking skills within each individual situation. Prioritization skills also involve the ability to prioritize what should be delegated and what should be performed by the nurse. For example, if the medical-surgical nurse has many patients who are due for medication administration and assessments, which ancillary staff cannot perform, these tasks may become priority for the nurse, while routine vital signs may be a priority delegation to the ancillary staff. Prioritization skills are a key part of effective and efficient patient care for the medical-surgical team.

Budgetary Considerations

Whether working at a non-profit healthcare facility or a for-profit facility, financial factors will always play a role in what is possible within the medical-surgical nursing setting. Because of this, nurses in both staffing and leadership roles should understand the budgetary considerations of their roles. Budgetary considerations refer to what money and resources are available versus what is needed to perform a particular role. Ideally, the medical-surgical nurse will be able to effectively perform their role within the budgetary constraints. Budgets may determine anything from how many nurses and other staff are hired onto a unit to which supplies are stocked for patient care.

When it comes to staffing, the budget can not only determine the number of nurses and ancillary staff that are available, but also the nurse-to-patient ratio. In situations where there are fewer staff to more patients, the medical-surgical nurses and ancillary staff will need to work extra hard to prioritize the needs of the patient and may also need to be more flexible with team dynamics. For better outcomes, however, the budget will allow for safe staffing that will decrease errors and improve patient care.

The budget may also determine what supplies are available and how many are available. Flexibility and creativity may be required if stock is low or if supplies are changed to meet budgetary needs. This ties into the concept of fiscal efficiency, or the ability to keep expenses on or below budget by minimizing waste in daily practice. Medical-surgical nurses must also be cognizant of being efficient with supply usage in order to preserve budget for other areas, such as staffing and quality improvement measures.

Career Development Relationships

Professional Engagement

Professional engagement refers to having dedication to and feeling fulfillment within a job or career. It is one of the key factors in maintaining longevity of quality nurses within the medical-surgical profession. Professional engagement can be created internally within the highly motivated nurse but can also be encouraged through positive leadership and a positive work environment. Leadership can encourage professional engagement by promoting a culture of safety and by ensuring that staff are comfortable within their roles and are able to meet their own needs through appropriate pay and benefits. Leadership may also provide positive feedback which can further improve engagement. Professional engagement can also be encouraged by positive relationships between

272

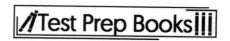
coworkers. Nurses are more likely to feel dedicated to their role when they feel safe, supported, and encouraged. Finally, and possibly most importantly, nurses are more likely to have increased professional engagement when they are able to engage positively with patients and see positive outcomes from their work.

Mentoring and Coaching Resources

Mentoring and coaching refers to the act of providing guidance and support to another. This can be done through the teaching and encouraging of new staff and nurses by more experienced staff and nurses. These resources are vital to integrating the newer generations of nurses into the medical-surgical profession and can promote further benefits such as a more positive work environment, improved care practices, and even career advancement. Nurses can be mentors and coaches at any stage of their professional career and can also have or need mentors and coaches at any stage. These mentor/mentee relationships can establish organically as one nurse guides and encourages another naturally as they work together and form a positive working relationship. Nurse leaders can also encourage mentorship through establishing mentoring programs by recruiting nurses and helping to match them with nurses who may need more support in their role.

Reflective Practice

Reflective practice refers to the act of looking back upon one's practice or work to understand a particular situation better and then using this reflection to improve their practice. Reflection can be more appropriate in certain situations, and understanding when and how to reflect is necessary for this practice to be successful. Reflective practice may also involve making changes to one's practice and then further assessing how those changes worked. In addition, reflective practice can be promoted by positive nurse leaders and mentors. Reflective practice can create better outcomes for patients when integrated into medical-surgical nurse practice.

There are many situations when the nurse may find that reflection is helpful and even necessary. Most commonly, reflective practice may be implemented following negative situations. If there are mistakes made during a procedure, complications following a procedure, or a patient expresses unhappiness with the care they have received, it can be beneficial to look back on what may have gone wrong. Identifying where a fallout may have happened and then considering how it could be avoided in similar situations in the future is a necessary form of practice improvement and education for the nurse. This can also be done in positive situations. When the nurse reflects on how actions taken in a situation were successful, those actions can then be further applied to promote more positive outcomes.

Once the medical-surgical nurse has reflected upon how a particular situation proceeded, the nurse can then take action to potentially implement changes for future situations. After these changes are implemented, reflective practice is further used to determine the successes and/or failings of said changes. The nurse may reflect on whether the changes made a difference in outcomes, and if these outcomes were better or worse than before the change was implemented. Here's an example of this: when a nurse reconstitutes a medication, he notices that the pressure in the bottle causes some of the medication to spray out when drawn up, leading to waste and the patient not receiving all of the medication. The nurse might try a new method of mixing and drawing up the medication, such as first drawing air out of the bottle to reduce the pressure. The nurse should then reflect on whether or not his new technique prevented medication waste. The nurse may even employ the knowledge and experience of those in leadership or mentor roles to help solve this problem. When nurse leaders and mentors promote a nonjudgmental environment that allows for constructive feedback and quality improvement, they can play a vital role in promoting reflective practice in the nursing profession.

Reflective practice is not always purely an individual action; it can involve the entire healthcare team. Often after a particularly difficult situation with unclear outcomes, the team may come together to debrief on what went well, what could have improved, and what to do moving forward. These can be especially common following situations

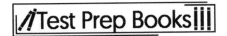
involving close teamwork and high levels of stress, such as codes or procedures with unexpected complications. However, reflective practice can also be applied to day-to-day activities and changes. Reflective practice can be an important part of quality improvement measures within a unit.

Roles and Responsibilities

For any team to be successful in a task, it is important that they have clear roles and responsibilities. Each role may have specific responsibilities attached to it. These roles may be important in the day-to-day management of the unit so that delegation and task management can be streamlined. However, establishing set roles and responsibilities is especially important when a high-stress emergency situation may occur. For example, if a patient is having a life-threatening emergency, it is important to know which nurse will be documenting interventions, which nurse will be assisting with interventions (such as CPR, medication administration, etc.), which nurse will provide communication with additional resources (e.g., doctors, house supervisors, etc.), and who may take on a leadership role directing the emergency situation. Establishing these roles before an emergency happens can reduce anxiety during the emergency and improve chances of success in overcoming the situation as a team.

While each team member on a medical-surgical unit may have individual roles and responsibilities, the roles and responsibilities of the individual nurse may change over time. As nurses gain more experience and knowledge, they may take on new responsibilities and leadership roles. For example, a nurse may gain a new skill and become a resource to the unit in being the expert on performing said skill. More knowledgeable and experienced nurses may become preceptors, mentors, or educators. Nurses may also choose to step into new roles. For instance, nurses may establish a practice council focused on making quality improvements to unit patient care practices.

Coaching and Learning Theories

When a new nurse joins a unit or when further education may be required, the nurse can refer to different coaching and learning theories in order to best assess the needs of the learner and where they are in their learning process. Within nursing, most learning theories relate to how the learner acts and how they express their thoughts and understanding. Five different theories that can be used are behaviorism, cognitive learning, constructivism, humanism, and connectivism. These may be used independently or interconnectedly depending on the learner and the learning situation, but when applied effectively, they can promote successful coaching and learning.

Behaviorism refers to the observable aspects of learning or the actions of the learner. This is most strongly applicable to teaching new skills. For example, the coach may demonstrate the skill to the learner and then observe the learner repeat the skill. Corrections may be made until the skill is demonstrated accurately. Nurse educators may use this method when new equipment is being introduced to ensure that all staff know how to use them properly. While this theory of learning is helpful for specific tasks, it does not go any deeper to show that the learner knows when to or why they should perform this skill.

Cognitive learning refers to more brain-based learning. This can be in the form of providing written resources or even classroom learning to better understand the fundamentals of something. Cognitive learning is generally demonstrated verbally or through testing to ensure that the learner has retained the new knowledge. However, this is mainly a demonstration of knowledge on a more surface level, such as regurgitation of facts or new policies. For example, the learner may be able to say that it is procedure to keep the head-bleed patient's head of the bed elevated but may not necessarily know why or be able to come to that conclusion on their own.

Constructivism is a theory that combines knowledge from behaviorism and cognitive learning and adds critical thinking and creativity to the mix. The learner may apply what they have learned to new situations or even create hypothetical situations to show understanding. This learning may be demonstrated through both verbalization and action. The learner may find a unique way to perform a skill that is more appropriate for a specific situation or may

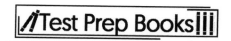

better advocate for a patient given their overall presentation rather than just hospital policy. In order to coach the learner through constructivism, it is important to ask the questions "why?" and "how would you act if...?"

The final two theories, humanism and connectivism, focus more on how the coach interacts with the learner than how to assess the learner's retention of knowledge. Humanism refers to the need to focus on the learner and find out what their goals and needs are. When the coach works to help the learner meet their goals, it increases the learner's sense of autonomy and pride in their work and accomplishments. This theory may not apply, however, if the learner's goals do not align with the needs or goals of the unit. Connectivism refers to identifying holes in the learner's knowledge and providing them with the resources to independently find answers. Examples of this could be showing the learner how to access the hospital or unit's policy and procedure databases, how to find medication references, and how to contact someone if they need help. This is especially important so that the learner feels they have the resources they need and know where to look if they don't know the answer once they no longer have a coach by their side.

Professional Empowerment

Professional empowerment refers to a professional's internal motivation to strive for excellence within their role. Within the nursing profession, this idea of excellence may mean becoming an expert in certain skills, advancing one's education or career station, or providing the best possible patient care experience to all who enter the hospital. Excellence may look different for each nurse. Some will find great motivation, for example, in staying within their current role and becoming competent mentors to their peers. Others may see excellence as advancing their education to management or advanced practice levels. All are valid and necessary for success within the nursing profession. While professional empowerment may look slightly different for each individual nurse, nurses can improve their own empowerment by setting professional goals and finding satisfaction in achieving their desired outcomes. Nurse leaders also promote professional empowerment by encouraging autonomy within roles and encouraging a positive environment dedicated to improvement and excellence.

Orientation Planning and Preceptor Best Practices

Orientation planning refers to the necessary preliminary step of preparing to orient new staff. Depending on available resources, this phase of precepting may be started by nurse educators and preceptors before new staff starts working or it may take place the first time the new hire and preceptor meet. The main point of orientation planning is to establish an idea of what the teaching goals and desired outcomes will be for the nurse entering a new role. Orientation planning should also establish an expected or desired timeline of how long precepting should take and when progress evaluations should take place.

Following the orientation-planning phase, preceptors should apply ongoing best practices in order to ensure the success of the new hire or preceptee. This begins with assessing the preceptee's current knowledge and learning style, as well as assessing how best to meet the goals established in the orientation plan. This may be a continuous assessment throughout the orientation phase or as the preceptee encounters new hurdles. Any feedback provided should be given in a respectful and timely manner. If there is not an immediate safety issue that needs to be corrected, offering feedback is generally best done when not in front of a patient or other staff that might make the preceptee feel humiliated or criticized. However, feedback should also be given soon enough that corrections can be made in the moment rather than after orientation is expected to be completed. It is also important to encourage the preceptee by showing them where their strengths lie and how they can contribute to the unit as a whole. Finally, preceptor best practices do not end when the preceptee has completed orientation. Providing continued support and mentorship throughout the nurse's career establishes an environment of support and growth.

275

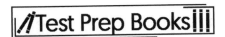

Career Development Resources

Medical-surgical nurses should strive to not only learn the advances in their fields, but to also self-reflect on the ways they learn best in order to make ongoing education a regular part of their careers. Continuing education refers to a range of activities that serve as post-graduate learning. These can be formal activities, such as coursework at an accredited university. Formal activities can also include online courses, seminars, workshops, conferences, and training that are relevant to one's field. Participants are often able to earn and document continuing education credits for formal continuing education activities; many fields and certifications require obtaining a certain number of continuing education credits over a period of time during one's career. Continuing education can also take place informally, such as through mentoring from someone who is further along their career trajectory or reviewing new literature that is relevant to one's field.

Since the medical and healthcare fields are always rapidly changing due to technological advances, new research, organizational and governmental regulations, and through continuous process improvements in healthcare delivery, nurses can expect to continue their education throughout the course of their careers. Consequently, the ability to learn new topics will be a necessary skill in order to remain a competent practitioner. Lifelong learning and continuing education are associated with improved patient outcomes, job satisfaction, personal validation and achievement, and obtaining skills that were not taught or available at the time that the nurse was enrolled in a formal education program. The most crucial association with lifelong learning activities is the improvement in quality of care. Incompetent or unaware nursing staff means a great deal of risk for the patient. By constantly striving to improve their knowledge and practical skills, nurses decrease the chance that they will be held liable for negligence or malpractice, and they are taking tangible actions to adhere to the ethical tenets of the healthcare profession.

While avenues to continue professional development in the nursing field may be formal (such as obtaining extra relevant degrees or certifications, publishing research, or enrolling in training offered by the nurse's workplace), many opportunities require intrinsic motivation, such as taking personal initiative to keep abreast of current relevant literature, consulting with mentors, or experiencing different responsibilities within the field. However, even with these varied opportunities and with the multitude of personal and professional benefits that engaging in lifelong learning activities bring, there are still some barriers for nurses. These include obstacles like disinterest, lack of time on the job or outside of the job to participate in activities, an inability to balance work and life needs with job demands, and lack of financial resources (to pay for educational activities and/or to take the time off to participate in them). In this regard, it is helpful for leadership and subordinate employees to work together to overcome these barriers.

Nurses who are in positions of leadership can help push for organizational support for development activities and promote a culture of top-down change and support. In the events that development activities are free or hosted by the nurse's workplace, it is imperative that the nurse realizes this is a valuable opportunity and take the time to attend and fully engage in the experience. This shows that such activities are in demand and valued, and is likely to make affordable and accessible professional development activities part of the workplace culture.

Professional Development

Professional Nursing Practice and Individual Competencies

Professional nursing practice includes behaviors and norms that are expected to be demonstrated by the successful nurse. These behaviors include demonstrating effective communication and teamwork, placing the patient first, and having an attitude of growth and positivity. This growth mentality is exemplified by improving and advancing individual competencies.

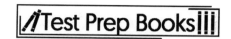

Effective communication may look different depending on the situation and the other participants the nurse is interacting with. For example, when communicating with peers, the nurse may be respectful but will likely be able to use technical terminology that is understood amongst peers. Communication with those in a leadership position may be slightly different—less relaxed than with peers and with an increased level of professionalism. Communication with patients may also be different, as the nurse will need to assess the patients' healthcare knowledge and show a level of care while providing education. Finally, situations may change how the nurse communicates effectively. Communication in an emergency situation may be more concise and require more of a closed loop than day-to-day problem solving with a team.

Effective teamwork is essential to a functioning healthcare facility and medical-surgical unit. Care of a single patient may involve multiple nurses, ancillary staff, and doctors. The professional nurse understands these roles and works within the team effectively to promote positive patient outcomes.

Finally, a nurse shows professional behaviors through putting the patients first and exemplifying a positive, growth-oriented attitude. Nurses must act as advocates for their patients, prioritizing their needs and safety within their role. Negative attitudes do not encourage a safe environment for nurses or patients. As the patient may be in a frightening and unfamiliar world on the medical-surgical unit, positivity can provide the patient with a feeling that they are in capable hands. Additionally, nurses who advance in their skills and competencies are more likely to have greater satisfaction within the profession and are able to provide more skilled care to patients. It is generally expected that as a nurse advances in their career, they become more competent, moving from novice to expert and potentially taking on new roles as their individual competency improves.

Professional Behaviors

Professional behaviors in nursing are meant to advance both the profession of the individual and also create better opportunities within nursing as a whole. Networking and participation in professional organizations are necessary to create connections between nurses and to provide professional opportunities that would not be possible without working together.

Networking refers to the act of forming relationships and contacts that could potentially provide one with future opportunities. This can be done on the unit between fellow nurses, by maintaining a positive relationship with leadership, and also by seeking outside relationships through professional organizations and community events. Networking requires forming a bond, but also expressing one's personal goals so that others within the relationship know how to help if an opportunity arises. Networking might help a nurse move up into a leadership position or find another job within their profession if change is needed. Working together in this way can help improve career satisfaction and stability within the nursing profession.

Similar to networking, participation in professional organizations allows nurses to work together to form a community and make improvements within the profession. One example that is common in some states and healthcare facilities is participation in nursing unions. When working in unions successfully, nurses can advocate for improved staffing standards, higher pay, and better work environments. This can improve career satisfaction, nursing job retention, and the level of care available to patients. Nurses can also get involved in practice counsels meant to improve quality of care on their unit and in their hospital. For example, a wound-care practice counsel could work together to track how certain interventions are affecting outcomes of patients with pressure sores and advocate for improvements to practice where needed. Finally, nurses can also participate in outside organizations, such as specialty organizations, to obtain continuing education, improve their personal practice, form bonds with others in the specialty, and even advocate for improved practice in the specialty as a whole.

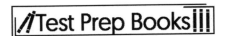

Clinical Judgment

Clinical judgment is the art of assessing and understanding what is happening in a particular medical situation and what actions should be taken based on this assessment. Clinical judgment develops with time, experience, and furthering education. The novice medical-surgical nurse may struggle to identify a disease process within a patient and need to ask more questions before acting, while a seasoned medical-surgical nurse may identify signs and symptoms quickly and take appropriate action. This advancement in clinical judgment comes from continued application of the nursing process and having more experience opportunities throughout one's career.

In its most fundamental and basic form, the nursing process generally refers to ADPIE (assess, diagnose, planning, implementation, and evaluation). Within this structure, the nurse will first assess the patient's presentation and then come up with an applicable nursing diagnosis. From there the nurse will create a plan of care, implement the plan, and then evaluate if the intervention was successful or not. As the nurse gains more experience, this process can become more efficient and effective with improved application of critical-thinking skills. In fact, the more experienced nurse may be able to jump more quickly from assessment to implementation and evaluation as they better understand a disease process or patient presentation within their clinical judgment.

While clinical judgment does come with time and experience, nurses must be proactive in working to improve it. Some nurses may be tempted to embrace comfort in their career, following doctors' orders with few questions and avoiding difficult situations whenever possible. These nurses may advance their clinical judgment for certain situations, but it is possible they will have difficulty thinking outside of the box when they are outside of their comfort zone. Nurses who push outside of their comfort zone, say "yes" to a more challenging patient assignment, continually ask questions of more clinically experienced individuals, and advocate for themselves to have further opportunities and educational experiences will be more successful in improving their clinical judgment.

Peer Review Methods

Peer review methods refer to the processes of assessing the validity and use of clinical articles, journals, studies, or nursing practices. The intent behind peer review is to ensure the integrity of the science behind the article or study and to ensure that practice is evidence based. The hope is to minimize harm from inaccurate or deceptive information. Peer review can be used in the academic setting and within the professional setting using several different methods.

Two forms of peer review within the academic setting are meant to emphasize anonymity. One is "single anonymized," where the author does not know who will be reviewing their article or study. This prevents the author from leaning the article's bias in favor of the reviewer and allows the reviewer to feel more comfortable providing negative feedback. The other is "double anonymized," where both the author and reviewer are anonymous in the review process to prevent bias in either direction. While these methods can be useful in reviewing academic articles and studies, it is important for nurses to be aware that the American Nurses Association does not consider anonymized peer review to be the standard of practice within the professional setting as it does not allow for accountability for either party.

Peer review methods that provide more transparency are open peer review and transparent peer review. Within open peer review, all parties are known to one another and accountability from all parties is encouraged. However, this method may discourage some reviewers from providing negative feedback. In order to encourage unbiased feedback, transparent peer review may be employed, in which the reviewer may choose whether or not to have their identity known. These methods can be applied both in the academic setting and within professional practice. A mentor may use open peer review with a mentee to provide feedback to ensure that their practice is evidence-based. On the other hand, a nurse may use transparent peer review when submitting a quality improvement form regarding an incident that had a negative outcome when it might not be appropriate or possible to provide negative feedback to a specific individual.

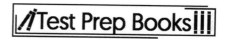

Educational Needs Assessment

An educational needs assessment is a goal-oriented assessment meant to better understand a person's level of knowledge, what they need to know, and how best to help them learn. Educational needs assessments are a useful tool in all levels of nursing practice and can be used between the nurse educator or preceptor and staff nurse as well as between the nurse and the patient.

In the mentor/mentee role, an educational needs assessment is meant to establish a baseline of the mentee's current knowledge and how best to help the mentee improve their knowledge and skills to meet unit expectations. This involves establishing the best learning styles and communication methods. This assessment often takes place during the orientation stage of a nurse's career or when a mistake is made to ensure that just culture is practiced.

In the nurse/patient role, an educational needs assessment is also necessary to establish a baseline understanding of the patient's knowledge and goals for their health. Not everyone enters the hospital with the same level of education or medical experience. This assessment is important to give the patient autonomy and to allow them to make informed decisions about their health.

Leadership

Regulatory and Compliance Standards

Regulatory and compliance standards mainly refer to the laws and policies that are in place to ensure safe and quality care within a healthcare facility. Specific requirements may vary from state to state. For example, some states require certain nurse-to-patient ratios, while others do not have any legal staffing requirements. There are also federal regulations, such as requirements for doctors and nurses to meet licensing standards and policies that protect patients, such as HIPAA (Health Insurance Portability and Accountability Act) and EMTALA (Emergency Medical Treatment and Labor Act). Hospitals may be monitored for compliance by government officials and by independent accrediting bodies depending on availability and resources of the hospital. It is important for nurses to understand these regulatory and compliance standards to maintain their licensure, avoid potential legal action, and maintain the health and safety of their patients.

The Joint Commission

The Joint Commission (TJC) is an international, independent review entity with the mission of ensuring that healthcare facilities operate by and maintain the highest quality standards for care. They accredit organizations based on a stringent set of standards and monitor accredited facilities on two- or three-year cycles. Safety goals are reviewed, and often revised, annually to reflect the most current research and best practice principles.

Organizational Structure

Organizational structure refers to the framework an organization uses to allot power and responsibilities to its employees and those in leadership positions. While this structure may differ, an example of an organizational structure would be the Chief Nursing Officer (CNO) as top nursing leader making overall organizational decisions for nursing staff, nurse managers running individual departments or units, house supervisors acting as resources for the entire hospital, charge nurses acting as resource and leadership for individual shifts on a unit, and then staff nurses generally following the leadership of the previously listed individuals. Each role has different expectations of responsibility, and facilities will often provide a guide to employees on the hierarchy of the organization's structure and what to expect from each role. This guide can also act as a way to understand what resources are available and to know which person to ask for help. For example, it might be more appropriate to ask the unit nurse manager about scheduling and days off than to ask the CNO. However, the CNO may be the person to go to when a practice council wants to recommend a facility-wide change. It is important for nurses to understand the organizational

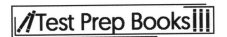

structure of their facility in order to best advocate for themselves and their patients and to best understand expectations of their own roles.

Shared Governance

Shared governance is a theoretical model used in the nursing profession to promote high quality care and a healthy work environment. Shared governance combines the inputs and skills of both superiors and subordinate staff to hold nursing professionals accountable for their work. This model also aims to nurture collaborative efforts to providing care that is safe, effective, and considered valuable by the patients. It promotes high levels of cooperation and aims to foster respect between all employees in a hierarchical structure, believing that this leads to improved worker productivity and satisfaction, and consequently, better service delivery. Ways to implement shared governance in a medical setting include defining collaborative efforts and boundaries between different professional roles, soliciting input from all staff members, regular in-person meetings where all members feel comfortable sharing opinions, ideas, and concerns, and reliable modes of communication outside of meetings. Shared governance is associated with stronger feelings of responsibility, group collaboration, and professional support in the work setting.

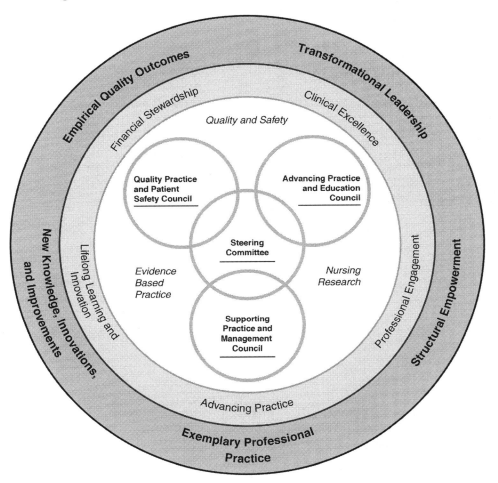

Shared Decision-Making

Shared decision-making refers to the practice of collaborating between the healthcare provider(s) and the patient to decide what is best for the patient. The healthcare provider does not sway the patient against their own wishes and shows respect for the patient's decisions. This process requires open, honest communication between the

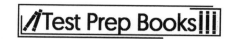

healthcare team and the patient. This also requires an assessment of the patient's healthcare literacy to ensure that the patient is making informed decisions. The nurse's role within shared decision-making is to build a relationship of trust so that the patient feels open to express their health autonomy. The nurse must also act as an advocate for the patient, assisting them to express their needs, desires, and values to what may be a diverse and complicated healthcare team. Shared decision-making may be difficult when the patient has values or makes decisions that do not align with what the nurse or rest of the healthcare team may choose, but it is important to respect patient autonomy.

Nursing Philosophy

Nursing philosophy refers to a definition of what is considered to be the most important aspect or aspects of nursing practice and its foundation. Many great nursing scholars have established changing ideas of what the philosophy of nursing is meant to be. Florence Nightingale's philosophy of nursing focused on the improvement of environmental factors to improve patient health. Jean Watson, on the other hand, focused more on the belief that the most important aspect of nursing is caring for patients. Similarly, Ernestine Wiedenbach encouraged providing for the individualized needs of each patient, and Virginia Henderson believed in helping patients achieve their highest level of independence and self-care. Modern nursing philosophy and practice may include all or most of these sentiments depending on the patient, the situation, and even the specific nurse. It is important for medical-surgical nurses to determine which philosophy or philosophies best fit their practice to provide the best outcomes for their patients. It is also important to be aware that nurses from different backgrounds with different values and experiences may have slightly different beliefs on which nursing philosophy is best for their practice. These differences working together can benefit the nursing profession as a whole, providing different perspectives that may better meet patient needs.

Leadership Models

When taking on a leadership role, a nurse may choose from different models of leadership to determine which style or method is best for a particular situation or group being lead. Some of these models include transformational, servant, autocratic, laissez-faire, democratic, and transactional.

Transformational leadership is goal- or improvement-centered leadership. This form of leadership is ideal for leaders in a preceptor, mentor, or nurse educator role, as transformational leaders work to inspire others toward their goals. Similarly, the servant leader is focused on the individualized needs of the team members.

Within an autocratic leadership role, the person in the leadership position takes little input from others and makes the vast majority of decisions. This leadership model may not go over as well in certain units for the day-to-day operations, as it discourages feedback from staff. However, this model is ideal in emergency situations when there is a need for efficiency in decision-making.

Democratic leadership is a more collaborative leadership model, in which the leader may ask staff for feedback on how best to approach change or other decisions. This model is best when applying quality improvement measures, as the leader can take advantage of the knowledge, experience, and perspectives of a variety of individuals. However, this model may not always be possible due to organizational expectations or goals.

Within a laissez-faire leadership model, the leader is more hands-off, allowing for experienced staff to work with little instruction or feedback from the leader. This may be a common leadership model for the general day-to-day flow of the unit and allows those in leadership to focus on other tasks than micro-management of daily work.

Transactional leadership is more focused on completion of a specific task or reaching a short-term goal. This is best when deadlines need to be met. Examples of these are when continuing education credits need to be completed by

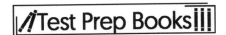
a certain date or when the hospital is preparing for a visit from an accrediting body. This leadership model ensures that staff are prepared and that needed tasks are completed.

Nursing Care Delivery Systems

Nursing care delivery systems refer to the different methods or structures used to decide roles and responsibilities in the care provided to patients. Some of the different care delivery systems include functional nursing, team nursing, primary nursing, and total patient care or individual nursing. These different systems depend on resources available in an organization, staff abilities, and the goals of specific patient care. Each hospital system may use a combination of these nursing care delivery systems to provide the best care possible.

Functional nursing is a very task-oriented nursing care delivery system. There is generally one primary or leading nurse who then delegates tasks to other nurses. For example, one nurse may administer medications, one may perform wound care, and one may focus on dietary needs. This care delivery system may be less common in the medical-surgical setting, but it is possible that hospitals will have staffed nurses to focus on certain specialized tasks, such as wound care, to ensure increased quality of those specific tasks. However, if this method is applied for all care of the medical-surgical patient, care may become disjointed, as each nurse is task-focused rather than understanding the whole patient care continuum.

The team nursing method of nursing care delivery involves a team leader—someone who is responsible for all patients—assigning a group of nurses to a group of patients. The assigned nurses are then responsible for ensuring that all patient care is completed, and they may delegate tasks to ancillary staff as needed. This method is helpful in environments that encourage flexibility. For example, if one nurse is needed with a particularly acute patient for an extended period of time, the other nurses in the group can take on the care of the other patients. This delivery method can be more common in emergency departments but can also be applied to medical-surgical nursing when there is a need. Care in this method is more individualized than in functional nursing, but the nurses may have less contact with specific patients and patients may struggle to know who is responsible for their care.

Total patient care (or individual) nursing is likely the care delivery system most commonly seen in medical-surgical nursing. Within this system, there is a head nurse in charge of a unit of patients, who then assigns each nurse on the unit a group of patients who will be the focus of their care for that specific shift. The assigned nurse is responsible for the planning and delivery of care to these patients, delegating tasks as needed.

Finally, in a primary nursing structure of care delivery, one specific nurse is assigned to a specific patient from admission to discharge. The nurse may delegate the care of the patient when the primary nurse is not available at the hospital, but all care responsibilities fall to the primary nurse. This nursing care delivery system allows for a much stronger relationship between nurse and patient, as well as improved continuity of care. However, this method is rare, as there are generally not enough nurses available to make this system possible at most hospitals.

Change Management

Change is an inevitable part of healthcare and medical-surgical nursing. New best practices may be discovered. Budgets may require cutbacks of certain resources or allow for new advancements in resources and practices. However, change can be difficult to accept within a professional environment, and this can make implementation even more difficult. If the staff does not know change is coming or why it is even necessary, they may become resistant to the change and prevent its success. This is why it is important for nurse leaders to manage change in a way that will be successful for all who are involved. One useful model for implementing and managing change is ADKAR (awareness, desire, knowledge, ability, reinforcement).

Within the ADKAR model, "awareness" refers to the need to ensure that staff are aware that change is coming. If a change is suddenly required of staff without warning, they have lost some autonomy within their role in the team.

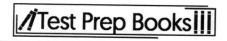

They are much more likely to oppose the change they did not know was coming and had no chance to prepare for. Because of this, leadership should provide staff with knowledge of the change before it is implemented, allowing staff time to feel prepared and to potentially contribute to its implementation.

"Desire" refers to the practice of convincing the staff that the change is both wanted and necessary. Staff will be more likely to participate in change implementation if they believe that the change is needed and will be beneficial to them. Staff that believe change is unnecessary or even a hindrance to their practice may be resistant and get in the way of progress made in implementing the change.

"Knowledge" refers to the need to provide staff with knowledge of how to make the change happen. Providing more information on what the change is, why it is necessary, and what is expected of them increases the staff's chances of accepting the change. This can be done through continuing education opportunities, meetings, fliers, and even in-service training as applicable.

"Ability" refers to making use of the staff's knowledge to implement the change. This may be from the new knowledge about the change discussed above or it may also include previous knowledge and experiences that may apply to making the change a success. For example, the nurse leader may encourage feedback from those within the staff on how to employ the change or even create a committee dedicated to ensuring success with the change. When staff feel they have contributed to the change, they are less likely to resist it, and the change is more likely to take place.

Finally, once the change has been implemented, "reinforcement" may be necessary to ensure that the change remains in place and continues to be successful. This may mean reminders if staff fail to follow through with the change, or it may mean further assessment to see how the change has affected the unit as a whole.

Recruitment and Retention

Recruitment refers to the act of bringing in and hiring new staff to a facility or unit. Retention refers to keeping staff long term. A balance between the two is necessary to maintain sufficient and safe staffing. There are several strategies nurse leaders can use to recruit and retain quality staff. Monetary incentives can be helpful for both recruitment and retainment. Sign-on and relocation bonuses may help recruit new staff from other locations. Offering quality benefits, retention bonuses, and retirement plans that increase over time can help with both recruiting and retention. Outreach programs through recruitment teams, job advertisements, and recruitment incentives for current staff can also help bring in new staff. However, the best way to bring in new staff and also retain staff is to promote a positive work environment with cohesive staff and supportive leadership. Nurses who enjoy their place of employment will stay and also encourage others to join them.

Employee Engagement

Employee engagement refers to an employee's passion for their job and for their place of employment. Those with a positive attitude about their job are more likely to stay in it and to perform their job well. There are several ways nurse leaders can improve employee engagement. One is by promoting a sense of purpose. Reminding nurses and other staff that what they do on a daily basis makes a difference and providing specific examples of positive outcomes can help staff feel that sense of purpose in their work. Another way to promote employee engagement is by encouraging opportunities for growth. Providing opportunities to learn advanced skills, take on leadership roles, and continue education can bring a new spark into a person's passion for their job. Finally, one of the main ways that leadership can encourage employee engagement is through ongoing and supportive communication. Ensuring that employees know the goals of the organization or unit, allowing them to participate in change processes, and ensuring that employee needs are being met are key to ensuring that employees remain engaged.

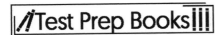

Staff Advocacy

Professionally, nurses advocate for policies that support and promote the practice of all nurses with regard to access to education, role identity, workplace conditions, and compensation. The responsibility for professional advocacy requires nurses to provide leadership in the development of the professional nursing role in all practice settings that may include acute care facilities, colleges and universities, or community agencies. Leadership roles in acute care settings involve participation in professional practice and shared governance committees, providing support for basic nursing education by facilitating clinical and preceptorship experiences, and mentoring novice graduate nurses to the professional nursing role. In the academic setting, nurses work to ensure the diversity of the student population by participating in the governance structure of the institution, conducting and publishing research that supports the positive impact of professional nursing care on patient outcomes, and serving as an advocate to individual nursing students to promote their academic success. In the community, nurses assist other nurse-providers to collaborate with government officials to meet the needs that are specific to that location.

Conflict Management

Conflict can be inevitable when humans work together. This can be especially true in high-stress environments like healthcare. Nurse leaders must work to identify potential causes of conflict and handle them head-on. This can start with conflict mitigation, through ensuring a safe environment for open and respectful communication. When conflict does arise, it is important for the nurse leader to communicate with all parties involved, working to understand the values of the individuals involved and what has caused the conflict. When appropriate, the nurse leader should facilitate communication between the conflicting individuals and work with them to find answers to the problem. Further education should be provided in instances where this is the cause of conflict. Above all, nurse leaders should lead by example, showing respect to all employees and encouraging them to do the same for one another.

Financial Stewardship

Financial stewardship refers to taking on the responsibility of using another person's or organization's finances and resources and doing so in a responsible and wise manner. In nursing, this refers to not causing undue financial hardship to the patient. It is important to be mindful of how patient care can affect the patient financially and how finances may affect a patient's decisions about their care. On the most basic level, nurses should be careful not to be wasteful of things like medications or supplies that patients may be charged for. Additionally, nurses should advocate for patients when an unnecessary procedure or treatment is being encouraged. It is important to listen to the patient's concerns about cost and work within the interdisciplinary team to find ways to reduce costs when possible while still providing quality care. Nurse leaders can also improve financial stewardship by implementing programs to decrease costs in areas of efficiency, supplies used, and resource management.

Disaster Planning and Management

Disaster Management

A disaster emergency refers to any event that may bring a large influx of patients into the medical setting, such as a natural disaster or a mass casualty situation. They tend to be events marked by horror, calamity, and chaos, and nursing staff play a vital role in managing the complex mental, emotional, and physical demands of a community.

All healthcare organizations will have internal standards and resources in place for responding to a disaster. These may be tailored to the geographical area; for example, a coastal healthcare facility may have specific guidelines for hurricane events, while a Midwestern facility may have specific guidelines for tornado events. Additionally, guidelines may be amended as new potential threats arise. For example, if an infectious disease outbreak is

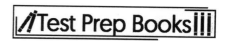
occurring in a certain area within the country, all healthcare facilities may implement standards to follow for that specific disease. Staying current on emerging threats, knowing the facility's capacity for treatment during a time of crisis, and planning for vulnerable populations (such as young children and the elderly) are crucial components of disaster preparation that allow medical staff to anticipate potential risks and the logistics of responding to them.

If a disaster does occur, nursing staff should utilize the tools prepared to navigate the event. This may require setting up workstations outside of the usual spaces, managing crowds, triaging incoming patients, working with assistive personnel, keeping patients calm, and determining the flow of treatment. It will be imperative for staff to cooperate in teams, follow a chain of command, and remain in constant communication with one another. Actual response to the disaster may encompass procedures like triaging existing patients, providing care as needed, and referring more serious cases to the appropriate medical staff member.

Recovery begins as the disastrous event ends and can last for a long time. It accounts for providing a safe space for patients to heal, promoting a sense of calm in the community, providing basic needs to patients (such as food and shelter), and evacuating stable patients as needed. As patients' initial injuries heal, managing infections becomes vital. Patients may return with post-traumatic stress, depression, fear, anxiety, or suicidal tendencies. Through all this, nursing staff must also learn to support themselves and their colleagues so that they may healthfully tend to the needs of the rest of the community.

Mass Casualty

Healthcare systems must develop procedures for mass casualty events that cause surges in patient admittance. Mass casualty events can quickly result in understaffing and other resource depletion. Examples include natural disasters, pandemics, acts of terrorism, and situations of extreme violence. A disaster management plan that integrates all available healthcare resources in a region (such as large hospitals, small medical offices, and volunteer healthcare personnel) can support a coordinated and comprehensive response. Communities should proactively ensure that such a plan exists and can be logistically deployed well before a mass casualty event occurs.

Several best practice frameworks, including the National Response Framework and the National Incident Management System, can be adapted locally to promote coordinated responses in the case of patient surges. The CDC has developed a resource calculator for various mass casualty events that helps a hospital system predict how many patients will be seen in the first hour after a specific type of event and the rate at which patients may arrive thereafter. This modeling tool can also help healthcare systems predict what resources may be needed after specific events and prepare a localized plan accordingly. Factors to consider may include from where to call additional personnel, the amount of personal protective equipment to have on hand, plans for triaging patients, methods for establishing makeshift healthcare centers, and addressing community recovery after the mass casualty event.

Mass casualty events not only affect the physical health and well-being of a community; they also take a psychological toll on community members and first responders. Community recovery may include mental health services for first responders, financial aid from the state or federal government, and long-term health supports for community members directly involved in the event. Healthcare systems can prepare for mass casualty events by regularly drilling their proposed plan and using these sessions to identify gaps that may be present during a real event. Gaps that present themselves in real situations include disproportionate admittance to a single hospital (e.g., the one closest to the scene of the event), language barriers, back-up staff that are unable to serve, widespread contamination, miscommunication, or harm caused to healthcare facilities themselves. For example, in many natural disasters, healthcare facilities may lose power or become inaccessible.

Natural Disasters

Natural disasters refer to destructive events resulting in property and infrastructure damage; injuries to people, animals, and livestock; and ecological devastation. Natural disasters are often mass casualty incidents. They include events such as hurricanes, floods, earthquakes, avalanches, blizzards, landslides, volcanic activity, tornados, heat

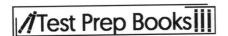

waves, wildfires, and windstorms. Medical facilities normally have protocols in place to address potential natural disasters that could occur in the surrounding geographic area. These protocols address not only organizational procedures to follow in the event of a natural disaster, but also how to house and/or evacuate victims of specific types of natural disasters. For example, a coastal hospital will likely have procedures in place for hurricanes and flooding, while a hospital near a fault line will likely have procedures in place for an earthquake.

Consider the importance of the nurse's adaptability to crises with reference to assisting patients and families impacted by natural disasters. Upon deployment to an area destroyed by torrential rains and subsequent flooding, a nurse could encounter families in need of not only immediate medical care, but ongoing crisis intervention. In conditions such as these, patients are often overwhelmed by their physical pain as well as concerns for how to meet their basic needs for food, shelter, and clean water. Disaster relief relies on medical triage to determine the appropriate level of care needed by patients and is typically assessed based on a four-tier model:

- Black/blue is reserved for the deceased.
- Red is reserved for immediate care such as chest wounds or gunshots.
- Yellow is reserved for those with stable wounds or head injuries.
- Green is reserved for minor injuries such as fractures or burns.

In this situation, the nurse must be prepared to rapidly assess the patient's level of injury and the most expedient treatment needed for stabilization and move on to the next case within minutes. Does the patient or anyone in the family maintain a specific medication regimen to manage chronic illnesses? Have any doses of required medications been missed? Are any assistive devices such as hearing aids or canes needed? It is important to note that the nurse will need to focus on the medical stabilization of patients in this stage rather than delving into psychosocial and emotional trauma.

During disaster-relief efforts, nurses are normally dispatched to both acute care and follow-up care zones. Once immediate medical needs are addressed, patients are transferred to a safe holding area. This space is set aside for psychosocial triage, where patients' basic emotional and physical needs are met. Social workers and chaplains are readily available to debrief survivors. Consider the example of a nurse working with a family impacted by the previous illustration. Having lost their home and belongings and facing recovery from minor injuries, they have been transferred to the holding area for processing.

The nurse in this example would receive a brief synopsis from triage, but only regarding injuries and treatment. In this stage, the nurse would obtain a brief social history, information on chronic disease, and feasible relocation options. Then, the nurse will need to begin guiding the patients through processing the emotional trauma of the incident. Are all family members accounted for? Does anyone in the family unit manage any mental health conditions that have been triggered? What, if any, legal or illegal substances are used or abused by anyone in the family unit? These questions are to help determine if the survivors' emotional responses are directly related to the recent trauma.

Responses to acute traumatic events often mirror the typical response of those who have experienced chronic trauma. The nurse must also assess patients for underlying mental health conditions that may have been exacerbated. In this instance, the most appropriate nursing diagnosis would include ineffective coping. Typical nursing interventions would require the nurse to work with the patient to access previously successful ways of navigating traumatic events, presenting viable options for the next steps, and allowing the patient the time to process the best response to the traumatic event.

Fire

RACE is an acronym used for fire safety purposes. It stands for Rescue, Alarm, Contain, Extinguish. It advises users to "RACE to safety" by *R*emoving themselves and others from dangerous fire situations; *A*ctivating available fire alarms

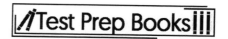

and alerting emergency services; *C*ontaining the area housing the fire by closing windows, doors, and other entry points; and attempting to *E*xtinguish the fire if it does not pose a direct threat to the user. PASS is an acronym used when employing a fire extinguishing device. It stands for Pull, Aim, Squeeze, Sweep. Users should pull the pin that allows the extinguisher to work, aim at the base of the fire, squeeze the lever that controls the flow of the extinguishing substance, and sweep the device in long strokes across the flames until the fire is extinguished or emergency services have arrived.

Hospital Incident Command Structure

Hospital incident command structure refers to the structure of command in place to coordinate the handling of an emergency situation. This can be a collaboration between many departments, both within an individual hospital and when working with outside organizations, such as emergency services and government. Depending on the severity of the emergency incident, this command structure may even go all the way up to the federal level. These emergencies can be natural disasters, such as storms or earthquakes, or caused by humans, such as terrorist attacks or mass shootings. Whatever the cause may be, it is important for the hospital to have an incident command structure and for staff to understand what to do in these scenarios.

Generally speaking, the incident command structure comprises the head command, who is then in charge of leading those responsible for things like logistics, operations, finances, and communication. The goal is to be able to bring in any available resources to react to emergency events. The person in command is also responsible for planning ahead so that the hospital and any involved community organizations are prepared, possibly even preventing potential emergencies from happening. After the response to the emergency, the command will then work on hospital and community recovery, working to rebuild to the normal state of affairs that was present prior to the event.

During an emergency event, it is expected that the roles of individuals involved may change depending on the needs of the incident command. Nurses who normally work at the bedside may be responsible for tasks such as decontamination of HAZMAT patients, triaging mass casualties, or even assisting with the flow of patients or visitors. Nurses must also be prepared to potentially take on more roles than usual due to limited resources to meet a greater need.

In order to prepare for emergency events, it is the nurses' responsibility to understand the hospital incident command structure and know generally what is expected of them in these situations. Nurses should know how they will be contacted or how emergency information will be relayed to them. They should also know what roles they may have to perform and should expect to be flexible depending on needs. Finally, the best way to be prepared is to participate in available practice drills and be a part of the incident command planning process.

Practice Quiz

1. Which action should the nurse delegate to the unlicensed assistive personnel (UAP)?
   a. Obtain sterile equipment
   b. Document early detection education
   c. Provide discharge teaching
   d. Prepare an incident report

2. At minimum, which sets of standards and guidelines should all perioperative nurses familiarize themselves with?
   a. FDA and EPA standards and guidelines
   b. OSHA and ANA standards and guidelines, in addition to the guidelines of the state in which they work
   c. HHS and DPH standards and guidelines for the country and state in which they work
   d. CDC standards and guidelines

3. When should the nursing team monitor for changes to regulatory guidelines and recommendations?
   a. Annually
   b. Quarterly
   c. Only when it contradicts the facility's policies and procedures
   d. Constantly

4. A nurse is a member of a peer review committee at a hospital. The committee is tasked with reviewing a case in which a nurse has been accused of providing substandard care to a patient who ultimately suffered harm. The reviewing nurse is a longtime friend of the accused nurse, and the two have worked together for many years. The committee has been unable to come to a consensus on the appropriate action to take. What is the best course of action for the reviewing nurse in this scenario?
   a. Removing themselves from this case due to their personal relationship with the accused nurse
   b. Advocating for the accused nurse and presenting evidence in their favor
   c. Making an unbiased decision based on the evidence presented, despite their personal relationship with the accused nurse
   d. Abstaining from voting and allowing the other members of the committee to make the decision

5. A nurse is concerned about the current nursing care delivery system, which relies on traditional task-oriented nursing care. The nurse believes that this system does not provide optimal care for patients, particularly those with complex medical needs. They are considering advocating for a different nursing care delivery system. What is the most appropriate nursing care delivery system for a patient with complex medical needs?
   a. Task-oriented nursing care
   b. Functional nursing care
   c. Team nursing care
   d. Patient-centered nursing care

See answers on the next page.

Answer Explanations

1. A: Choice *A* indicates an action that aligns with the scope of practice of the unlicensed assistive personnel (UAP), which can safely be delegated by the nurse. Choices *B*, *C*, and *D* indicate actions that should be carried out by the nurse, as they align with the scope of practice of the nurse and not with the scope of the UAP.

2. B: Nurses across disciplines are held accountable to the standards and guidelines established by the Occupational Safety and Health Administration, American Nursing Association, and the specific state guidelines where they are licensed and employed. They aren't held accountable individually to any guidelines of the Food and Drug Administration, the Environmental Protection Agency, the Department of Health and Human Services, or the Centers for Disease Control, making Choices *A*, *C*, and *D* incorrect.

3. D: In order to maintain professional accountability, the nursing staff should constantly monitor for changes to regulatory guidelines and recommendations. Subscribing to journals is a great way to stay informed of these changes. If the changes contradict the facility's policies or procedures, the nurse should have their manager to review the impact.

4. A: Peer review committees are responsible for evaluating the quality of care provided by their peers and determining appropriate actions when substandard care is identified. To ensure that the process is fair and unbiased, it is important for committee members to avoid conflicts of interest, including personal relationships with the nurse being reviewed. Choices *B* and *C* would compromise the integrity of the peer review process by creating a conflict of interest. Choice *D* is not the best course of action, as it still allows the nurse to participate in the discussion and influence the outcome of the committee's decision.

5. D: Patient-centered nursing care is an approach to care delivery that prioritizes the patient's needs and preferences. This model focuses on individualized care, shared decision-making, and collaborative communication among patients, families, and healthcare providers. Patient-centered care is particularly important for patients with complex medical needs who require individualized attention and comprehensive care plans. Choices *A* and *B* are less comprehensive approaches to care that may not meet the needs of patients with complex medical needs. Choice *C* is a collaborative approach to care delivery but may not provide the level of individualized care needed for patients with complex medical needs.

Practice Test #1

1. The nurse is assessing the abdomen of a 30-year-old female patient with appendicitis. Which finding is the nurse most likely to assess?
    a. Soft abdomen
    b. Periumbilical pain
    c. Absent bowel sounds
    d. Abdominal pulsations

2. Which assessment data is of greatest concern when present in a patient with pneumonia?
    a. Capillary refill greater than three seconds
    b. 9,000 white blood cells per microliter
    c. Respiratory rate of twenty breaths per minute
    d. Productive cough

3. Which intervention should the nurse NOT include while maintaining seizure precautions for a patient with epilepsy?
    a. Padded side-rails
    b. Suction by the bedside
    c. Side-rails down
    d. Ambubag in room

4. A 19-year-old college student who presents with sudden onset of headache that is associated with neck stiffness and fever has been admitted to the hospital. In caring for the patient with meningitis, the nurse understands that which of the following observations is correct?
    a. The presence of a skin rash eliminates the diagnosis of viral meningitis.
    b. Brain herniation after lumbar puncture is more common in immunosuppressed patients.
    c. The CSF protein level is decreased in bacterial meningitis.
    d. The MCV4 vaccine has dramatically decreased the incidence of meningitis in patients in long-term care facilities.

5. While working with a withdrawn patient, how should the medical-surgical nurse respond?
    a. Enable the patient to establish the pace
    b. Remain the lead of the conversation
    c. Include short, quick movements
    d. Discourage verbal expression of anxiety triggers

6. The medical-surgical nurse provides patient education before administering a new treatment for a patient with myasthenia gravis. Which description provided by the nurse accurately describes the reason for administering immunosuppressive therapy for this patient?
    a. It decreases autoantibody production.
    b. It promotes excretion of autoantibodies.
    c. It increases autoantibody production.
    d. It blocks autoantibody receptors.

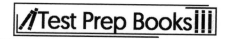

7. The nurse is caring for a patient in the medical-surgical unit who has manifestations of diverticulitis. The patient asks the nurse to explain the difference between diverticulosis and diverticulitis. Which of the following statements is correct?
   a. Diverticulosis rarely occurs in adults.
   b. Diverticulitis is associated with chronic NSAID use.
   c. The initial treatment for diverticulitis is surgery to remove the affected bowel segment.
   d. The patient's age at onset of diverticulosis is associated with the risk of diverticulitis.

8. Which condition does the medical-surgical nurse attribute the patient's painful reddish-purple blistering rash to?
   a. Lupus erythematosus
   b. Vitiligo
   c. Stevens-Johnson syndrome
   d. Lyme disease

9. Which treatment intervention should be implemented in the plan of care for a patient with acute renal failure?
   a. Sulfonylureas
   b. Intravenous contrast studies
   c. Bed rest
   d. High-protein diet

10. Which analgesic, a dye known to numb pain within the urinary tract, should the medical-surgical nurse administer while caring for the patient with a urinary tract infection?
   a. Meperidine
   b. Phenazopyridine
   c. Naprosyn®
   d. Ceftriaxone

11. How long should the medical-surgical nurse auscultate the apical heart rate while completing a focused assessment?
   a. 15 seconds
   b. 30 seconds
   c. 60 seconds
   d. 120 seconds

12. A patient overdosed on acetaminophen after retrieving it from their visitor's purse during visiting hours. While providing emergent care with the code response team, which medication should the nurse administer to counteract the effects of this poisoning?
   a. Atropine
   b. Acetylcysteine
   c. Naloxone
   d. Flumazenil

13. The nurse is caring for a patient with a non-ST elevation myocardial infarction (NSTEMI). Using the Thrombolysis in Myocardial Infarction (TIMI) tool, which of the following categories would the nurse NOT assess?
   a. Age
   b. ST deviation on ECG
   c. Left bundle branch block
   d. Prior aspirin intake

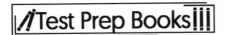

14. While caring for a 54-year-old patient with rheumatoid arthritis and long-term corticosteroid use, which side effect does the medical-surgical nurse consider?
   a. Hypotension
   b. Weight loss
   c. Hyperglycemia
   d. Thickening skin

15. The nurse is caring for a patient who was admitted 3 hours after sustaining electrical burns. The patient is awake, alert, and oriented, and vital signs are BP 136/70, HR 86, normal sinus rhythm, T 97.6 °F, pulse oximetry 97 percent, respiratory rate 18. The patient's skin is intact with one area of redness over the anterior chest wall. Two hours after admission, the patient is in cardiac arrest. What is the most likely cause of this complication?
   a. Hypovolemic shock
   b. Hypoxia
   c. Myocardial perforation
   d. Myonecrosis of skeletal muscle

16. Which of the following test results is consistent with pulmonary edema of a non-cardiogenic origin?
   a. Chest x-ray with bilateral pulmonary infiltrates
   b. Elevated blood levels of B-type natriuretic peptide (BNP)
   c. ABG analysis revealing hypoxemia
   d. A pulmonary artery wedge pressure of 12 mmHg

17. The medical-surgical nurse notes jugular vein distention during a head-to-toe physical assessment of a 63-year-old patient. Which cause does the nurse consider may be responsible for this finding?
   a. Right-sided heart failure
   b. Decreased pressure in circulation in lungs
   c. Fluid volume deficit
   d. Hypotension

18. The nurse is caring for a patient with congestive heart failure and is reviewing their medications with them during medication teaching. The patient expresses concern about their potassium level after recalling an issue with low potassium when prescribed a diuretic in the past. Which medication does the nurse explain is a potassium-sparing diuretic during this teaching?
   a. Lasix® (furosemide)
   b. Demadex® (torsemide)
   c. Aldactone® (spironolactone)
   d. Microzide® (hydrochlorothiazide)

19. To detect cholecystitis in a child with sickle cell disease, the nurse should be alert for which assessment finding?
   a. Localized abdominal tenderness
   b. Generalized abdominal pain
   c. Left upper quadrant pain
   d. Rebound abdominal tenderness

20. Which of the following is an indication for the placement of a vena cava filter to prevent pulmonary embolism (PE)?
   a. Pregnancy
   b. Documented recurrent PE
   c. Active smoking history
   d. Age less than 65 years

21. Which phase of the nursing process provokes the nurse to prioritize diagnoses?
   a. Assessment
   b. Analysis
   c. Planning
   d. Implementation

22. The nurse is caring for a 52-year-old female patient with metabolic syndrome. Which of the following is the nurse NOT likely to assess?
   a. Low HDL cholesterol level
   b. High triglyceride level
   c. Fatty deposits on the upper back
   d. History of a stroke

23. The nurse is developing a teaching plan for a patient with newly diagnosed type 2 diabetes. Which of the following symptoms of hyperglycemia would the nurse include?
   a. Tremors, fatigue, dizziness
   b. Excessive urination, excessive thirst, confusion
   c. Anxiety, blurred vision, headache
   d. Slurred speech, sweating, fainting

24. Which interventions should the medical-surgical nurse include while implementing a plan of care for a patient experiencing a dysautonomia flare?
   a. Promote sustained increased activity
   b. Reduce sodium intake
   c. Eat 2-3 large meals per day
   d. Administer corticosteroid

25. The nurse is teaching a patient about modifiable risk factors for aneurysm formation. Which of the following risk factors would NOT be included in this teaching plan?
   a. Smoking
   b. Cocaine use
   c. Hypertension
   d. Age

26. The nurse is assessing an 87-year-old patient admitted with a urinary tract infection. The nurse notes that the patient is confused. The patient's daughter reports that prior to being admitted to the hospital, her mother lived alone and was able to manage her apartment and perform her own self-care. The nurse understands that this patient is most likely exhibiting manifestations of which of the following conditions?
   a. Delirium
   b. Dementia
   c. Alzheimer's disease
   d. Agitation

27. A 33-year-old female has been admitted to the hospital after complaining of vomiting blood. Which description of the hematemesis indicates an active upper GI bleed?
   a. Coffee ground
   b. Bright red
   c. Large amount
   d. Small amount

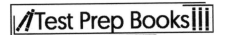

28. Which sound should be assessed using the bell of the stethoscope for proper detection?
    a. Bruit
    b. Inspiratory wheeze
    c. S2 heart sound
    d. Stridor

29. The medical-surgical nurse is caring for a 48-year-old patient assessed to have an elevated white blood cell count following anesthesia. What is the normal range for white blood cells in a healthy adult patient?
    a. 2,000-3,000/μL
    b. 4,000-11,000/μL
    c. 15,000-16,000/μL
    d. 21,000-36,000/μL

30. The nurse identifies a patient care safety risk while rounding on the unit at the start of shift. Which member of the care team should the nurse elevate this concern to?
    a. Director of nursing
    b. Charge nurse
    c. Chief nursing officer
    d. Nursing supervisor

31. The medical-surgical nurse is evaluating the patient's understanding of ways to reduce their risk of colon cancer post discharge. Which statement made by a patient supports a clear understanding of the plan for wellness?
    a. "I will have an annual endoscopy."
    b. "I will eat more produce from my garden."
    c. "I will go on daily jogs."
    d. "I will eat more red meat from my local butcher."

32. Tensilon has been administered to treat an acute relapse in a patient with myasthenia gravis. The attached tracing is consistent with the expected response in which form of crisis?

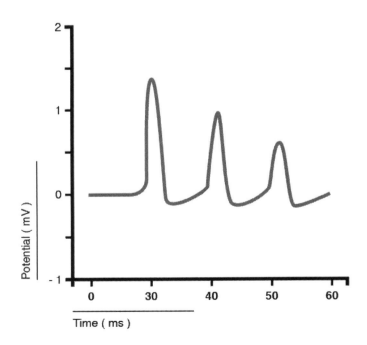

294

    a. Tensilon is not an effective treatment for either form of crisis.
    b. The tracing is consistent with the Tensilon response in a myasthenic crisis.
    c. The tracing is consistent with the Tensilon response in a cholinergic crisis.
    d. Tensilon will improve the muscle function in both forms of crises.

33. A 7-year-old male presents with hypoxia, hoarseness, fever, agitation, dysphagia, drooling, and complaints of a sore throat. What is the most likely diagnosis for this patient?
    a. Laryngotracheobronchitis
    b. Acute tracheitis
    c. Acute epiglottitis
    d. Bronchiolitis

34. The nurse is caring for a patient with manifestations of peptic ulcer disease. Which of the following statements is correct?
    a. Stomach pain begins 20 to 30 minutes after eating.
    b. The condition is associated with an increased risk of malignancy.
    c. Endoscopy is used to establish hemostasis.
    d. Chronic NSAID use is the most common etiology.

35. Which intervention should the medical-surgical nurse implement in the plan of care for a 53-year-old patient with acromegaly?
    a. Explain that the bone enlargement is temporary and will reverse
    b. Monitor for signs of diabetes mellitus, such as polyuria and polydipsia
    c. Reschedule pituitary surgery for when acromegaly has subsided
    d. Provide family teaching regarding the expectation for the patient's hands and feet to shrink

36. A patient has had three separate blood pressure readings of 138/88, 132/80, and 135/89, respectively. The nurse anticipates the patient to be categorized by the physician as which of the following?
    a. Prehypertensive
    b. Normal
    c. Stage 1 hypertension
    d. Stage 2 hypertension

37. Which psychosocial assessment findings does the medical-surgical nurse suspect will indicate a need for patient transfer to inpatient psychiatry once medically stable?
    a. Anhedonia
    b. Alcohol abuse
    c. Hopelessness
    d. Inability to care for self

38. The nurse is receiving reports at the beginning of the shift. One of the patients is being taken for emergency surgery for obstructive shock. Which of the following findings are characteristic of obstructive shock?
    a. Jugular vein distention, peripheral edema, and pulmonary congestion
    b. Decreased urine output, increased BUN, and increased creatinine
    c. Chest pain, fatigue, and lightheadedness
    d. Problems with coordination, blurred vision, and partial paralysis

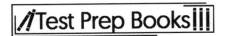

39. While evaluating a neurological plan of care, the medical-surgical nurse reviews the patient's cranial nerve function. Which cranial nerve is responsible for gag and swallow?
    a. Glossopharyngeal
    b. Hypoglossal
    c. Facial
    d. Trigeminal

40. The nurse is caring for a 62-year-old woman with myalgia, fever, dyspnea, and decreased breath sounds. To assist with a more rapid diagnosis for possible viral pneumonia, the nurse should prepare the patient for which of the following tests?
    a. Pulmonary function tests
    b. Blood cultures
    c. CT scan
    d. Rapid antigen testing

41. During an ECG, the nurse observes an abnormally lengthened PR interval (greater than 0.3). The nurse recognizes this finding as a characteristic of which of the following?
    a. Sinus rhythm
    b. Junctional rhythm
    c. Mobitz type I heart block
    d. Mobitz type II heart block

42. Which of the following would the nurse expect to assess in a patient with Guillain-Barré syndrome who has cranial nerve involvement?
    a. Core muscle weakness
    b. Respiratory muscle weakness
    c. Limb weakness
    d. Eye muscle weakness

43. After a patient complains of chest pain, which priority action should the nurse complete FIRST?
    a. Assess vital signs
    b. Ask questions regarding the radiation of pain
    c. Start an IV with normal saline
    d. Page the cardiologist

44. Which of the following statements is true?
    a. As fluid levels decrease, electrolyte levels increase.
    b. As fluid levels increase, electrolyte levels increase.
    c. As fluid levels osmose, electrolyte levels diffuse.
    d. As fluid levels homogenize, electrolyte levels dissipate.

45. The medical-surgical nurse percusses the patient's lungs during a focused assessment. Which sound aligns with a normal finding?
    a. Tympany
    b. Hyperresonance
    c. Dullness
    d. Resonance

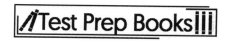

46. The medical surgical nurse assesses the patient to have shortness of breath while in a recumbent position. How should the nurse document this finding?
    a. Orthopnea
    b. Dyspnea
    c. Tachypnea
    d. Bradypnea

47. During morning report, the oncoming nurse learns from the outgoing night nurse that a 38-year-old patient has been requesting discharge all night. Upon walking into the patient room to meet them after report, the patient exclaims, "I want to go home now!" Which action should the nurse implement first?
    a. Page the physician for a consult for potential discharge
    b. Report suspected patient neglect to the nurse manager
    c. Administer a PRN medication for anxiety
    d. Explore the patient's reasoning for requesting discharge

48. The nurse is caring for a 24-year-old woman in her first trimester of pregnancy who has been experiencing moderate vaginal bleeding. The nurse understands that which of the following factors is true regarding first trimester spontaneous abortions?
    a. Young maternal age increases the risk.
    b. Type 2 diabetes is a common cause.
    c. Moderate exercise increases the risk.
    d. Chromosomal abnormalities are the most common cause.

49. Nurses are responsible for which of the following elements of informed consent?
    a. Identification of alternatives to the planned procedure
    b. Description of associated risks and benefits
    c. Explanation of the planned procedure or diagnostic test
    d. Assessment of the patient's understanding of the information that is provided

50. Which action is considered a dependent nursing intervention?
    a. Bedbound care
    b. Infection control
    c. Health education
    d. Tube feeding

51. An 18-year-old female patient is complaining of worsening wheezing, shortness of breath, and a cough over the past twelve hours. She has a history of asthma and has been using her albuterol metered-dose inhaler (MDI) every ten minutes for the past two hours. She's given supplemental oxygen, both albuterol and ipratropium (Combivent®) via nebulizer, and methylprednisolone IV in quick succession. Shortly afterwards, she complains of anxiety, develops hand tremors, and her pulse increases from 80 to 120 beats per minute (bpm). Which treatment is most likely responsible for her anxiety, tremors, and tachycardia?
    a. Supplemental oxygen
    b. Albuterol
    c. Ipratropium
    d. Methylprednisolone

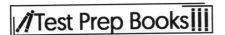

52. After receiving opposing opinions from interdisciplinary team members regarding a patient's care, what should the medical-surgical nurse do next to navigate this situation?
    a. Collect clinical data affecting the dilemma
    b. Phone Quality Assurance and establish a collaborative meeting
    c. Elevate this problem to the charge nurse
    d. Page the physician to request an ethics consult

53. Which finding gathered in the patient's history is a risk factor for a cerebrovascular accident?
    a. Male gender
    b. Diabetes mellitus
    c. Caucasian race
    d. Hypotension

54. What is the therapeutic reference range for carbamazepine, an anti-epileptic agent?
    a. 1-3 mg/L
    b. 4-12 mg/L
    c. 18-22 mg/L
    d. 26-29 mg/L

55. Which position should the medical-surgical nurse help a patient into for pain management of acute appendicitis?
    a. High Fowler's position
    b. Fetal position
    c. Prone position
    d. Supine position

56. What ethical principle sets forth that the nurse must maintain truthful engagements with their patient?
    a. Justice
    b. Veracity
    c. Nonmaleficence
    d. Beneficence

57. The patient with primary hypertension is being treated with medications to reduce blood volume and lower systemic vascular resistance. Which of the following medication combinations should the nurse anticipate for the patient?
    a. A diuretic and a calcium channel blocker (CCB)
    b. A diuretic and an angiotensin-converting enzyme (ACE) inhibitor
    c. An angiotensin II receptor blocker (ARB) and morphine
    d. A diuretic and a beta-blocker

58. Which food item consumed by a patient taking phenelzine sulfate, a monoamine oxidase inhibitor, concerns the medical-surgical nurse because it is contraindicated and must be avoided with this treatment?
    a. Sausage
    b. Cottage cheese
    c. Chicken
    d. Egg

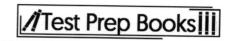
59. While implementing a plan of care for a patient with heart failure, how should the nurse address activity?
   a. Increase activity and limit time in bed
   b. Remain on bed rest
   c. Alternate rest and activity
   d. Ambulate to the bathroom only

60. The nurse is providing discharge education for a 66-year-old patient with type 2 diabetes who has had a TIA. Which of the following patient statements indicates that the teaching has been effective?
   a. "There is nothing I can do to change my risk for another episode."
   b. "The best thing I can do is to keep my A1C level below 6.5 like my doctor said."
   c. "I only have type 2 diabetes, so that doesn't affect my blood vessels."
   d. "I'm glad I don't have to take insulin to fix this."

61. A 39-year-old Hispanic-American patient visits with her husband and her young child during unit visiting hours. The medical-surgical nurse ensures not to stare or overtly admire her young child as this could be interpreted as giving the "evil eye." Understanding cultural considerations to care, what may this belief lead the patient to feel?
   a. Her child will become weak and ill.
   b. Her child is unusually short in stature.
   c. Her child will become lucky.
   d. Her child is too attractive.

62. A 55-year-old male is undergoing an endoscopy to discover the source of his hematemesis. The gastroenterologist encounters an active, bleeding lesion. What procedure using the application of heat to seal the lesion will probably be used next?
   a. Banding
   b. Biopsy
   c. Angioplasty
   d. Cauterization

63. Which ethical principle guides the medical-surgical nurse's actions while guaranteeing that the patient with the most critical condition receives priority treatment?
   a. Hedonism
   b. Virtue ethics
   c. Act deontology
   d. Utilitarianism

64. Which response should the nurse make when a patient with advanced pancreatic cancer and a poor prognosis asks why she is receiving chemotherapy?
   a. "Your chance of remission is increased with chemotherapy."
   b. "There is always the chance that chemotherapy can cure your cancer."
   c. "Chemotherapy will keep your cancer from advancing further."
   d. "Chemotherapy is being used to help manage your pain."

65. When should nurses participate in professional development activities?
   a. Only if required by the facility
   b. Whenever possible
   c. Only when compensated
   d. Whenever a JCAHO audit is suspected

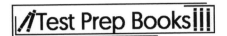

66. A patient in the medical-surgical unit collapses while taking a walk around the floor. The nurse identifies the condition as cardiopulmonary arrest, and resuscitation efforts are started. The nurse understands that, in addition to CPR, defibrillation, and the ACLS protocol, the most important factor for patient survival is which of the following?
   a. Administration of oxygen
   b. Establishing IV access
   c. Inserting a Foley catheter
   d. Time between the collapse and the start of resuscitation efforts

67. Which of the following statements by a patient with type 2 diabetes indicates that more teaching is needed?
   a. "My pancreas produces insulin, but my body isn't able to use it effectively."
   b. "I need to maintain an ideal body weight."
   c. "I need to cut down on carbohydrates in my diet."
   d. "I will need to take insulin for the rest of my life."

68. The nurse is caring for a patient who is being evaluated for a small-bowel obstruction. The nurse understands that which of the following assessment findings is consistent with this condition?
   a. pH 7.32, PCO_2 38, HCO_3 20
   b. Serum osmolality 285 mosm/kg
   c. Serum sodium 128 mmol/L
   d. Lower abdominal distention

69. While undergoing warfarin anticoagulant therapy, a 71-year-old patient experiences an elevated INR and signs and symptoms of over-anticoagulation. Which antidote should the medical-surgical nurse administer?
   a. Vitamin K
   b. Protamine
   c. Ethanol
   d. Amyl nitrate

70. When gathering narrative information regarding the patient's perceived outcome of an intervention, the medical-surgical nurse uses the communication technique known as back channeling. Which phrase is an example of this communication cue?
   a. "Go on."
   b. "Can you clarify?"
   c. "Slow down."
   d. "Repeat that."

71. The nurse is answering an HIV-positive patient's questions about the differences between the HIV-1 and HIV-2 viruses. Which information would the nurse tell this patient?
   a. HIV-2 is highly transmissible.
   b. HIV-1 is the dominant strain worldwide.
   c. HIV-2 is well-studied and highly understood.
   d. HIV-1 is the weaker virus strain.

72. The nurse is monitoring the intracranial pressure of a 36-year-old patient who was in a motor vehicle accident resulting in trauma to the head. Which of the following measurements does the nurse recognize as a normal intracranial pressure reading of an adult in the supine position?
   a. 5 millimeters of mercury
   b. 10 millimeters of mercury
   c. 18 millimeters of mercury
   d. 22 millimeters of mercury

300

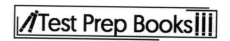

73. The nurse is caring for a diabetic patient who reports that he has been experiencing tremors, fatigue, and dizziness. Which blood glucose level would the nurse expect in this patient?
    a. 58 milligrams per deciliter
    b. 120 milligrams per deciliter
    c. 180 milligrams per deciliter
    d. 220 milligrams per deciliter

74. While establishing a treatment plan for a patient newly admitted to the medical-surgical floor from the emergency department, which understanding regarding discharge planning should the nurse consider?
    a. Discharge planning starts at admission.
    b. Discharge planning starts after all providers have met with the patient.
    c. Discharge planning starts once an official discharge diagnosis has been charted.
    d. Discharge planning starts after significant progress towards wellness has been established.

75. The nurse in the medical-surgical unit is caring for a patient who had a seizure today for the first time. The patient said that she noticed a strange odor just prior to "not feeling well." Vital signs are BP 120/74, HR 76, and an oral temperature 97.8°F. The patient has no complaints of pain and no recent history of viral or bacterial illness. A friend witnessed that seizure and stated that the muscular movement lasted about thirty seconds. The patient was incontinent during the seizure but did not suffer any injuries. The patient recovered without any further manifestations of seizure activity. The nurse understands that which of the following interventions is most appropriate for this patient?
    a. Obtain laboratory analysis of recreational drug use.
    b. Institute oral therapy of AEDs.
    c. Prepare the patient for an immediate lumbar puncture for CSF analysis.
    d. Obtain an EEG and an MRI.

76. Which statement made by the patient displays understanding of the self-administration of Advair-Diskus® post discharge?
    a. "I will use my inhaler to relieve sudden, unprovoked breathing issues."
    b. "I will use my inhaler before and after exercise."
    c. "I will use my inhaler every morning and evening."
    d. "I will use my inhaler when I develop a tight chest and cough."

77. A patient is being discharged from the hospital with the diagnosis of peripheral vascular disease with intermittent claudication. Which of the following information should be discussed with the patient prior to discharge?

       I. Avoid tight clothing.
       II. Wear compression stockings.
       III. Avoid airplane travel.
       IV. Minimize exercise.

    a. I and II only
    b. I and III only
    c. I, II, and III only
    d. I, II, III, and IV

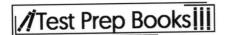

78. A 60-year-old ex-smoker presents with a complaint of increasing shortness of breath over the past 24 hours. He has a medical history conducive of chronic obstructive pulmonary disease (COPD). He is administered supplemental oxygen, albuterol via nebulizer, methylprednisolone IV, and a dose of azithromycin IV. Which of these therapies has been clinically proven to decrease the risk of treatment failure and death?
   a. Supplemental oxygen
   b. Albuterol
   c. Methylprednisolone
   d. Azithromycin

79. A 19-year-old patient was admitted to the medical-surgical unit with a fever of 104.1, sore throat, and small white spots inside their mouth. On the second day of hospitalization, a rash of flat red spots breaks out, and the patient is tested for measles. Which precautions should the medical-surgical nurse implement for this patient while awaiting the confirmation of illness?
   a. Standard
   b. Contact
   c. Droplet
   d. Airborne

80. A patient presents with the complaint of fever and shortness of breath. During the physical examination, the nurse observed a petechial rash on both hands and a recent nipple piercing on the right chest. The patient reported being on a corticosteroid for a respiratory infection. These findings alert the nurse to the possibility of which of the following?
   a. Endocarditis
   b. An autoimmune disease
   c. Pneumonia
   d. Heart failure

81. Which precautions should the medical-surgical nurse engage in while caring for a patient with herpes zoster that is classified as disseminated infection?
   a. Standard
   b. Reverse isolation
   c. Contact
   d. Airborne and contact

82. Which of the following disinfecting agents is highly effective in small amounts, one of the strongest disinfectants used in healthcare institutions, relatively safe for workers, and powerful in low temperatures?
   a. Sodium peroxide
   b. Sodium Hypochlorite
   c. Formaldehyde
   d. Hydrogen peroxide

83. Consent is not required in which situation?
   a. Pediatric procedure
   b. Invasive procedure
   c. Routine procedure
   d. Emergent procedure

84. Which diet would a patient with Meniere's disease likely benefit from?
    a. Low carbohydrate
    b. High fat
    c. Low sodium
    d. High protein

85. Goals of care conversations are used at the end of life to do which of the following?
    a. Collaborate with experts
    b. Keep the focus on what the patient wants
    c. Support families during a difficult time
    d. Get the patient into palliative care

86. Aria is a nurse who primarily works with breast cancer patients. She is working with a new patient who will be undergoing chemotherapy, and Aria is waiting for physician's orders as to how the patient's treatment plan will proceed. The physician arrives and seems distressed. She quickly reviews the new patient's file and tells Aria that the first chemotherapy treatment can take place the following day. Then the physician hurries off. What would be the best course of action for Aria in order to ensure her new patient begins treatment as soon as possible?
    a. Make sure that she receives written and signed orders from the physician on a chemotherapy order form.
    b. Follow up with the physician to ask if anything is wrong in the physician's personal life.
    c. Check with the patient if the patient is available for an appointment the next day and if the patient has reliable transportation to and from the facility.
    d. Begin treatment on the patient now, as the patient is already at the center and Aria is a seasoned nurse who knows how to proceed with the patient's treatment.

87. The medication reconciliation process includes which of the following components?
    a. Prescriber of medication
    b. Use of recreational drugs
    c. Only prescription medications
    d. Location of patient's preferred pharmacy

88. The nurse caring for a patient post lung lobectomy detects a chest tube air leak when assessing the water-seal chamber after surgery. Which response by the nurse is appropriate at this time?
    a. Call the provider to report the concern.
    b. Document the finding in the patient's chart and continue to monitor.
    c. Elevate this finding to the nursing supervisor.
    d. Initiate a rapid response to obtain support.

89. The nurse caring for a patient post cardiac catheterization will perform which specific intervention to monitor for the development of life-threatening dysrhythmias?
    a. Keep the patient flat on their back for at least six hours postprocedure.
    b. Take regular vital signs, especially heart rate and blood pressure.
    c. Regularly observe the patient's ECG via cardiac monitoring, according to facility protocol.
    d. Regularly observe the incision site, looking for bruising, swelling, and redness.

90. Which of the following is a characteristic of a good hand-off?
    a. One-way communication
    b. Repetitive and brief
    c. Specific
    d. Involves multiple care providers

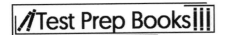

91. Which symptom should be reported to the FDA as an ADR?
    a. Intractable vomiting following oral chemotherapy
    b. Acute cirrhosis secondary to self-induced acetaminophen overdose
    c. Intervention is required to prevent permanent damage following the reported ADR
    d. Alteration of the pharmacotherapeutic plan is required due to the reported ADR

92. The nurse manager of a busy unit continuously incorporates a charismatic leadership style, despite the challenging work environment. Which description aligns with the manager's style of leadership?
    a. Follows rules closely and avoids flexibility in action
    b. Incorporates eloquent communication that inspires junior staff to admire them
    c. Commits to the growth of each team member through high emotional intelligence and advanced conflict-resolution skills
    d. Judges team members on performance, while offering little support

93. When is root cause analysis used?
    a. When anything goes wrong in the medical setting
    b. When there are adverse events or close calls
    c. When the doctor orders one
    d. Only when a patient death or serious injury occurs

94. A nurse is developing a plan of care for a patient population that is culturally diverse. Which statement correctly identifies the appropriate nursing actions?
    a. The nurse follows the standard protocol for the predominant culture of the community.
    b. The nurse focuses on the cultural needs of the largest group in the population.
    c. The nurse Identifies and acknowledges self-biases and addresses the needs of the patient.
    d. The nurse meets the needs of the group according to personal values and beliefs.

95. Which of the following statements is consistent with the QESN competencies?
    a. Using systems thinking increases collaboration.
    b. Systems thinking is the goal of all nursing competencies.
    c. Successful application of all QESN nursing competencies will improve patient safety.
    d. The ability to use systems thinking is dictated by the nurse's level of basic nursing education.

96. The American Hospital Association's Patient Care Partnership mandates which of the following?
    a. How hospitals communicate with families
    b. Responsibility for caring for terminal patients
    c. A decision-making partnership between patients and the healthcare system
    d. Access to affordable insurance for everyone

97. Which of the following choices is most consistent with nurses' responsibilities for advocacy?
    a. Notify the nursing supervisor of any conflict to assure resolution of the patient issue.
    b. Considering the patient's point of view and being prepared to support and explain the point of view as needed.
    c. Provide comprehensive documentation of the patient's care in the EHR.
    d. Understand all relevant laws associated with the nursing care of the patient.

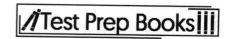

98. When working with adult learners, it is important for the nurse to incorporate which concept into their lesson plan and teachings?
    a. Relate teachings to real-life experiences.
    b. Assume the patient has no prior knowledge of the topic.
    c. Maintain authority and control of the patient during education.
    d. Keep objectives fluid and subjective.

99. Hospital-wide decisions and committees involving client rights in a healthcare setting should include which of the following groups?
    a. Administrative heads of the hospital
    b. Doctors and nurses
    c. Medical staff, administration, patients, and family members
    d. Administration and doctors

100. The medical-surgical nurse is working with a certified nursing assistant (CNA) to help provide care for a 55-year-old patient who is morbidly obese. Which of the following tasks would be appropriate to delegate to the CNA to perform independently?
    a. Giving an oral pain medication that has already been scanned
    b. Inserting a new peripheral IV
    c. Repositioning the patient in bed
    d. Recording output from a foley catheter

101. The nurse is receiving new medication orders from the patient's medical team during rounds. Which action can help reduce medication errors?
    a. Request a verbal order.
    b. Use standard medical abbreviations when possible.
    c. Read back and verify new orders received.
    d. Rely on paper charting to double-check for error.

102. Two nurses get into an argument during their shift about restocking the supply room and go to the charge nurse to intervene. What is the first step of conflict resolution the charge nurse should instruct them to take?
    a. Present their sides of the argument.
    b. Come to a compromise.
    c. Discuss their disagreement in detail.
    d. Dismiss their argument as non-productive.

103. A patient has died while they have family members in the room. Which of the following is NOT an appropriate action for the nurse to take immediately after death?
    a. Continue to refer to the patient by their name after death.
    b. Assist with arrangements for funeral or burial facilities.
    c. Escort the family out of the room to begin post-mortem care.
    d. Encourage grieving and communication for the family.

104. The nursing unit recently discovered a high rate of UTIs amongst post-op patients. As a result, nurses have begun removing indwelling foley catheters within 24 hours after surgery, instead of 48 hours, to try to reduce the rate of UTIs. This nursing unit is at which stage of a problem-solving strategy?
    a. Evaluation of solution
    b. Development of solutions
    c. Identification of the problem
    d. Implementation of solution

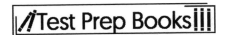

105. While creating an evidence-based practice guideline, a nurse is conducting research and wants to use research that has the highest level of evidence, level A. From which of the following studies should the nurse draw information?
   a. Meta-analysis
   b. Randomized-control trial
   c. Integrative interviews
   d. Cohort study

106. A patient who is recovering from a stroke requests the incorporation of acupuncture in their care and recovery. What is the most appropriate response from the nurse?
   a. Tell the patient it is not recommended to start acupuncture because it is dangerous.
   b. Explain that acupuncture does not work and should not be added to their care.
   c. Suggest that the patient starts acupuncture care twice weekly in place of PT.
   d. Discuss the safety of incorporating acupuncture into the patient's current care regimen with the medical team.

107. Utilitarianism can place a limit on which other ethical principle?
   a. Autonomy
   b. Beneficence
   c. Nonmaleficence
   d. Justice

108. When the nurse is documenting a task that is delegated, which piece of information are they NOT required to include?
   a. What task was completed
   b. Location where the task was completed
   c. When the task was completed
   d. Duration in which the task was completed

109. While discussing treatment plans for a patient with a stage IV pressure ulcer, the nurse works with a doctor, a nurse practitioner, a wound care nurse, and a registered dietitian. On which type of team is this nurse working?
   a. Primary medical team
   b. Secondary medical team
   c. Intradisciplinary team
   d. Interdisciplinary team

110. The nurse is caring for a patient from China who speaks Mandarin as their first language. They have just received news that their cancer has returned and they will need to restart chemotherapy. When the nurse comes in the room to try to speak with the patient, they are looking away and are closed off to discussing their feelings with the nurse. What is the most appropriate response by the nurse?
   a. Encourage the patient to maintain eye contact for better communication.
   b. Suggest therapeutic techniques so they can work on expressing their feelings.
   c. Contact the patient's family so they can offer their support and help to the patient.
   d. Use an interpreter to let the patient know the nurse is there to answer any questions.

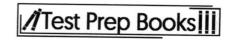

111. Along with standard precautions, transmission-based precautions are used with patients with known or suspected infection with highly transmissible pathogens. What are the three categories of transmission-based precautions?
    a. Surface, droplet, and contact
    b. Contact, droplet, and airborne
    c. Surface, airborne, and contact
    d. Airborne, droplet, and surface

112. ChloraPrep® is a commonly used chlorhexidine gluconate-based skin prep solution. For which patient is ChloraPrep solution contraindicated?
    a. The 47-year-old with a documented allergy to povidone iodine
    b. The patient who has open venous stasis ulcers on the left lower extremity and is undergoing left leg revascularization
    c. The patient with an intact left groin who is having a left groin hematoma evacuation
    d. The open-heart surgery patient who has no open areas noted on the chest

113. Amy is a nurse practitioner that has begun her shift. Using her designated log-in, she signs into a mobile clinical workstation and reviews how many patients are scheduled for appointments with her during this shift. She notices that her first patient has already been checked in by the front-desk staff, so she logs out of the workstation and greets her patient. Once roomed, Amy logs back into the room's clinical workstation and pulls up the patient's medical history and chief complaint to review with him. The patient mentions he has a new allergy to NSAIDs, which Amy documents in his electronic medical record. Later, the patient goes to the clinic's pharmacy to pick up a prescription that Amy ordered. The pharmacist is able to note the patient's updated allergy information and double-checks that the patient's prescription won't cause any issues. He also provides the patient with a patient portal log-in so that the patient can order a refill when he's out of his current medication. What primary tool is the medical organization effectively utilizing to streamline processes, improve documentation, and enhance accessibility to care?
    a. Healthcare information technology
    b. Paper charting documentation
    c. A nearby pharmacy
    d. A customer-service oriented pharmacist

114. A 75-year-old patient has been admitted to the hospital with multiple bruises and a broken hip. During the nurse's assessment, they observe that the patient's bruises are not consistent with the explanation of a fall, and the nurse suspects that they may be a victim of elder abuse. What is the most appropriate action for the nurse to take if they suspect elder abuse in a hospital setting?
    a. Confronting the family or caregiver about the suspected abuse
    b. Documenting the suspected abuse and reporting it to the appropriate authority
    c. Keeping the suspected abuse to themselves
    d. Talking to the patient about the suspected abuse and trying to get them to confirm it

115. Which of the following is critical for a medical facility to establish prior to a natural disaster ever occurring?
    a. A hurricane evacuation plan
    b. A temporary morgue
    c. Interim chain of command
    d. Storage of extra PPE

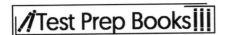

116. Douglas is a nurse in a dermatology clinic. He notices during some surgical procedures that the hand sanitization station is in a difficult location for many team members to reach and that waiting while everyone washes and sanitizes their hands before placing their gloves on before a procedure can take up to 45 minutes. The clinic is often delayed during their daily schedule. Douglas speaks with the clinic manager and proposes moving the hand sanitization station to a more common area. After a month, he documents that the overall clinic delay time has decreased by approximately 20 minutes per day. What is this an example of?
   a. WHO global sanitization efforts
   b. JHCO regulations
   c. Quality improvement
   d. A common dermatology clinic issue

117. Which is an example of how an electronic health record (EHR) improves patient outcomes?
   a. By reducing medical errors due to misinterpretation of handwriting
   b. By increasing the time a nurse spends researching the patient's disease process
   c. By decreasing the interdisciplinary team's access to patient information
   d. By discouraging the use of built-in systems in preventing treatment errors

118. The nurse is providing discharge instructions for a 54-year-old patient with newly diagnosed type 2 diabetes who was admitted yesterday for hypoglycemia. Which of the following statements made to the patient best indicates the nurse's understanding of health literacy?
   a. "Including carbohydrates in your diet that have a low glycemic index will cause a more steady increase in your blood glucose."
   b. "Some of the signs and symptoms of hypoglycemia include tachycardia, diaphoresis, confusion, irritability, and pallor."
   c. "Your doctor will take a blood test every three months, called the A1C, which tells them how well your diabetes is under control."
   d. "Ozempic® is a once-weekly subcutaneous injection for type 2 diabetes that may also help with weight management."

119. The nurse understands that all of the following are appropriate times to call the organ procurement organization (OPO) EXCEPT:
   a. As soon as possible once imminent death is recognized
   b. As soon as possible once the nurse has notified the family of the intent for organ retrieval
   c. As soon as possible once the provider has determined brain death
   d. As soon as possible once the provider has determined cardiac death

120. The nurse is administering medications to a 72-year-old patient who was admitted two days ago for COPD exacerbation. Before leaving the room, the patient states, "Thank you so much, you've been so helpful and patient with me. Not like that night nurse! She's been so rude! I don't want her in my room anymore." Which of the following actions by the nurse is most appropriate in this situation?
   a. Telling the patient that all of the nurses on the unit are helpful and kind, and it's probably just a misunderstanding
   b. Finding the night shift nurse and asking her why she made the patient upset
   c. Apologizing to the patient and telling them that they will relay the information to the nurse manager
   d. Apologizing to the patient, asking for more details, and attempting to alleviate the situation

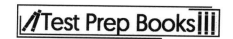

121. A 55-year-old patient with a history of heart disease is admitted to the hospital with chest pain. The doctor recommends an invasive procedure, but the patient is hesitant and wants to discuss alternative options. In this situation, the nurse understands that all of the following are ways to promote patient advocacy EXCEPT:
    a. Providing accurate information about the recommended procedure and alternative options
    b. Encouraging the patient to consent to the doctor's recommended treatment for the betterment of their health
    c. Respecting the patient's autonomy and right to make their own medical decisions
    d. Facilitating open communication between the patient and the doctor

122. The nurse is caring for an 85-year-old patient with a history of congestive heart failure and Alzheimer's disease who is currently being combative. Per the doctor's orders, the nurse places the patient in restraint mitts to prevent self-injury. Several hours later, the patient passes away. Why must the nurse report this death to the Centers for Medicare and Medicaid Services (CMS)?
    a. The patient had Alzheimer's disease.
    b. The patient had congestive heart failure.
    c. The patient was being combative prior to death.
    d. The death occurred while the patient was in restraints.

123. Which of the following steps is most important for the nurse to take in order to support patient- and family-centered care?
    a. Looking for educational materials, such as brochures or videos, which explain patient-centered care and how it can benefit the patient
    b. Involving the patient and their family in decision making by asking for their input and preferences
    c. Utilizing online resources, such as patient-centered care websites or forums, to learn from other healthcare professionals and patients
    d. Reaching out to the hospital's patient advocacy department to see if they have any resources or programs available

124. A 63-year-old patient was admitted to the medical-surgical unit for management of hypertension and chronic obstructive pulmonary disease (COPD). They have a history of smoking, diabetes, and high cholesterol. The nurse has obtained the patient's health history from both the patient and their family members. What is the primary reason for the nurse to obtain a health history from multiple sources?
    a. To verify accuracy of information
    b. To save time
    c. To satisfy legal requirements
    d. To comply with hospital policy

125. A 68-year-old patient was recently discharged from the medical-surgical unit after an appendectomy two days before. The patient lives alone and has a history of congestive heart failure, hypertension, and diabetes. During their hospital stay, they experienced multiple complications, including wound infection and difficulty managing their blood sugar levels. The healthcare team is concerned about the patient's risk for hospital readmission. Which of the following is a risk factor for readmission for this patient?
    a. Living alone
    b. History of hypertension
    c. History of congestive heart failure
    d. Recent appendectomy

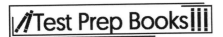

126. A 45-year-old patient was admitted yesterday for asthma exacerbation. The patient lives in a low-income area and works multiple jobs to support themselves and their two children. They also report difficulty affording their medications and managing their symptoms while juggling work responsibilities. Which of the following is an example of a social determinant of health (SDOH) that may be affecting this patient's ability to manage their asthma?
   a. The patient's asthma diagnosis
   b. The patient's occupation
   c. The patient's inability to manage their symptoms
   d. The patient's difficulty affording medications

127. A 72-year-old patient who is postoperative day one after undergoing hip replacement surgery has a patient-controlled analgesia (PCA) device to manage their pain, which they are instructed to use as needed. The nurse is alerted that the PCA device is not functioning properly, and the medication is not being delivered. Which of the following is the appropriate initial action by the nurse when troubleshooting the PCA device for this patient?
   a. Discontinuing use of the PCA device
   b. Assessing the patient's pain level and providing alternative pain management
   c. Checking the connections of the PCA device and repositioning as needed
   d. Contacting the healthcare provider for an order to change the medication

128. A new graduate nurse is responsible for documenting the vital signs and medication administration times of their patients in the electronic health record (EHR). The charge nurse has recently noticed that their documentation is often incomplete and inconsistent. Which of the following is an appropriate coaching technique for the charge nurse to use when working with the new graduate nurse to improve their documentation performance in the EHR?
   a. Confronting and criticizing the nurse for their incomplete documentation
   b. Providing positive feedback on the documentation that is accurate and complete
   c. Reporting to the nurse manager that additional training on EHR documentation is required
   d. Disregarding the incomplete documentation and focusing on more important aspects of care

129. A 65-year-old patient who was diagnosed with stage IV pancreatic cancer was referred to an oncologist who provided them with chemotherapy and radiation therapy. Despite the treatment, the cancer has metastasized, and the patient's condition is deteriorating rapidly. The family is concerned about their end-of-life care and wants to ensure that they receive appropriate care. What is the most appropriate step in the continuity of care for this patient?
   a. Transferring the patient to hospice care
   b. Scheduling a palliative care consultation
   c. Referring the patient to a support group
   d. Discussing advanced care planning with the patient's family

130. A 70-year-old patient who was admitted to the hospital for a right hip replacement surgery has a history of hypertension, hyperlipidemia, and type 2 diabetes. The surgical team, nursing staff, physical therapist, and dietician are involved in his care. Which interprofessional team member is responsible for managing the patient's postoperative pain through assessment, administration, and monitoring?
   a. Surgeon
   b. Nurse
   c. Physical therapist
   d. Dietician

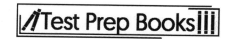
131. A 75-year-old patient who was admitted to the hospital for a left hip fracture has a history of osteoporosis and mild cognitive impairment. The patient's daughter, who is the primary caregiver, is concerned about their care and wants to be involved in the decision-making process. What is the best approach to providing patient/family-centered care for this patient?

    a. Providing the daughter with a copy of the hospital's policies and procedures
    b. Scheduling a family conference with the patient's healthcare team
    c. Advising against the daughter's involvement to avoid interfering with patient care
    d. Limiting communication with the patient's daughter to ensure patient confidentiality

132. A nurse has just received report from the previous shift and has four patients that require their attention:

    Patient 1: A 70-year-old patient with a history of congestive heart failure (CHF) who has been admitted with shortness of breath and increasing edema in their lower extremities. Their vital signs are currently stable.

    Patient 2: A 50-year-old patient with a diagnosis of acute renal failure who requires frequent hemodialysis treatments. They are currently hypotensive and tachycardic.

    Patient 3: A 60-year-old patient with a diagnosis of acute pancreatitis who is experiencing severe abdominal pain and vomiting. They are also tachycardic and have a low-grade fever.

    Patient 4: A 55-year-old patient with a history of type 2 diabetes who has been admitted with an infected foot ulcer. They require frequent wound care and intravenous antibiotics.

Which patient should the nurse prioritize first?

    a. The patient with CHF
    b. The patient with acute renal failure
    c. The patient with acute pancreatitis
    d. The patient with an infected foot ulcer

133. A nurse manager has been tasked with allocating resources for a medical-surgical unit consisting of 20 beds and a diverse patient population, including post-surgical patients, patients with chronic illnesses, and patients with complex medical conditions. Which of the following actions should the nurse manager take to ensure fiscal efficiency on the unit?

    a. Increasing the number of experienced nurses on the unit
    b. Purchasing the latest technology and equipment for patient care
    c. Implementing a waste reduction program to minimize unnecessary expenses
    d. Increasing the number of support staff, such as housekeeping and dietary aides

134. A new graduate nurse is assigned to a 50-year-old patient who has been admitted with a diagnosis of acute myocardial infarction (AMI). The nurse realizes that they have limited knowledge and skills related to the care of a patient with AMI. Which of the following actions should the nurse take to provide the best care for this patient?

    a. Delegating care to other staff members who have more experience in caring for patients with AMI
    b. Providing basic care to the patient and avoiding tasks that require specialized knowledge and skills
    c. Collaborating with the interdisciplinary team, engaging in ongoing professional development, and seeking guidance from experienced colleagues to enhance knowledge and skills in caring for patients with AMI
    d. Following the routine care plan without making any changes based on the patient's condition

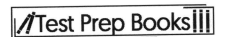

Practice Test #1

135. A medical-surgical nurse has recently taken on a leadership role on their unit and is responsible for mentoring and coaching new nurses. Which action should the nurse take to provide effective mentoring and coaching for new nurses who are overwhelmed and unsure how to provide the best care for their patients?
   a. Leaving the new nurses to work independently and providing feedback after the shift
   b. Giving the new nurses a task list and instructing them to follow the unit's policies and procedures
   c. Providing the new nurses with a comprehensive orientation to the unit's policies and procedures, and reviewing the patients' care plans together
   d. Assigning the new nurses to care for patients who are less complex and who require minimal monitoring

136. A medical-surgical nurse is caring for a patient who underwent a complicated surgery for a gastrointestinal disorder. The patient's postoperative course has had multiple complications, including a wound infection, fever, and electrolyte imbalances. The nurse has been caring for this patient for several days and is starting to feel overwhelmed and frustrated by the lack of progress. Which of the following actions by the nurse best demonstrates the use of reflective practice in this situation?
   a. Taking a break from the patient's care to clear their head and reduce stress
   b. Consulting with colleagues to get their input on the best course of action
   c. Reviewing their own actions and thought processes to identify any biases or assumptions that may be impacting their care of the patient
   d. Blaming other members of the healthcare team for the patient's lack of progress

137. A nurse is caring for a patient who suddenly develops chest pain and becomes unresponsive. The patient's family is present and is demanding immediate action. Which of the following actions should the nurse take first in this situation?
   a. Administering medications and performing procedures to stabilize the patient's condition
   b. Directing other members of the healthcare team in the management of the emergency
   c. Communicating with the patient's family and providing emotional support
   d. Activating the emergency response system

138. A nurse educator has been assigned to mentor a new nurse who is struggling with time management and prioritization skills. The nurse has expressed a desire to improve, but is feeling overwhelmed and frustrated. Which of the following learning theories is most appropriate for the nurse educator to use in the coaching and mentoring of this nurse?
   a. Cognitive Load Theory
   b. Social Learning Theory
   c. Experiential Learning Theory
   d. Transformative Learning Theory

139. A charge nurse on a busy medical-surgical unit notices that one of their team members is struggling with confidence and assertiveness in communicating with other members of the healthcare team. The charge nurse wants to empower this nurse to advocate for their patients and participate fully in the interdisciplinary care team. Which of the following strategies is the most appropriate for promoting professional empowerment in this nurse?
   a. Assigning the nurse to take charge of a complex patient case and present it at interdisciplinary rounds
   b. Providing the nurse with written resources and articles on assertive communication techniques
   c. Encouraging the nurse to participate in shared governance committees and other professional development opportunities
   d. Offering the nurse a financial incentive to speak up in interdisciplinary team meetings

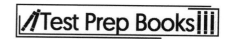

140. A nurse preceptor is responsible for orienting a new graduate nurse to the medical-surgical unit. The new nurse is enthusiastic and eager to learn but has expressed anxiety about transitioning from the classroom to the clinical setting. Which of the following actions by the nurse preceptor is most important for ensuring a successful orientation experience for the new graduate nurse?
    a. Providing the nurse with a detailed orientation binder containing unit policies and procedures
    b. Assigning the nurse to shadow experienced nurses for the first week of orientation
    c. Conducting frequent check-ins with the nurse to assess their progress and provide feedback
    d. Assigning the nurse to take on a full patient load on their second day of orientation

141. A nurse who has been working in a medical-surgical unit for several years is interested in furthering their education and career. Which of the following is the most effective career development resource for a nurse who is seeking professional development?
    a. Job shadowing opportunities
    b. Self-paced online courses
    c. Hospital-based continuing education programs
    d. Industry conferences and networking events

142. A nurse is interested in advancing their career through professional networking and involvement in professional organizations. Which of the following is a benefit of participating in a professional organization as a nurse?
    a. The opportunity to receive promotions and salary increases
    b. The ability to access free continuing education courses
    c. The chance to connect with other professionals and stay up to date on industry trends
    d. The opportunity to work on innovative research projects

143. A nurse has been asked to participate in a peer review process for a colleague who has been receiving complaints from patients and their families. The nurse is unfamiliar with the peer review process and the methods used to evaluate the quality of care provided by their colleague. Which of the following methods is an appropriate method for conducting a peer review of a nurse's clinical practice?
    a. Conducting an informal interview with the nurse to discuss their clinical practice
    b. Observing the nurse's clinical practice and documenting any deviations from best practices
    c. Reviewing the nurse's patient records and interviewing patients and their families
    d. Documenting the nurse's work experience and educational background

144. A medical-surgical nurse notices that a colleague has not been washing their hands before and after patient care. When the nurse confronts the colleague, they admit that they have been skipping hand washing because they are short-staffed and they need to save time. Which regulatory and compliance standard is violated in this scenario?
    a. The Joint Commission accreditation standards for infection control
    b. The Occupational Safety and Health Administration (OSHA) standards for workplace safety
    c. The Health Insurance Portability and Accountability Act (HIPAA) privacy and security rule
    d. The National Council of State Boards of Nursing (NCSBN) standards of nursing practice

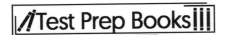

145. A nurse is caring for a 45-year-old patient who has just been diagnosed with an advanced stage cancer. The patient is in a state of shock, and their family members are emotional and demanding of constant attention. As the day progresses, the patient's family members become increasingly agitated and start to make unreasonable demands on the nursing staff, including requests for unnecessary procedures and medications. Why is having an effective organizational structure important in this scenario?

    a. To ensure that the nursing staff is properly trained and competent to deal with complex medical conditions
    b. To facilitate effective communication and coordination between members of the nursing team
    c. To ensure that patients receive prompt and appropriate medical treatment and interventions
    d. To enable nurses to make independent decisions without seeking approval from superiors

146. A nurse is caring for a patient who has recently been diagnosed with a serious chronic illness. The patient is struggling to come to terms with their diagnosis and is unsure about the best course of treatment. The patient's family members are also involved in the decision-making process and have strong opinions about what the patient should do. What is the most important factor in facilitating a shared decision-making process with this patient and their family?

    a. Ensuring that the patient is fully informed about their diagnosis and treatment options
    b. Advocating for the patient's best interests and preferences
    c. Encouraging the patient and family members to consider all available options
    d. Ensuring that the patient and family members understand the risks and benefits of each treatment option

147. A nurse is caring for a patient who has strong religious beliefs that conflict with some of the medical treatments recommended by their healthcare team. The patient is refusing certain treatments based on their religious beliefs, and their family members are also pressuring the healthcare team to respect the patient's wishes. Which of the following actions by the nurse is most important in order to uphold nursing philosophy principles in this scenario?

    a. Confronting the patient and their family members about their beliefs and insisting they follow the medical treatments recommended by the healthcare team
    b. Providing evidence-based care and adhering to medical guidelines
    c. Maintaining a non-judgmental attitude and respecting the patient's beliefs
    d. Fostering a strong therapeutic relationship with the patient and their family

148. A 56-year-old patient with a history of chronic pain and substance abuse is admitted to the hospital for a surgical procedure. The patient is noncompliant with the prescribed pain medications, frequently requesting higher doses and becoming agitated when their requests are denied. The patient is also known to have a history of aggressive behavior towards healthcare providers. Which nursing care delivery system would be most appropriate for managing a patient with a history of substance abuse and aggressive behavior?

    a. Team nursing
    b. Case management nursing
    c. Total patient care
    d. Functional nursing

149. A healthcare organization is implementing a new electronic medical record (EMR) system, and the nursing staff is expected to complete training and begin using the new system within the next month. However, one nurse is resistant to change and expresses frustration with having to learn a new system, stating that they have always used paper charts and do not see the need for an electronic system. The nurse is a seasoned staff member who has been with the organization for over 20 years. Which stage of the change management process is the nurse in, based on the ADKAR model?

    a. Awareness
    b. Desire
    c. Knowledge
    d. Ability

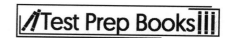

150. A large urban hospital is experiencing high turnover rates among its nursing staff. Despite offering competitive salaries and benefits, many nurses are leaving the organization for other facilities or non-clinical settings. The hospital administration has identified the need to address the root causes of nursing turnover and is considering implementing several strategies to alleviate the issue. Which of the following is a common reason for high turnover in nursing, and what strategy would be most effective for the administration to use?

    a. Inadequate staffing levels; offering overtime opportunities to existing staff

    b. Limited opportunities for career advancement; offering tuition reimbursement for continuing education

    c. Poor work-life balance; offering flexible work schedules and on-site childcare

    d. Negative organizational culture; increasing salaries and benefits

Answer Explanations #1

1. B: One of the classic findings in a patient with appendicitis is periumbilical pain that may progress to the right lower quadrant. Because the patient with appendicitis may develop peritonitis, the nurse would expect to assess a rigid abdomen rather than a soft abdomen; therefore, Choice *A* is not correct. Choices *C* and *D* are not correct because they are not typical assessment findings in the patient with appendicitis.

2. A: Choice *A* is a significant concern when assessed in a patient with pneumonia and requires priority intervention post assessment. Choices *B*, *C*, and *D* are not causes for concern in a patient with this illness at this time. Choices *B* and *C* are within normal range. Choice *D*, while potentially concerning outside of pneumonia, is a normal finding for this illness and encouraged during active illness to support movement towards wellness and a resolution of symptoms.

3. C: Choice *C* should NOT be implemented for a patient with epilepsy. Side-rails should be up to discourage patient falls during seizure activity. Choice *A* provides additional protection from injury. Choices *B* and *D* include equipment that should be ready for use in case it is needed during a seizure. The nurse should support the patient into a side-lying position and maintain their airway.

4. B: The risk of brain herniation is higher in patients who are immunosuppressed, over sixty years old, have a history of recent seizure activity, or have a disease of the CNS. A CT scan may be done prior to the lumbar puncture in this patient population; however, instituting antibiotic therapy to prevent morbidity remains the priority intervention. Bacterial meningitis is associated with a characteristic erythematous rash. However, depending on the causative organism, rashes may also be present with viral meningitis; therefore, the presence or absence of the rash cannot differentiate between the two conditions, which means that Choice *A* is incorrect. The protein level of the CSF is elevated, not decreased, in bacterial meningitis. The inflammatory response resulting from the bacterial infection alters the blood-brain barrier, which allows the leakage of protein from the blood into the subarachnoid space, causing marked increase in the protein level of the CSF; therefore, Choice *C* is incorrect. The meningococcal vaccine, MCV4, is effective against meningococcal meningitis and has decreased the incidence of the disease among college students and military personnel who typically reside in close quarters. Residents of long-term care facilities are protected against pneumococcal meningitis by the PPSV; therefore, Choice *D* is incorrect.

5. A: Choice *A* is a supportive intervention to establish effective communication with a withdrawn patient. Choice *B* should be avoided as it may encourage the patient's withdrawn behavior. Choice *C* should be avoided as it may produce heightened anxiety that induces further withdrawn behavior. Choice *D* should be avoided as it encourages the patient to withhold information about their symptoms, which impairs the communication process as well as treatment planning.

6. A: Choice *A* provides an accurate explanation of the mechanism of action of immunosuppressive therapy agents and should be included in the nurse's patient education. Choices *B*, *C*, and *D* are not true to the basic principles of this therapy's action and should not be included in the education provided to a patient with myasthenia gravis.

7. D: There is evidence that patients who are diagnosed with diverticulosis before the age of fifty have a greater risk for episodes of diverticulitis, which may be due to an unidentified difference in the infective process, living longer, or delays in seeking care for the initial episode. The presence of diverticulosis is age-dependent, affecting less than 5 percent of individuals less than forty years old and up to 65 percent of individuals over eighty years old; therefore, Choice *A* is incorrect. Diverticulitis is caused by infection of the diverticula due to impacted fecaliths and other cellular debris, which results in overgrowth of normal colonic bacteria with progression to an inflammatory process that is responsible for the clinical manifestations of the acute attack. Therefore, Choice *B* is incorrect. Initial episodes of diverticulitis are treated with bowel rest, antibiotics, and IV fluids. Emergency surgical intervention of an

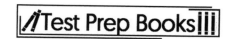

initial attack is required only for severe manifestations, and an elective colectomy is recommended after three episodes of diverticulitis; therefore, Choice *C* is incorrect.

8. C: Choice *C*, a serious disorder of the skin and mucous membranes, aligns with the nurse's assessment of a painful, reddish-purple, blistering rash. Choice *A* represents a possible butterfly-shaped rash on the face. Choice *B* represents a rash of lost pigment. Choice *D* represents a possible rash in a bull's-eye pattern secondary to a tick bite.

9. C: Choice *C* is a supportive intervention that should be implemented in the plan of care for a patient with acute renal failure. Choices *A*, *B*, and *D* all should be avoided in this patient's treatment plan.

10. B: Choice *B* is a dye known to numb pain within the urinary tract and is administered as an analgesic for pain management for a patient experiencing a urinary tract infection. Choices *A* and *C* represent analgesics; however, neither fit this description or this need for a patient with a urinary tract infection. Choice *D* indicates a medication used for the treatment of urinary tract infection but that does not provide pain management. It is an antibiotic rather than an analgesic.

11. C: Choice *C* represents the length of time that the medical-surgical nurse must auscultate the apical heart rate while completing a focused assessment. Choices *A* and *B* are too short in length, thereby limiting the assessment. Choice *D* is longer than necessary and not typical. Auscultating longer than a minute would only be indicated if the nurse was unable to obtain a clear finding after auscultating for a full minute or if additional considerations warranted further review.

12. B: Choice *B* should be administered to the patient to counteract the effects of the acetaminophen overdose. Choices *A*, *C*, and *D*, while all antidotes for a variety of medications, would not prove effective in reversing the progression of acetaminophen poisoning.

13. C: Left bundle branch block is not assessed using the TIMI tool with a diagnosis of NSTEMI, although it is a category scored with a diagnosis of ST elevation myocardial infarction (STEMI). The TIMI tool for patients with NSTEMI provides a score in seven categories: age, risk factors, a prior coronary artery stenosis, ST deviation on ECG, prior aspirin intake, presence and number of angina episodes, and elevated creatinine kinase or troponins.

14. C: Choice *C* is an expected side effect of long-term corticosteroid use and should be assessed by the medical-surgical nurse. Choices *A*, *B*, and *D* are not associated with the long-term use of this medication and would not cause the nurse to suspect these issues. Expected side effects of long-term use of this medication include hypertension, weight gain, and thinning of the skin.

15. D: Although electrical shock may not result in visible burns on the skin, extensive damage to skeletal muscle tissue can result in myonecrosis of the muscle cells. This damage leads to the release of large amounts of potassium from the cell, resulting in hyperkalemia. Potassium levels in excess of 8.5 mEq/L will cause lethal cardiac arrhythmias; therefore, Choice *D* is correct. Hypovolemic shock can potentially contribute to cardiac complications. However, there is no evidence of hypovolemia in this discussion; therefore, this is an unlikely cause of the cardiac arrest, and Choice *A* is incorrect. The patient's oxygenation is normal, and the patient is alert and oriented; therefore, hypoxia is an unlikely cause of the cardiac arrest, so Choice *B* is incorrect. Cardiac perforation is a possible consequence of electrical burns. However, in this discussion, more than five hours has elapsed since the injury, and this lethal consequence is most commonly evident immediately after the injury occurs; therefore, Choice *C* is incorrect.

16. D: Pulmonary edema can be of cardiogenic or non-cardiogenic origin. There is no single test to differentiate whether the cause of pulmonary edema is cardiac or noncardiac. Bilateral pulmonary infiltrates and hypoxemia are nonspecific symptoms and can occur in both. A pulmonary artery wedge pressure < 18 mmHg is consistent with pulmonary edema of non-cardiogenic origin.

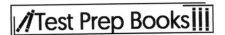

17. A: Choice *A* is responsible for the jugular vein distention as it induces bulging veins as the blood accumulates. Choices *B*, *C*, and *D* do not cause jugular vein distention as pressure is reduced in all of these choices. Jugular vein distention is a sign of increased central venous pressure and presents itself as a visible bulging vein in the neck.

18. C: Aldactone® (spironolactone), Choice *C*, is a potassium-sparing diuretic and supports the patient's concern regarding their potassium level at this time. This medication does not encourage the excretion of potassium via urine. Lasix® (furosemide) and Demadex® (torsemide) are loop diuretics and Microzide® (hydrochlorothiazide) is a thiazide diuretic. These medications do not specifically target conserving potassium in the body to address the patient's concern arising from their history. Therefore, Choices *A*, *B*, and *D* are incorrect.

19. B: Chronically ill children may not present with the typical manifestations of cholecystitis, such as colicky epigastric pain that radiates to the right upper quadrant. The chronically ill child with sickle cell disease may present with generalized abdominal pain. Therefore, Choices *A*, *C*, and *D* are not correct.

20. B: Vena cava filters are also known as inferior vena cava (IVC) filters or Greenfield filters. They are used to prevent a pulmonary embolism (PE). Indications for the placement of a vena cava filter include:

- An absolute contraindication to anticoagulants
- Survival after a massive PE and a high probability that a recurrent PE will be fatal
- Documented recurrent PE

21. C: Choice *C* provokes the nurse to prioritize diagnoses while developing a nursing plan and setting goals. Choice *A* involves a review of subjective and objective data. Choice *B* involves interpreting signs and symptoms to identify the patient's needs. Choice *D* involves providing patient education and carrying out procedures.

22. C: Metabolic syndrome, also called Syndrome X, is the presence of comorbid cardiovascular and insulin-related conditions. Those with metabolic disease may have excess belly fat, not excess fat on the upper back. Choices *A* and *B* are incorrect since patients with metabolic syndrome must have three or more of the following conditions: hypertension, elevated fasting blood glucose levels, low HDL cholesterol, high triglycerides, and excess belly fat. Patients with this disorder are typically overweight or obese and are at an increased risk for organ failure, heart attack, and stroke.

23. B: Hyperglycemia occurs when the patient's blood sugar level is greater than 200 milligrams per deciliter. Common symptoms of hyperglycemia include polyuria (excessive urination), polydipsia (excessive thirst), nausea, abdominal pain, fruity-scented breath, and confusion. Choices *A*, *C*, and *D* describe symptoms of hypoglycemia.

24. D: Choice *D* is a supportive intervention for a patient experiencing a dysautonomia flare. This condition causes substantial drops in blood pressure, which can be controlled via corticosteroid use. Choice *A* causes risky blood pressure fluctuations and should be avoided. Choice *B* promotes further reduction in blood pressure; therefore, the nurse should encourage an increased intake of sodium. Choice *C* encourages postprandial syncopal episodes and should be avoided.

25. D: While individuals over forty years of age are at increased risk for aneurysm formation, age is a nonmodifiable risk factor and would not be included in the teaching plan for modifiable risk factors. Smoking, cocaine use, and hypertension are all modifiable risk factors for aneurysm formation.

26. A: An acute situation, such as a urinary tract infection, may lead to delirium, a condition marked by confusion and agitation. Delirium is transient and resolves once the cause is eliminated, such as successfully treating a urinary tract infection. Choice *B* is not correct since dementia is a chronic condition in which the patient experiences reduced cognition over time. Choice *C* is not correct since Alzheimer's disease is a form of dementia and develops over time. Choice *D* is not correct since a patient who is agitated demonstrates acute anxiety and may be verbally abusive.

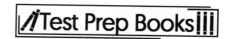

27. B: Bright red blood that is being vomited usually indicates an active upper GI bleed. Coffee ground blood indicates the blood has been sitting in the stomach for a while, indicating a slower bleed. The amount of blood, whether large or small, does not indicate active bleeding necessarily. For instance, a large bleed that has not fully manifested itself might result in a relatively small amount of blood vomited.

28. A: Choice *A* should be assessed using the bell of the stethoscope for detection. Choices *B*, *C*, and *D* should be auscultated with the diaphragm of the stethoscope. The bell supports auscultation of low frequency sounds, while the diaphragm filters low sounds out. The bell is helpful for detecting abnormal heart sounds and bruits.

29. B: Choice *B* represents the normal range for white blood cells in a healthy adult patient. Choices *A*, *C*, and *D* are outside of the normal range and would indicate a potential problem requiring further assessment by the medical-surgical nurse at this time. Choice *A* is below normal range. Choices *C* and *D* are above normal range.

30. B: Choice *B* indicates the appropriate team member for the nurse to elevate a patient care safety risk to. Choices *A*, *C*, and *D* fall higher in the nursing chain of command; therefore should not yet be prompted to handle this concern at this time.

31. B: Choice *B* represents an understanding of ways to reduce colon cancer risk post discharge. Increasing fruits and vegetables in the diet is one way to support a reduction in risk. Choice *A* is incorrect because this invasive routine is not supported. Choice *C* is incorrect; exercise does not directly correlate to a reduction of risk. Choice *D* is incorrect, as red meat is associated with a heightened risk of colon cancer.

32. B: Tensilon is used in myasthenic crisis to improve muscle function affected by deficient cholinesterase inhibitor levels; however, the improvement is temporary. Tensilon administration results in improved muscle function in myasthenic crisis; therefore, Choice *A* is incorrect. Tensilon effectively treats a myasthenic crisis. However, it will not improve a cholinergic crisis and may worsen the symptoms; therefore, Choices *C* and *D* are incorrect.

33. C: This scenario depicts the classic triad of symptoms of acute epiglottitis, including hypoxia, drooling and dysphagia. Acute epiglottitis is most often caused by *Haemophilus influenzae* type B. Direct visualization reveals that the epiglottis appears cherry red in color. Treatment includes antibiotic therapy, analgesic-antipyretic agents, and emergency airway management. Laryngotracheobronchitis (classic croup) is a common viral illness that primarily affects children and toddlers from six months to three years of age. The parainfluenza viruses (types 1, 2, and 3) account for 80 percent of all cases. Presenting symptoms include a barking cough, wheezing, tachypnea, and tachycardia. Treatment is symptomatic and includes corticosteroids, racemic epinephrine, and mechanical ventilation. Tracheitis is the inflammation of the trachea caused most commonly by *Staphylococcus aureus*. Children under the age of fifteen are most commonly affected. Antibiotic therapy and anti-pyretic medications are used. Mechanical ventilation is rarely necessary. Bronchiolitis is an inflammation of the bronchioles caused by the respiratory syncytial virus. It most commonly affects children under the age of two. Its diagnosis is based on clinical examination and the disease is self-limiting.

34. C: Endoscopy is used to diagnose the condition and to cauterize hemorrhagic sites. The treatment algorithm for peptic ulcer disease recommends surgical intervention if two endoscopic attempts at hemostasis are unsuccessful. The pain related to peptic ulcer disease does not begin until the ingested food has reached the duodenum; therefore, the pain does not begin for two to three hours after a meal, while the onset of pain with gastric ulcers is 20 to 30 minutes after a meal. Choice *A* is incorrect. Gastric ulcers are associated with an increased incidence of malignancy, not peptic ulcers; therefore, Choice *B* is incorrect. NSAID use is a commonly associated cause of peptic ulcer disease. However, even excluding patients who use NSAIDs, more than 60 percent of the cases of peptic ulcer disease are related to *H. pylori* infection; therefore, Choice *D* is incorrect.

35. B: Choice *B* is a likely condition associated with acromegaly. The medical-surgical nurse should be aware of this association and monitor for signs and symptoms of diabetes mellitus, such as polyuria and polydipsia. Choice *A* is

319

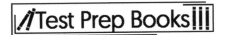
incorrect, as the patient's bone enlargement is permanent. Choice C is incorrect, as the patient needs to engage in surgery as soon as possible. Choice D is incorrect, as the patient's hands and feet will grow larger.

36. A: Prehypertension is defined as systolic pressures ranging between 120 and 139 mmHg or diastolic pressures between 80 and 89 mmHg. Normal blood pressure is less than 120/80 mmHg. Stage 1 hypertension ranges from 140 to 159 mmHg systolic or 90 to 99 mmHg diastolic. Stage 2 hypertension is greater than or equal to 160 mmHg systolic or greater than or equal to 100 mmHg diastolic.

37. D: Choice D supports suspicion for the need to transfer the patient to inpatient psychiatry once medically stable. Reasons for acute inpatient psychiatric hospitalization include danger to self, danger to others, and gross inability to care for self. Psychosocial symptoms warrant the need for a psychiatric consult to evaluate continuation of care options. Choices A, B, and C may each be present symptoms of the patient's mental illness but not reason enough for inpatient care. Patient presentations outside of the needs listed here for acute inpatient stabilization can be referred for outpatient management.

38. A: Jugular vein distention, peripheral edema, and pulmonary congestion are characteristics of blood volume backing up due to an obstruction. Decreased urine output, increased BUN, and increased creatinine are signs of renal failure. Chest pain, fatigue, and lightheadedness are signs of an MI. Problems with coordination, blurred vision, and paralysis are symptomatic of a stroke.

39. A: Choice A represents the cranial nerve responsible for the patient's reflex to gag and swallow. Choice B is responsible for tongue movements. Choice C is responsible for taste. Choice D is responsible for jaw movements.

40. D: Viral pneumonia, commonly caused by RSV, parainfluenza virus, and adenovirus, may be diagnosed by chest x-ray and viral cultures. Rapid antigen testing is now also being used for diagnosis and has the advantage of shortening the time for diagnosing this infection. Choices A, B, and C are incorrect, as these tests are not used to either diagnose viral pneumonia or shorten the diagnostic time.

41. C: In second-degree heart block, specifically Mobitz type I, the PR interval is lengthened and greater than 0.20. The PR interval for a normal sinus rhythm is 0.12–0.20. In a junctional rhythm, the impulse starts at the AV node, so the P wave is absent. In Mobitz type II second-degree heart block, the P waves are not followed by the QRS complex. The atria and ventricles are asynchronously contracting.

42. D: The patient with Guillain-Barré syndrome with cranial nerve involvement may exhibit weakness or paralysis of the eye muscles, facial drooping, diplopia, dysphagia, and pupillary alterations.

43. A: The nurse must first assess the patient's vital signs before continuing on with subsequent actions. Therefore, Choice A is correct. Choices B, C, and D are all relevant interventions, but they lack the priority in the case of the patient complaining of chest pain. Once the vital signs have been assessed, the nurse should follow the nursing process to proceed with further care options.

44. A: Since electrolytes need to be suspended in a certain amount of liquid to move optimally and carry out their intended function, fluid level in the body is important. As fluid levels increase beyond a state of fluid-electrolyte balance, electrolyte levels will decrease, since there is too much fluid present. If fluid levels are too low, such as in a state of dehydration, there will be too many electrolytes per unit of fluid, which also prevents the electrolytes from carrying out their intended function.

45. D: Choice D demonstrates a normal finding when auscultating the patient's lungs. Choice A is a normal finding over the stomach, not the lungs. Choice B is not a normal finding, as it is indicative of air hyperinflation, such as with asthma. Choice C is normal over dense areas such as the liver, not over the lungs.

320

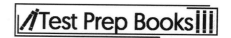

46. A: Choice *A* is correct as this finding represents the shortness of breath that is present specifically in a recumbent position. Choice *B* identifies difficulty breathing. Choice *C* identifies elevated breathing rate. Choice *D* correlates with decreased breathing rate.

47. D: Choice *D* designates the appropriate first action to be implemented by the nurse in response to the patient's request for discharge. Exploring the patient's reasoning for discharge is patient-centered and allows the nurse to gather additional information to formulate a clear understanding of the present issue(s) before deciding on next steps. Choice *A* may be an appropriate second step, depending on the patient's response to the original inquiry in step one. Choices *B* and *C*, while potential actions that may be necessary at some point, are not priorities in this situation.

48. D: Chromosomal abnormalities of the fetus are the most common cause of early spontaneous abortions. Other factors that increase the risk include advanced maternal age, type 1 diabetes, renal disease, severe hypertension, thyroid dysfunction, anatomical defects of the uterus, illicit drug use, smoking, alcohol abuse, and non-ASA NSAID use; therefore, Choices *A* and *B* are not correct. Moderate exercise is not a risk factor for spontaneous abortion.

49. D: While the physician is legally responsible for satisfying all elements of informed consent, nurses are ethically responsible for assessing the patient's ability to process and understand the implications of informed consent. Nurses protect the patient's autonomy by raising these questions and concerns. The remaining elements of informed consent are required of the physician, rather than the nurses.

50. D: Choice *D* is a dependent nursing intervention as it requires a provider's order to carry out. Choices *A*, *B*, and *C* are all within the nursing scope to initiate and are therefore considered independent nursing interventions. A third classification, interdependent intervention, involves nursing and collaborative specialties providing care measures.

51. B: The scenario depicts an episode of status asthmaticus. Common pharmacological agents used to treat this condition include albuterol (short-acting Beta-2 agonist), ipratropium (anticholinergic), and methylprednisolone (corticosteroid). Her new symptoms (anxiety, tremors, and tachycardia) are all common side effects which can be attributed to albuterol. Anticholinergics can induce side effects such as dry mouth, blurred vision, and constipation. Corticosteroids (if used for longer than two weeks) can have side effects such as weight gain, osteoporosis, thinning of skin, cataracts, easy bruising, and diabetes. She should be switched to the short-acting Beta-2 agonist levalbuterol because it's as effective as albuterol but without the alarming side effects.

52. A: Choice *A* indicates the priority action in navigating a dilemma of opposing opinions within the interdisciplinary team. Choices *B*, *C*, and *D* are actions that may or may not need to happen depending on what is found when collecting clinical data.

53. B: Choice *B* is correct as diabetes mellitus increases one's risk of a cerebrovascular accident due to pathologic changes in blood vessels. Choices *A*, *C*, and *D* are not considered risk factors for cerebrovascular accident.

54. B: Choice *B* indicates the therapeutic reference range for serum carbamazepine. Choices *A*, *C*, and *D* represent serum medication ranges outside of therapeutic limits. The therapeutic range is measured by fluorescence polarization immunoassay.

55. B: Choice *B* should be supported by the nurse, as it brings the knees to the chest and typically encourages some pain relief in acute appendicitis. Choices *A*, *C*, and *D* represent positions that would likely exacerbate the patient's pain symptoms and should not be encouraged at this time.

56. B: Choice *B* aligns with the ethical principle to maintain truthful engagements. Choice *A* aligns with ethical fairness. Choice *C* aligns with refraining from harm. Choice *D* promotes doing right by the patient.

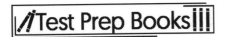

57. B: The diuretic reduces blood volume, and the ACE inhibitor reduces SVR by interfering with the RAAS. An ARB reduces systemic vascular resistance, but morphine is used to treat pain. The diuretic reduces blood volume, but a beta-blocker increases myocardial contractility. The diuretic reduces blood volume, but a CCB works by increasing myocardial contractility.

58. A: Choice *A* is correct as sausage is a high tyramine-containing food and must be avoided by the patient taking a monoamine oxidase inhibitor, such as phenelzine. Foods rich in tyramine need to be avoided in order to prevent tyramine levels in the blood from becoming critically high and leading to a hypertensive crisis. Choices *B*, *C*, and *D* are not considered high tyramine-containing foods and are not contraindicated for the patient at this time.

59. C: Choice *C* represents the appropriate level of activity for the patient with heart failure. Alternating rest with activity supports a reduced cardiac workload. Choice *A* would encourage a higher level of activity than the patient's condition can maintain. Choices *B* and *D* place unnecessary restrictions on the patient's activity.

60. B: The elevated glucose levels associated with both type 1 and type 2 diabetes result in atherosclerosis, or wall thickening of the small arterioles and capillaries, which alters the circulation in the brain, retina, peripheral nerves, and kidneys. These changes are cumulative and irreversible; however, long-term control of the serum glucose level as measured by the A1C can limit the progression of this process. Current research indicates that the optimum A1C level is patient-specific. In this discussion, the patient knows his personal A1C target and understands the association between the elevated glucose levels and the occurrence of the TIA; therefore, Choice *B* is correct. Two of the ABCD^2 score categories are modifiable risk factors. Maintaining the systolic and diastolic blood pressure and blood glucose level as defined by the A1C within normal limits may lower the risk of a repeated attack. The patient should be encouraged to make the necessary lifestyle changes, including smoking cessation, dietary modifications, exercise participation, and compliance with the medication regimen that may include antihypertensive and glucose-lowering agents. Choice *A* is incorrect. There are differences in the pathophysiology between type 1 and type 2 diabetes; however, the complications are similar. In type 2 diabetes, hyperglycemia and insulin resistance contribute to increased low-density lipoproteins and triglycerides and decreased levels of high-density lipoproteins and alterations in microvasculature; therefore, Choice *C* is incorrect. To prevent further damage to the vascular system and reduce the risk of recurrent TIAs, the use of insulin may be necessary to control hyperglycemia as evidenced by the A1C level; therefore, Choice *D* is incorrect.

61. A: Choice *A* identifies the patient's potential fear regarding the consequence of the nurse's actions. Giving what is perceived to be the "evil eye" may induce significant worry that the patient's child will become weak and ill and can even lead to fears that the child may die. Choices *B*, *C*, and *D* represent concerns of staring outside of the definition of this cultural consideration.

62. D: The gastroenterologist will likely use cauterization, an application of heat, to seal the bleeding lesion. Banding is a procedure used to help stop bleeding in esophageal varices. Biopsy is where tissues are removed for histological analysis. Angioplasty is performed in cardiac catheterizations and involves balloon inflation and stent placement to open up occluded blood vessels.

63. D: Choice *D* includes bringing about the greatest good for the greatest number of people, which is what the medical-surgical nurse does when prioritizing patient care. Choices *A*, *B*, and *C*, while all ethical considerations, do not align with the nurse's actions at this time.

64. D: In advanced stages of cancer, even when the prognosis is poor, chemotherapy may be able to manage pain and suffering. Choices *A*, *B*, and *C* are not correct, because the chance of remission, cure, or halting the advance of cancer in advanced stages of cancer with a poor prognosis is low, and the nurse should not give the patient false hope.

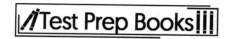

65. B: Nurses should participate in professional development activities whenever possible, balancing time and job demands. These activities may be within the facility or outside the organization. This participation helps maintain professional accountability.

66. D: Time between the collapse and the start of resuscitation efforts is the most important factor in patient survival. Administering supplemental oxygen is a component of resuscitation efforts. Establishing IV access is an essential component of resuscitation efforts. Inserting a Foley catheter to drain the urinary bladder is not related to survival.

67. D: In type 2 diabetes, the pancreas produces insulin, but the body does not use it effectively. This type of diabetes may be treated with oral anti-diabetic medications and, in some cases, insulin. However, many people can control their type 2 diabetes through lifestyle changes, such as losing weight and eating less carbohydrate-rich and sugar-laden foods, making Choices A, B, and C incorrect.

68. C: Small-bowel obstruction is associated with severe fluid and electrolyte losses. The normal serum sodium level is 135 to 145 mEq/L; therefore, Choice C is indicative of deficient serum sodium and severe alterations in fluid balance. Small-bowel obstruction is manifested by metabolic alkalosis due to the loss of acids with vomiting. Choice A is consistent with metabolic acidosis, not alkalosis, and is therefore incorrect. As noted, small-bowel obstruction is associated with fluid volume deficits; however, the reported serum osmolality at 285 mosm/kg is within the normal range for serum osmolality (275–295 mosm/kg); therefore, Choice B is incorrect. Abdominal distention in large-bowel obstruction most commonly occurs in the lower abdomen, while abdominal distention in the small bowel most commonly occurs in the epigastric or upper abdominal area; therefore, Choice D is incorrect.

69. A: Choice A is the antidote to be given to a patient experiencing over anticoagulation to halt the progression of this process. Choices B, C, and D, while antidotes for a variety of medications, will not work for this issue.

70. A: Choice A is a back channeling communication cue that signals to the patient that the nurse is actively listening and would like the patient to continue with their narrative. Choices B, C, and D, while all potentially useful communication cues, do not meet the description of back channeling.

71. B: Of the two types of human immunodeficiency virus (HIV), HIV-1 is the dominant strain among global cases. HIV-2 is not highly transmissible, so Choice A is not correct. Since HIV-2 is poorly understood, Choice C is not correct. HIV-1 is the more severe strain

72. B: In an adult lying in the supine position, a normal intracranial pressure reading ranges from 7 to 15 millimeters of mercury. Therefore, Choices A, C, and D are incorrect.

73. A: Since tremors, fatigue, and dizziness are manifestations of hypoglycemia, the nurse would expect to see a low blood glucose level. Since a normal blood glucose level is 70 to 130 milligrams per deciliter, 58 milligrams per deciliter is consistent with hypoglycemia. Choice B is not correct since 120 milligrams per deciliter is a normal blood glucose level. Choice C is not correct since 180 milligrams per deciliter is above normal. Choice D is not correct since a blood glucose level greater than 200 milligrams per deciliter is considered hyperglycemic.

74. A: Choice A indicates an accurate understanding of the discharge process. Discharge planning starts upon admission to ensure that resources are allocated appropriately, interventions align with an established treatment plan, and an ultimate safe discharge outcome is recognized. Choices B, C, and D do not represent a clear understanding of treatment planning for the discharge process.

75. D: The appropriate response to an initial unprovoked seizure episode—one that is not related to a specific cause such as head trauma—is to identify any abnormal electrical activity of the brain with an EEG and any anatomical lesions in the brain with MRI. There is no indication of substance abuse in the patient's history, which means that

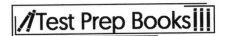

this assessment would not be a priority for this patient at this point; therefore, Choice *A* is incorrect. General guidelines indicate that AED therapy should be delayed until a second unprovoked seizure episode occurs and after the initial EEG and MRI studies are completed; therefore, Choice *B* is incorrect. The patient's history does not support the possibility of infection as the precipitating event for this seizure activity, which means performing the invasive lumbar puncture would not be indicated; therefore, Choice *C* is incorrect.

76. C: Choice *C* is correct, as the patient should use their Advair-Diskus inhaler routinely, twice per day. The patient appropriately understands that this inhaler is not designed for rescue breathing relief when they share that they will use it every morning and evening. Choices *A*, *B*, and *D* represent responses that align with inhalers indicated for rescue relief and are not appropriate for this medication.

77. A: Avoiding tight clothing and wearing compression stockings are appropriate. Although prolonged sitting should be avoided, airplane travel itself is not contraindicated. Exercise should be continued with frequent rest periods as needed. The occurrence and severity of claudication can be decreased with regular exercise.

78. D: This scenario depicts a moderate to severe acute exacerbation of COPD. Azithromycin is a macrolide antibiotic. In clinical trials, the use of antibiotics in individuals with a moderate to severe exacerbation of COPD diminishes the risk of treatment failure and death. Oxygen and albuterol target dyspnea. In clinical trials, the administration of oral corticosteroids fairly early in the midst of a COPD exacerbation decreased the need for hospitalization.

79. D: Choice *D* involves the appropriate plan for reducing the spread of measles. It is important for the nurse to understand that measles requires airborne precautions and that proactive initiation is required once this illness is suspected. The nurse should NOT wait to start this precaution until the confirmation is received. Choices *A*, *B*, and *C* provide inadequate protection against the transmission of measles.

80. A: Fever and petechial rash are signs of endocarditis. Body piercings and corticosteroids are among the risk factors for developing endocarditis. Autoimmune conditions vary, but the most frequent presenting symptoms are fatigue and body aches. Pneumonia presents with fever, chills, and cough. Heart failure (HF) is not associated with a petechial rash or a fever.

81. D: Choice *D* represents the proper infection control practices to reduce the transmission of herpes zoster for the patient with classified disseminated infection. Both airborne and contact precautions are necessary during this phase of illness. Choices *A*, *B*, and *C* would provide improper infection control and increased risk.

82. B: Sodium hypochlorite is the only commonly used disinfecting agent that possesses all of the listed characteristics. Sodium peroxide is a cleaning agent commonly found in laundry detergents and other household cleaning items but is typically not used in medical settings. Formaldehyde and hydrogen peroxide don't possess all the qualities listed, though they're commonly used in medical settings.

83. D: Emergent procedures are the only exception when it comes to requirement of consent prior to procedure. Consent for pediatric patients is given by the patient's parent or legal guardian. Surgery is a type of invasive procedure. Routine procedures fall under Universal Protocol guidelines.

84. C: Choice *C* should be limited in the diet of a patient with Meniere's disease. Sodium leads to a buildup of water, which can contribute to an increase in inner-ear fluid and exacerbation of symptoms. Choices *A*, *B*, and *D* do not directly lead to an improvement in symptoms of this condition.

85. B: Goals of care conversations are held to keep the focus on what the dying patient wants at the end of their life.

86. A: All chemotherapy orders must be written orders received from a physician on the proper form. Even if

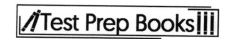

scheduling is available, the patient is prepared, the physician is present, and Aria feels comfortable performing the procedure, chemotherapy administration cannot occur without the written physician orders.

87. B: Use of recreational drugs should be included in the medication reconciliation process. The prescriber of the current medications is not relevant during the reconciliation process. Prescription medication, as well as over-the-counter medications, supplements, and vitamins, should be noted. The patient's preferred pharmacy is not included in the medication reconciliation process.

88. B: Choice *B* represents an appropriate response to this finding, as it is normal for air to leak until the lung incision heals and is sealed. Choices *A*, *C*, and *D* all involve the nurse elevating this finding as a point of concern, which would be inappropriate at this time. The nurse should document this normal finding, and then continue to monitor the patient's chamber and incision.

89. C: Observing and recording the patient's heart rhythm via ECG is the specific intervention necessary to monitor for the development of dysrhythmias post cardiac catheterization. All of the other interventions listed are correct post-cardiac catheterization care but not specific to dysrhythmias. The nurse will keep the patient flat to assist with incision healing, take regular vital signs such as heart rate and blood pressure, and monitor for bleeding and hematoma at the incision site to evaluate the patient's overall stability.

90. C: A good hand-off provides information that is accurate, clear, and specific. A good hand-off allows for open discussion between the perioperative nurse providing information about the patient and the nurse who is receiving the patient. Poor communication during a hand-off increases the risk for errors and poor patient outcomes.

91. C: An event that requires intervention to prevent permanent damage is considered to be an adverse drug reaction (ADR) by the FDA. Intractable vomiting following chemotherapy is identified as an expected side effect of the treatment and is not reportable as an ADR; therefore, Choice *A* is incorrect. Harmful self-inflicted behaviors are not identified as ADRs by the FDA; therefore, Choice *B* is incorrect. The American Society of Healthcare Pharmacists has proposed that any unexpected or undesired outcome that requires the alteration of the drug dosage should be defined as an ADR. However, currently, the FDA defines the outcomes more narrowly. Therefore, Choice *D* is incorrect.

92. B: Choice *B* incorporates the characteristics witnessed within the charismatic leadership style. Choice *A* incorporates characteristics of the bureaucratic leadership style. Choice *C* incorporates characteristics of the transformational leadership style. Choice *D* incorporates characteristics of the transactional leadership style.

93. B: The root cause analysis is used when there is an adverse event, a sentinel event, or close call in the medical setting. It can also be used when there is a concern about a process due to repeated errors, when there is a possibility of serious errors, and when there are high-cost errors.

94. C: Nurses must acknowledge their own biases and recognize that those biases will affect their ability to provide culturally sensitive care. Standard protocols related to cultural beliefs and practices are an imperfect solution to the problem of culturally sensitive care because they are not individualized to the specific patient. Meeting the needs of the largest group in a population generally means that the cultural needs of the minority groups within the population are not met. As previously stated, culturally competent care results when caregivers first consider their own biases and the possible effect of those beliefs on patient care. If nurses base their care only on their own beliefs, the patient's beliefs and practices will be ignored.

95. C: The QESN competencies were originally identified to improve patient safety in response to research that indicated that nearly 100,000 people died each year as a result of provider errors. The QESN competencies refer to nursing activities and are often used as the basis for undergraduate nursing curricula. Systems thinking is the process by which nurses meet the competencies, and attainment of this ability is an incremental process based on

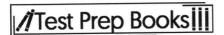

nurses' continuing education and clinical experiences. Although systems thinking is associated with the QESN competencies, and the use of systems thinking has improved patient outcomes, the basic assumption of the QESN competencies was improved patient safety as a result of expert nursing care.

96. C: The American Hospital Association's Patient Care Partnership document mandated a decision-making partnership between the healthcare system and the patient, facilitating patients' efforts to determine their own future. This decision-making partnership highlighted the responsibilities of the healthcare system to fully communicate treatment options and the plan of care and mandated a change in care patterns and nursing practices.

97. B: Sharing, supporting, and explaining the patient's point of view are activities that are consistent with advocacy. The remaining choices contribute to good professional practice but are not specifically related to the concept of advocacy.

98. A: When working with adult learners, it is important for the nurse to relate the teachings to real-world experiences. This acknowledges patients' prior knowledge and experience and helps provide a more robust teaching and understanding that adult learners can utilize. Choice B is incorrect because the nurse should not assume the patient has no prior knowledge, as this can come off as belittling and limit the extent to which the nurse can teach. Instead, the nurse should assess the prior knowledge the patient has and tailor the teaching level and material accordingly. Choice C is incorrect because by maintaining authority and control, the nurse does not allow the patient to be involved in learning and may invalidate concerns they have. This approach may also come off as disrespectful when trying to educate adult learners. Instead, the nurse should have a professional and collaborative approach. Choice D is incorrect because keeping objectives fluid and subjective may make it more difficult for patients to understand the goals they are trying to reach and more difficult for the nurse to assess their learning. Objectives should be clear, measurable, and goal focused.

99. C: When committees are being constructed to make hospital-wide changes regarding client rights, it is best to involve not only administrative and medical staff, but also patients and their family members, since these matters directly concern them. Additional feedback can be gained from patients and family members through surveys, feedback cards, and follow-up appointments. Choices A, B, and D are incorrect because they do not include all groups of people that should be involved in decisions regarding client rights.

100. D: It is appropriate for the nurse to delegate the task of recording output to a certified nursing assistant (CNA). Certified nursing assistants can also be delegated other routine care such as recording intake/output, vital signs, and activities of daily living as appropriate. The nurse should be able to assess if each task is necessary, appropriate, and within the CNA's scope of practice. Choice A is incorrect because passing medication is outside of the regular scope of a CNA's practice. The nurse should pass this medication if it was scanned and charted under their name and license. Choice B is incorrect because inserting a new IV is outside of the regular scope of practice for a CNA. Some facilities may allow training for CNAs for additional skills, so the nurse should be familiar with the policies at their facility. Choice C is incorrect because, although it is within the scope of practice for a CNA to reposition a patient, it is not appropriate to ask a CNA to independently reposition an obese patient. This task can cause injury to the CNA and patient; instead, the nurse should either assist the CNA or ensure the CNA has additional help.

101. C: Any new orders should be read back to the provider to verify they are correct, and any additional questions or concerns should be addressed at this time. Choice A is incorrect because verbal orders should be avoided when possible, as there is a higher possibility of error. Instead, electronic orders or clearly legible handwritten orders should be used first. Choice B is incorrect because medical abbreviations should be avoided to help reduce the likelihood of medication errors. Choice D is incorrect because the nurse should rely on the electronic medical record to double-check orders and reduce incidences of medication error. Using electronic methods allows for medication barcodes and scanning, which is an additional check to decrease error.

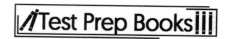

102. A: The first step of conflict resolution should be for both sides to present their side of the disagreement calmly and professionally. This allows whoever is mediating the conflict to understand the opinions of both sides. Choices *B* and *C* are incorrect because these steps come later in conflict resolution. After presenting the sides of the argument, the disagreement should be discussed in detail, eventually coming to a compromise or some negotiation or re-evaluation. Choice *D* is incorrect because disagreements should not be dismissed. Using conflict resolution can help teams grow and build better communication.

103. C: Following a patient's death, the family members should not be immediately asked to leave the room. The family should be allowed to stay in the room with the patient to grieve, process their emotions, and participate in care if safe and appropriate. Choices *A, B,* and *D* are incorrect because these are appropriate actions for the nurse to take to help provide support to the family and remain respectful to the patient.

104. D: This team is now at the implementation stage of problem-solving because their team is actively using their possible solution by removing catheters within 24 hours of surgery. Choice *A* is incorrect because evaluation would be the next step in this process and would include the team seeing if this is an effective strategy in reducing UTIs. In this scenario, the nursing team has already identified a problem, in this case high UTI rates, and developed a possible solution of removing catheters earlier in the post-op period; therefore, Choices *B* and *C* are also incorrect.

105. A: Evidence is usually graded on a letter scale, with A being the highest level of evidence. The type of research with the highest level of evidence is a meta-analysis. Choice *B* is incorrect because a randomized-control trial is the second highest level of evidence, level B. Choices *C* and *D* are incorrect because integrative interviews and cohort studies have a moderate level of evidence and are both level C.

106. D: When a patient requests complementary therapies, the nurse should not discourage or immediately deny their request. Instead, this request should be discussed with the medical team to ensure it is safe and will not interfere with their current prescribed therapy and recovery. Choice *A* is incorrect because the nurse should not deny the request and state it is dangerous until it can be further reviewed. Choice *B* is incorrect because, in addition to denying their request without further review, many complementary therapies are tied to cultural and religious practices and denying their benefit may be offensive and insensitive. Choice *C* is incorrect because, before starting new complementary therapy such as acupuncture, benefits and risks should be reviewed. Additionally, complementary therapy should not take the place of prescribed therapies and should be used in conjunction with traditional therapies and medications.

107. A: Utilitarianism is defined as providing the greatest good for the greatest number, which can limit the autonomy of the individual. Therefore, Choices *B, C* and *D* are incorrect.

108. B: The location where the task was completed is not a required piece of documentation when delegating a task. In charting this would often be redundant to include, as the patient's room or location would automatically be linked in their health record. Choices *A, C,* and *D* are incorrect because these are the three essential components to include in charting when a task is delegated.

109. D: A team that is made of healthcare professionals from multiple disciplines, such as doctors, specialized nurses, nurse practitioners, and dietitians is an interdisciplinary team. Choices *A* and *B* are incorrect because they are not types of medical teams that a nurse works on. Choice *C* is incorrect because an intradisciplinary team is made up of members that are all from the same profession or discipline. In the healthcare setting, nurses will work on both intradisciplinary and interdisciplinary teams and should be comfortable in both settings.

110. D: Using a hospital interpreter helps bridge language barriers and helps increase a patient's understanding of their medical care. Patients who come from certain Asian cultures do not outwardly express their emotions and grief and may appear stoic. It is important that the nurse still offers a line of respectful communication so the patient can ask questions and process this news as they feel appropriate. Choice *A* is incorrect because patients

327

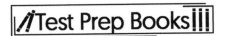

from Asian cultures may not maintain eye contact as a sign of respect, and this cultural preference should be understood and respected by the nurse. Choice *B* is incorrect because patients from Asian cultures may see it as a sign of weakness to express their feelings or grief. The nurse should be respectful of how the patient wishes to process and show their emotions in relation to their cultural beliefs and traditions. Choice *C* is incorrect because patients who are sick may feel a sense of shame and want to hide their illness from their families; the nurse should respect the patient's wishes and only contact the patient's family if the patient directly asks them to.

111. B: Transmission-based precautions are classified in three ways: contact, droplet, and airborne. Surface precautions are not an example of transmission-based precautions.

112. B: ChloraPrep is an alcohol-based chlorhexidine gluconate solution. Alcohol-based solutions are contraindicated on open wounds. ChloraPrep is safe for the patient with a povidone iodine allergy. It is indicated for use on intact skin areas (such as left groin and chest).

113. A: The use of mobile work stations, electronic medical records, integrated clinic and pharmacy systems, and patient portal systems all indicate a medical organization that's fully utilizing healthcare information technology. The online practices illustrated in the case are helping the providers access, document, and maintain patient files more efficiently. The case also illustrates how online systems allow an interdisciplinary team to work together to deliver treatment that the patient needs. Paper charting systems aren't relevant to this case. The proximity of the pharmacy and the demeanor of the pharmacist is a benefit for the patient, but these aren't recurring themes presented in the case.

114. B: The most appropriate action for the nurse to take if they suspect elder abuse in the hospital setting is to document the suspected abuse and report it to the appropriate authority, such as the hospital's elder abuse hotline or the local protective services agency. Choices *A*, *C*, and *D* can put the patient at risk and potentially compromise the investigation into the suspected abuse.

115. C: An interim chain of command provides a hierarchy of order for staff to follow in the event of a regional emergency. It may involve people from sister facilities or other first response agencies. A documented and recognized chain of command specific to this context minimizes the risks from communication issues or new processes during a vulnerable time. Hurricane evacuation plans may be important for coastal facilities where hurricanes are likely, but they are not necessary for all facilities (e.g., a Midwestern location) and could be a waste of time and resources. Therefore, Choice *A* can be eliminated. A temporary morgue is a waste of cost and space until it is actually needed, so Choice *B* can be eliminated. While hospitals may want to have a secure plan for procuring extra PPE if the need arises, storing them unnecessarily can also be a waste of money and storage space; therefore, Choice *D* can be eliminated.

116. C: Positive changes in workflow processes are considered quality improvement projects, as they allow for better healthcare delivery. In this case, hand sanitization is more likely to be efficiently completed, and overall waits and delays are reduced for the clinic as a whole, as a result of Douglas's proposed change. Quality improvements are often small changes that can make a large impact. The other options aren't applicable, as the WHO isn't conducting this type of sanitization initiative, JHCO doesn't implement such changes, and this case isn't understood to be a common dermatology clinic issue.

117. A: EHRs have been shown to reduce (and even prevent) medical errors due to misinterpretation of handwriting. EHRs also allow built-in systems designed to prevent treatment errors. EHRs do not relate to the time spent researching a disease process.

118. C: It is recommended that educational materials and instructions be provided at no higher than a fifth-grade level, and the nurse should never assume that a patient can understand medical terms. Choices *A*, *B*, and *D* all contain more complex words, such as *glycemic*, *diaphoresis*, and *subcutaneous*. Choice *C* is the only answer that

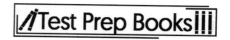

uses simple terminology. The nurse can also assess health literacy by using the teach-back method to clarify the patient's understanding of the instructions provided.

119. B: Choices *A*, *C*, and *D* are all appropriate times for the nurse to call the organ procurement organization. However, the nurse is never responsible for contacting the patient's family regarding organ donation. This will be the OPO's responsibility.

120. C: In this scenario, it would be best to relay the information to the nurse manager for them to handle it further. It is not the primary nurse's responsibility to manage patient/provider conflicts; therefore, Choice *D* is incorrect. Nurse managers are trained in conflict management and will have the effective tools necessary to de-escalate these types of situations. Choices *A* and *B* would be inappropriate as they are dismissive and confrontational, respectively.

121. B: Choices *A*, *C*, and *D* are all actions that support patient advocacy. Choice *B* does not encourage the patient to make their own medical decisions; therefore, it is incorrect.

122. D: Per CMS regulatory requirements, all patient deaths that occur while in restraints or seclusion must be reported. Reporting is also required if the death occurs within 24 hours of restraint/seclusion removal. Choices *A*, *B*, and *C* are not reportable criteria for CMS.

123. B: While these are all acceptable actions that the nurse can take to support patient and family-centered care, Choice *B* is most important in the clinical setting. The patient and family should always be involved in daily rounding and should have a say in treatment decisions that are being made. Choices *A*, *C*, and *D* are supplemental resources that the nurse can utilize.

124. A: Obtaining a health history from multiple sources, including the patient and their family members, can help to ensure the accuracy of the information gathered. Patients may not remember all details of their medical history or may not understand the significance of certain symptoms, whereas family members may have a more complete picture of the patient's health status. Additionally, patients may not disclose sensitive information to the nurse during the initial interview, but a family member may be able to provide this information. Saving time, satisfying legal requirements, and complying with hospital policy, as in Choices *B*, *C*, and *D*, are all important aspects of the nursing profession, but they are not the primary reasons for obtaining a health history from multiple sources.

125. A: Patients who live alone have an increased risk of readmission because they may have difficulty managing their symptoms and taking their medications as prescribed without assistance. Additionally, they may not have someone to monitor their condition or recognize when they need to seek medical attention. While hypertension and congestive heart failure are both chronic conditions that may increase the risk of readmission, neither is the primary factor for this patient's case; therefore, Choices *B* and *C* are incorrect. Choice *D* is not a risk factor for hospital readmission.

126. B: Social determinants of health are the physical, social, and economic conditions that impact health outcomes, such as income, education, and housing. In this example, the patient's occupation is an example of an SDOH, as working multiple jobs can make it difficult to manage their asthma and afford treatment. While the patient's asthma diagnosis is an important factor in their overall health status, as in Choice *A*, it does not specifically address the challenges they face in managing their condition due to social circumstances. Choices *C* and *D* can both be affected by social determinants of health but are not examples of SDOH themselves.

127. C: In this case, the nurse should first check the connections of the PCA device and reposition as needed to ensure proper delivery of medication to the patient. Choices *A*, *B*, and *D* may be appropriate actions if the issue cannot be resolved through assessment and troubleshooting.

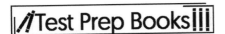

128. B: Coaching for documentation performance improvement is an important part of professional development for new nurses. The charge nurse should focus on providing positive feedback on the documentation that is accurate and complete, while also providing constructive feedback on areas that need improvement. Criticizing the new nurse for incomplete documentation or reporting directly to the nurse manager, as in Choices *A* and *C*, can be demotivating and counterproductive. Choice *D* may lead to inaccurate or incomplete records, which can negatively impact this patient's care.

129. B: A palliative care consultation can help relieve this patient's symptoms and give spiritual and emotional support to the patient and the family. Choice *A* is too early because hospice care is usually recommended when patients have a life expectancy of less than six months. Choice *C* is incorrect because while support groups can be helpful for patients and their families, palliative care can provide more immediate and individualized support. Choice *D* is incorrect because while advanced care planning is an important part of end-of-life care, it would be more appropriate if discussed later, as the patient's condition changes.

130. B: Pain management is an important part of postoperative care, and nurses play a key role in managing patients' pain. Nurses are responsible for assessing and documenting pain, administering pain medications as ordered, and monitoring patients for side effects and adverse reactions. This is not the responsibility of the surgeon, physical therapist, or dietician; therefore, Choices *A*, *C*, and *D* are incorrect.

131. B: A family conference with the patient's healthcare team can provide an opportunity to discuss the patient's care, ask questions, and provide input into the decision-making process. While policies and procedures are important, Choice *A*, they may not address the patient's specific concerns or needs. Choices *C* and *D* are not consistent with patient/family-centered care.

132. B: It is essential to prioritize patients based on the severity of their conditions to ensure that the most critical patients receive timely intervention. Hypotension and tachycardia can indicate impending shock and require immediate intervention to stabilize the patient's condition; therefore, Choice *B* is the correct answer. Choice *A* should be the second priority, as the patient is symptomatic and requires management to prevent further deterioration. Choices *C* and *D* are important, but their conditions are not as immediately life-threatening as the other two patients.

133. C: Fiscal efficiency involves optimizing resource utilization and minimizing unnecessary expenses. By implementing a waste reduction program, the nurse manager can identify and minimize waste, reducing expenses and improving fiscal efficiency. Choices *A*, *B*, and *D* may improve patient care but may not necessarily lead to fiscal efficiency.

134. C: By engaging in interprofessional collaboration, pursuing ongoing professional development, and seeking guidance from experienced colleagues, the nurse is ensuring that the patient will receive the highest quality of care. Choices *A*, *B*, and *D* may not be sufficient to meet the patient's needs and may compromise the quality of care, leading to adverse patient outcomes.

135. C: As a nurse in a leadership role, it is important to provide effective mentoring and coaching to new nurses to ensure that they are competent and confident in their role. New nurses may feel overwhelmed and unsure about how to provide the best care for the patients, especially when they have multiple comorbidities and complex cases. Providing a comprehensive orientation to the unit's policies and procedures and reviewing the patients' care plans together can help the new nurses understand their roles, the expectations of the unit, and the patients' individualized needs. Choices *A* and *B* may not provide sufficient guidance and support. Choice *D* may alleviate the workload, but it does not address the underlying issue of the new nurses' need for mentorship and coaching.

136. C: Reflective practice involves critically examining one's own actions and thought processes to identify areas for improvement and growth. By reviewing their own actions and thought processes, the nurse can identify any biases

330

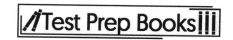

or assumptions that may be impacting their care of the patient. By identifying these factors, the nurse can work to address them and provide more effective care to the patient. Choice A may be helpful for reducing stress, but it does not address the underlying issue of the nurse's frustrations and lack of progress in the patient's care. Choice B can be helpful for getting input and support, but it does not necessarily involve reflective practice. Choice D is not reflective practice and does not address the underlying issues in the patient's care.

137. D: In an emergency situation, the nurse's first priority is to ensure that the patient receives timely and appropriate care. Activating the emergency response system can help ensure that the patient receives the necessary interventions and treatment quickly and effectively. Choices A, B, and C may be necessary, but they are not the nurse's first priority during an emergency situation.

138. C: Experiential learning theory suggests that people learn best through hands-on experiences and reflection on those experiences. By providing the new nurse with opportunities to practice time management and prioritization skills in a safe and supportive environment, and then reflecting on those experiences with the nurse educator, the new nurse will develop their skills and gain confidence in their abilities. Choice A is more focused on the way that information is processed and stored in the brain and is less relevant to coaching and mentoring of clinical skills. Choice B focuses on the role of social interactions in learning, and while this may be relevant in some contexts, it is not the most appropriate theory for this scenario. Choice D is more focused on helping individuals to change their beliefs and assumptions about the world and is less relevant to coaching and mentoring of clinical skills.

139. A: It is important for nurses to feel empowered to advocate for their patients and to participate fully in the interdisciplinary care team. Assigning a complex patient case to a nurse who is struggling with confidence and assertiveness can provide them with an opportunity to practice these skills in a safe and supportive environment while also demonstrating their competence and expertise to other members of the healthcare team. While Choice B may be helpful, it is not as effective as giving the nurse hands-on experience in a real-world situation. Choice C may not directly address the nurse's confidence and assertiveness in communicating with other team members. Choice D may be seen as coercive, can create a negative work environment, and may not be effective in promoting true empowerment.

140. C: It is important for preceptors to provide individualized support and feedback to new graduate nurses during the orientation process. This can include frequent check-ins to assess their progress, providing feedback, and addressing any concerns or questions they may have. By providing this support, the preceptor can help to ensure a successful orientation experience and set the new graduate nurse up for success in their role as a nurse. While Choice A may be helpful, it is not as effective as providing individualized support and feedback to the new graduate nurse. Choice B may not provide the new graduate nurse with the opportunity to develop their own skills and confidence. Choice D is neither realistic nor appropriate and could be overwhelming and detrimental to their orientation experience.

141. C: It is important for nurses who want to further their education and career to take advantage of career development resources such as hospital-based continuing education programs. These programs can provide the nurse with the education and training they need to advance their career while also meeting continuing education requirements. Additionally, these programs may be tailored to the specific needs of the nurse and the hospital, making them an effective and valuable resource for career development. Choice A may not provide the nurse with the specific education and training they need to further their career. Choice B may not be as effective as a structured program that is tailored to the needs of the nurse and the hospital. Choice D may be helpful for building connections and learning about new developments in the field but may not provide the specific education and training the nurse needs to further their career.

142. C: Participating in a professional organization as a nurse can be an excellent way to stay current with industry trends and connect with other professionals. These connections can provide valuable learning opportunities, foster

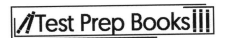

mentorship relationships, and open doors to new career opportunities. By participating in professional organizations, nurses can develop the professional behaviors necessary to become effective leaders and advance their careers. Choices *A*, *B*, and *D* are not the primary benefits of participating in a professional organization.

143. B: Observing the nurse's clinical practice and documenting any deviations from best practices is an appropriate method for conducting a peer review of a nurse's clinical practice. Choice *A* may not provide a complete picture of the nurse's clinical practices and may not capture any deviations from best practices. Choice *C* may provide valuable information but should be used in conjunction with observing the nurse's practice to ensure a comprehensive evaluation. Choice *D* does not provide information about the nurse's current clinical practice and performance.

144. A: The Joint Commission accreditation standards require healthcare organizations to implement infection control practices, including hand hygiene, to prevent the spread of infections in healthcare settings. Choice *B* is related to workplace safety and does not specifically address hand hygiene. Choice *C* is related to protecting the privacy and security of patients' health information and also does not apply to hand hygiene. While Choice *D* is related to the scope and standards of nursing practice and hand hygiene is a fundamental aspect of nursing practice, it is not the specific standard violated in this scenario.

145. B: Having an effective organizational structure lays the foundation for strong communication and coordination amongst the healthcare team. By establishing clear lines of communication and defining roles and responsibilities, the nursing team can collaborate to provide high-quality care to the patient. Without an effective organizational structure, the nursing staff may struggle to work together, leading to delays in treatment, confusion, and errors in patient care. Choices *A*, *C*, and *D* do not directly address the importance of organizational structure in this scenario.

146. B: Shared decision making involves the patient, family members, and healthcare providers collaborating together to make treatment decisions that are based on the patient's preferences, values, and concerns. As the nurse, it is important to facilitate this process by ensuring that the patient's voice is heard and that their preferences and concerns are taken into account. Advocating for the patient's best interests and preferences is essential to ensuring that the patient feels empowered to participate in the decision-making process and that the decision ultimately reflects their values and priorities. Choices *A*, *C*, and *D* do not fully capture the collaborative nature of shared decision making, as they are solely focused on providing the patient and family with pertinent information. While this is an important part of shared decision making, the nurse must also engage the patient in a conversation about their values, preferences, and concerns.

147. C: Nursing philosophy is based on a set of core values and beliefs that guide the practice of nursing. One of the core values of nursing is respect for patient autonomy, which includes respecting the patient's beliefs and values, even if they conflict with the nurse's own personal beliefs. In this scenario, it is important for the nurse to approach the situation with an open mind and to avoid judging the patient or their family members. By maintaining a non-judgmental attitude and respecting the patient's beliefs, the nurse can build trust and foster a therapeutic relationship with the patient, which can ultimately lead to better outcomes. Choice *A* is not appropriate in this scenario and goes against the core values of nursing philosophy. Choices *B* and *D* are important aspects of nursing philosophy, but they are not the most important to consider in this scenario.

148. A: Team nursing is a patient-centered approach that involves a group of healthcare providers working collaboratively to plan and implement patient care. This approach can be especially helpful when caring for patients with complex medical histories and challenging behaviors. Choices *B*, *C*, and *D* may not be the most efficient approaches for a patient with a history of substance abuse and aggressive behavior who may require the expertise and collaboration of multiple healthcare providers.

149. B: The ADKAR model is a change management framework that includes five stages: Awareness, Desire, Knowledge, Ability, and Reinforcement. The model suggests that in order for change to be successful, individuals must progress through each of these stages in order. In this scenario, the nurse is expressing frustration with having

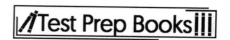

to learn a new system, indicating that they may not have a strong desire to change. In order to move forward with the implementation of the new EMR system, the nurse will need to progress through the remaining stages of the ADKAR model, including gaining knowledge about the new system, developing the ability to use it, and receiving reinforcement and support to sustain the change. Choice A is incorrect because the nurse is already aware that the organization is implementing a new EMR system. Choice C is incorrect because the nurse has not yet completed the training on the new EMR system, indicating that they may not have the necessary knowledge to use the new system. Choice D is incorrect because the nurse has not yet gained the ability to use the new EMR system, as they have not yet completed the necessary training.

150. C: While all of the answer choices can contribute to high nursing turnover rates, Choice C is the only answer choice with an appropriate and effective solution. Poor work-life balance is a common issue that can be alleviated through the implementation of work-life balance programs. These programs may include flexible scheduling options, on-site childcare, and wellness programs, which can help reduce stress and burnout among nursing staff. The solution in Choice A is incorrect because offering overtime opportunities to existing staff may exacerbate the issue and lead to further burnout. The solution in Choice B may not address the root causes of turnover. The solution in Choice D may not be enough to retain nurses if the underlying issues are not addressed.

Practice Test #2

1. The senior nurse of a unit has taken on an informal leadership role by functioning as a resource to meet the needs of the team. Leading by example, the nurse focuses on values and ethics, while continuously using foresight and empathy to advance the team. Which leadership style is this nurse displaying in their role?
   a. Servant
   b. Bureaucratic
   c. Laissez-faire
   d. Transactional

2. The nurse is caring for a 26-year-old female patient with abnormal uterine bleeding. Which of the following tests does the nurse anticipate will be obtained first?
   a. Pap smear
   b. Uterine biopsy
   c. Pelvic ultrasonography
   d. Pregnancy test

3. Which communication technique hinders the discussion between the nurse and the patient?
   a. Empathetic engagement
   b. Open-ended questions
   c. Nurse-focused answers
   d. Restating

4. The nurse is caring for a patient with diabetic ketoacidosis. Which of the following statements is consistent with the cause of this disorder?
   a. This condition results from having excess insulin in the body.
   b. Poor management of diabetes can cause this disorder.
   c. Reduced glucose ingestion can lead to this disorder.
   d. Taking too much oral anti-diabetic medication can cause this disorder.

5. Which action should the nurse include in the evaluation stage of the nursing process?
   a. Assess patient separate from views of goals
   b. Revise plan as needed
   c. Avoid modifying goals
   d. Maintain locus of control

6. Which symptom clinically supports the nurse's review of laboratory values suspecting uremic syndrome post systemic infection?
   a. Constipation
   b. Bloody diarrhea
   c. Low body temperature
   d. Increased urination

7. Which action should the medical-surgical nurse omit from the treatment plan for a patient struggling with hemorrhoids?
   a. Witch hazel
   b. Hydrocortisone cream
   c. Stool softeners
   d. Low fiber diet

8. Which of the OARS communication tools can potentially enhance the patient's self-efficacy?
   a. "Tell me more about that experience."
   b. "Are you saying that …?"
   c. "I understand your concerns."
   d. "Is there anything else that you would like to say?"

9. The nurse is caring for the 25-year-old male patient with an acute spinal cord injury at the C3 to C4 level. Which of the following manifestations is consistent with this injury?
   a. Vital capacity 45 percent of normal, hemoglobin 10.4 g/dL, heart rate 96 beats per minute
   b. Loss of somatic and reflex function, BP 160/90, effective cough effort
   c. Coarse and fine crackles bilaterally, heart rate 56 beats per minute, core temperature 96.7°F
   d. BP 104/60, urinary output 18 mL over the last 60 minutes, heart rate 120 beats per minute

10. A patient with iron deficiency anemia is unsure which foods to consume to support an improvement in health status. Which food option should the nurse explain would provide the least support for this condition?
    a. Beans
    b. Spinach
    c. Cheese
    d. Raisins

11. Which of the following interventions delegated by the licensed practical nurse (LPN) to the unlicensed assistive personnel (UAP) alerts the registered nurse (RN) to provide education on safe delegation?
    a. Removal of compression stockings
    b. Transfer of wheelchair-bound patient using device
    c. Application of over-the-counter numbing cream
    d. Documentation of vital signs

12. Which of the following manifestations is the nurse likely to assess in the patient with diabetic ketoacidosis?
    a. Alkalotic pH
    b. Ketones in the blood
    c. Fluid volume overload
    d. Hypoglycemia

13. During the nursing assessment, which data concerns the nurse regarding the patient's understanding of medication storage?
    a. Humira® stored in refrigerator
    b. Amoxicillin, reconstituted, stored on the bedroom dresser
    c. Furosemide stored in the hallway closet
    d. Insulin, unopened, stored in the bedroom closet

14. The nurse notices the site around the patient's peripheral IV has become puffy, cold, and tight. She suspects what has occurred?
    a. Infection
    b. IV infiltration
    c. Allergic reaction
    d. Nothing, this is a normal assessment of peripheral IV

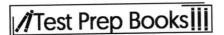

15. The nurse is providing discharge teaching for a patient recently diagnosed with Crohn's disease. Which of the following patient statements indicates the need for additional instruction?
   a. "I understand that once I get through this surgery, my disease will be cured."
   b. "I know that I have a risk for the development of arthritis."
   c. "I know that vitamin B-12 is important for me."
   d. "I will tell my doc if my pain localizes to the right lower quadrant of my abdomen."

16. When taking a history from a patient with unstable angina, the nurse would expect the patient to report which of the following findings?
   a. "My chest pain goes away when I rest."
   b. "I sometimes experience chest pain at rest."
   c. "Nitroglycerine always relieves my chest pain."
   d. "The chest pain only occurs when I walk too fast."

17. A 60-year-old male patient with a history of alcohol abuse and IV drug abuse presents with encephalopathy, ascites, and jaundice. Which organ of the abdomen does the nurse suspect is in failure?
   a. Kidney
   b. Liver
   c. Stomach
   d. Spleen

18. The medical-surgical nurse is preparing a patient's treatment plan prior to surgery. How many hours before surgery should the heparin drip be discontinued?
   a. 2 hours
   b. 6 hours
   c. 24 hours
   d. 48 hours

19. The medical-surgical nurse is preparing a patient's treatment plan prior to a colonoscopy. How many hours prior to the procedure should the patient be placed on total npo?
   a. 2 hours
   b. 6 hours
   c. 8 hours
   d. 12 hours

20. A nurse has been assigned to care for a patient who has a history of aggressive behavior and is known for being difficult to manage. The patient is currently experiencing significant pain and is demanding immediate attention. As the nurse approaches the patient to assess their condition, the patient becomes increasingly agitated and begins to verbally abuse the nurse, using profanity and threatening physical harm. Despite the nurse's attempts to de-escalate the situation, the patient continues to escalate and becomes physically aggressive. What is the best course of action for the nurse to take in this scenario to promote resiliency and well-being?
   a. Continuing to engage with the patient, using active listening and empathy to try and calm them down
   b. Responding to the patient's aggression with force, in order to establish control and prevent further escalation
   c. Retreating from the situation and seeking support from a colleague or supervisor
   d. Immediately calling for assistance from other staff members to help manage the patient

21. A medical-surgical nurse is caring for a female patient receiving chemotherapy. When the patient develops a low neutrophil level, which of the following instructions is a priority for the nurse to give the patient?
   a. Use a safety razor
   b. Take iron supplements
   c. Avoid crowds
   d. Drink plenty of fluids

22. The nurse is caring for a patient with heart failure following a myocardial infarction and is assessing the cardiac output. Which of the following statements describes the parameter being measured?
   a. Cardiac output is the vascular resistance in the pulmonary circulation.
   b. Cardiac output is the amount of ventricular stretch at the end of diastole.
   c. Cardiac output is the resistance the heart needs to overcome to pump blood to the body.
   d. Cardiac output is the volume of blood pumped by the heart in one minute.

23. What is the purpose of conducting an interdisciplinary 5 Whys Analysis?
   a. To report the near miss to the correct agency
   b. To identify the person at fault for an issue
   c. To understand the root cause of an incident
   d. To develop a chain of command for the elevation of a concern

24. What patient condition would require the medical-surgical nurse to wear a surgical mask?
   a. Severe acute respiratory syndrome
   b. Influenza B virus
   c. Asthma
   d. Chronic obstructive pulmonary disease

25. A 44-year-old male patient complains of chest pain and shortness of breath. Examination by the nurse reveals distended neck veins and muffled heart sounds. The patient's blood pressure is 80/55. The nurse should suspect which of the following?
   a. Cardiac tamponade
   b. Abdominal aortic aneurysm (AAA)
   c. Cardiopulmonary arrest
   d. Cardiogenic shock

26. Which member of the interdisciplinary team should the nurse consult with regarding patient dressing and hygiene aids?
   a. Physical therapist
   b. Social worker
   c. Occupational therapist
   d. Case manager

27. A 72-year-old patient was administered an IV push of furosemide indicated to reduce the edema secondary to renal impairment. Which finding post furosemide administration is an emergent concern for the medical-surgical nurse?
   a. Hypotension
   b. Pruritis
   c. Headache
   d. Agranulocytosis

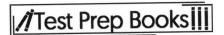

28. Which of the following drugs is often used for treatment of acute seizure activity?
   a. Memantine HCl
   b. Phenytoin
   c. Pregabalin
   d. Rifaximin

29. Which food item should the nurse encourage a patient to avoid because it would pose the greatest risk for someone with acquired immunodeficiency syndrome (AIDS)?
   a. Bok choy
   b. Rice
   c. Wheat crackers
   d. Blue cheese

30. Which intervention should the nurse include in a treatment plan for a patient with early dumping syndrome?
   a. Drink more fluids with meals
   b. Consume two larger meals per day
   c. Maintain low Fowler's position for 30 minutes post meals
   d. Decrease fiber intake

31. What serological marker indicates, with high specificity, that cardiac muscle tissue has been damaged and cell contents are being released into the bloodstream?
   a. Creatinine
   b. BUN
   c. Creatine kinase
   d. Troponin

32. Which intervention should the medical-surgical nurse avoid in the plan of care for a patient with acute Deep Vein Thrombosis (DVT)?
   a. Administer enoxaparin sodium subcutaneously
   b. Apply spontaneous compression devices
   c. Evaluate aPTT levels
   d. Provide continuous cardiac monitoring

33. While working with a patient with a poor swallowing reflex secondary to a neurological condition, the medical-surgical nurse is assessing the patient's ability to safely consume their breakfast. Which food item on the tray does the nurse recognize conflicts with this meal plan and should be removed?
   a. Beets
   b. Scrambled eggs
   c. Vanilla pudding
   d. Mashed potatoes

34. The nurse is caring for a patient with a fracture of the eighth rib on the right side of the chest. The nurse should assess the patient for possible injury to which underlying body structure?
   a. Bronchus
   b. Trachea
   c. Spleen
   d. Liver

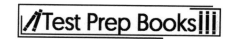

35. Which intervention should the medical-surgical nurse include in the plan of care for a patient with Alzheimer's disease?
    a. Limit physical activity
    b. Provide caprylidene medical food
    c. Perform activities of daily living in the evening
    d. Administer diphenhydramine for sleep

36. What statement made by the patient verbalizes understanding the education regarding safety precautions to take at home after being discharged from the hospital on oxygen for respiratory management?
    a. "I should switch from aerosol deodorant to a stick."
    b. "My cigarettes are safe to smoke as long as I smoke one at a time."
    c. "I must use an oven mitt while cooking on my gas stove."
    d. "I should switch from electric candles to flame-based ones."

37. A patient who is silently aspirating may exhibit which of the following signs and symptoms?
    a. Flat, red rash on the thoracic region
    b. Constant clearing of the throat
    c. Swollen lymph nodes on the neck
    d. Trouble remembering person, place, and time

38. Which action witnessed by the medical-surgical nurse prompts immediate education while working with an unlicensed assistive personnel (UAP)?
    a. The UAP took a blood sugar finger-stick reading.
    b. The UAP wore gloves while providing a bed bath.
    c. The UAP used sanitizer to clean hands after caring for a patient with *Clostridium difficile*.
    d. The UAP placed the connected Foley catheter bag below the patient's waist.

39. The nurse is caring for a patient with Cushing's disease. The nurse understands that dysfunction of which of the following glands causes this disorder?
    a. Thyroid gland
    b. Adrenal gland
    c. Pancreas
    d. Parathyroid gland

40. Which statement made by a woman with gestational diabetes indicates to the nurse that more teaching is needed?
    a. "I need to monitor my weight."
    b. "I need to watch what I eat."
    c. "I need to stay off my feet as much as possible."
    d. "I need to see my obstetrician regularly."

41. While facilitating nursing student education, which condition does the medical-surgical nurse discuss when describing post-renal causes of acute renal failure?
    a. Obstruction
    b. Rhabdomyolysis
    c. Acute pyelonephritis
    d. Systemic vasodilation

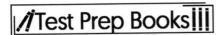

42. The nurse is caring for an 82-year-old man with acute bronchitis. In evaluating the effectiveness of therapy with a beta-2 agonist, the nurse would expect which assessment finding?
    a. Reduced or absent cough
    b. Reduced fever
    c. Improved breath sounds
    d. Decreased pain

43. A 50-year-old male presents with a cough producing rust-colored sputum, a fever (102° F), and shortness of breath. A complete blood count (CBC) reveals an elevated white blood cell count with predominant neutrophils. A chest x-ray reveals consolidation of the left, lower lobe of the lung. Blood cultures reveal gram-positive diplococci. What is the most likely cause of this patient's pneumonia?
    a. *Haemophilus influenzae*
    b. *Moraxella catarrhalis*
    c. *Streptococcus pneumoniae*
    d. *Staphylococcus aureus*

44. A 68-year-old woman with a history of gallstones is in the same-day surgery unit today for a cholecystectomy. This procedure will likely be performed using which technique that involves small incisions and minimal invasion?
    a. Laparoscopic
    b. Endoscopic
    c. Bronchoscopic
    d. Laparotomy

45. The nurse is caring for a 58-year-old man who has an active upper gastrointestinal bleed. The nurse notes a 10-millimeter drop in diastolic blood pressure when the man stands to urinate. The nurse estimates that which of the following volumes of blood loss is associated with this drop in diastolic blood pressure?
    a. 250 milliliters
    b. 500 milliliters
    c. 750 milliliters
    d. 1,000 milliliters

46. The medical-surgical nurse is reviewing laboratory results to assess the patient's ability to clot before surgery. Which prothrombin time test (PTT) result aligns with a normal range?
    a. 2 seconds
    b. 12 seconds
    c. 22 seconds
    d. 32 seconds

47. The medical-surgical nurse preceptor is educating the new nurse regarding safe antimuscarinic administration. Which patient is unable to receive antimuscarinic medications due to contraindication with their diagnosis?
    a. Patient with a peptic ulcer
    b. Patient with urinary incontinence
    c. Patient with angle-closure glaucoma
    d. Patient with reflux esophagitis

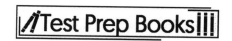

48. A 25-year-old male is transferred to the medical-surgical unit from the emergency department (ED) after blunt chest trauma. On initial evaluation, he had absent breath sounds over the right lung and tracheal deviation to the left. A chest x-ray revealed mediastinal shift to the left and depression of the right hemidiaphragm. What is the most likely diagnosis?
    a. Secondary spontaneous pneumothorax
    b. Bronchiolitis
    c. Tension pneumothorax
    d. Acute respiratory distress syndrome (ARDS)

49. The nurse is providing discharge instructions to a patient with Barrett's esophagus. Which statement by the patient indicates that more teaching is needed?
    a. "I am not at an increased risk for cancer."
    b. "I will need to take my corticosteroids, as prescribed."
    c. "I need to look at my lifestyle and make some changes."
    d. "I should report any heartburn or difficulty swallowing to my doctor."

50. Which of the following manifestations is considered to be a late sign of increased ICP?
    a. Mental confusion related to time
    b. Blurred vision
    c. BP of 170/40
    d. HR of 94 bpm

51. After taking a nurse-to-nurse report in the beginning of their evening shift, the medical-surgical nurse is reviewing laboratory results and surgical notes regarding their patient's emergency procedure from this afternoon. Which diagnosis correlates with an infection of the tissue that lines the inner abdominal wall?
    a. Iritis
    b. Dermatitis
    c. Cystitis
    d. Peritonitis

52. Which manifestation would the nurse expect to find in a patient with severe glycogenosis?
    a. Liver failure
    b. Kidney failure
    c. Respiratory failure
    d. Congestive heart failure

53. The nurse is caring for a patient with diabetes who is sweating and confused. Using a handheld blood glucose monitoring device, the nurse determines that the patient's capillary blood glucose level is 55 milligrams per deciliter. Which of the following intervention would the nurse NOT perform?
    a. Administer oral glucose
    b. Administer subcutaneous insulin
    c. Administer IV dextrose
    d. Administer parenteral glucagon

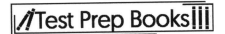

54. The nurse is caring for a patient with endoscopic evidence of esophageal varices. Which of the following statements correctly identifies the interventions associated with primary prevention of hemorrhage for this condition?
   a. Sclerotherapy ablation of the esophageal arteries
   b. Vasopressors to maintain the hepatic venous pressure gradient above 20 mmHG
   c. Transjugular intrahepatic portosystemic shunt implantation
   d. Endoscopic band ligation

55. The nurse is completing a shift assessment of a patient who had an unwitnessed fall yesterday afternoon in his hospital room. The nurse notices changes in her assessment since yesterday. Which of the following signs and symptoms does NOT directly support a diagnosis of increased intracranial pressure?
   a. Nausea
   b. Vomiting
   c. Headache
   d. Blurred vision

56. The nurse would expect a patient with urinary retention to report having experienced which of the following types of urinary incontinence?
   a. Stress incontinence
   b. Urge incontinence
   c. Overflow incontinence
   d. Functional incontinence

57. During nurse-to-nurse shift report, the oncoming medical-surgical nurse learns that the patient has a history of aggressive behavior. What action should the nurse prioritize in this patient's plan of care?
   a. Proactive seclusion
   b. Administer sedative medication
   c. Request that a social worker meets with the patient before the nurse
   d. Establish patient trust

58. The nurse is caring for a 66-year-old male patient with a history of warfarin therapy who presents with complaints of decreased sensation of the right lower and upper limbs, visual alterations, right hemiparesis, blurred vision, ataxia, nystagmus, and aphasia. The nurse expects to administer which of the following medications?
   a. Mannitol and vitamin K
   b. Warfarin and labetalol
   c. Alteplase and nitroprusside
   d. ASA and enalapril

59. The medical-surgical nurse is describing their professional role and function as defined by state law to their interdisciplinary peer. What term describes this set of guidelines?
   a. Nursing Process
   b. Scope of Practice
   c. Code of Ethics
   d. Nursing Care Plan

60. Which desired outcome is most appropriate for a patient with Marfan syndrome?
   a. Patient maintained adequate tissue perfusion.
   b. Patient remained free from self-harm.
   c. Patient maintained optimal gas exchange.
   d. Patient remained free from signs of infection.

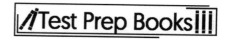

61. The 36-year-old patient's current orders include levothyroxine 88 µg PO daily. Which assessment by the nurse prompts patient education regarding levothyroxine administration?
    a. The patient reports that they take their medication in the afternoon, 30 minutes after consuming lunch.
    b. The patient reports that they take their medication at night, at least four hours after their last meal.
    c. The patient reports that they take their medication in the morning, 30 minutes before their first meal.
    d. The patient reports that they take their medication in the morning, 2 hours before consuming their first meal.

62. The medical-surgical nurse is evaluating the patient's progress related to pain reduction secondary to appendicitis. Which abdominal quadrant does the nurse ask the patient to rate their pain in?
    a. Right lower quadrant (RLQ)
    b. Left lower quadrant (LLQ)
    c. Right upper quadrant (RUQ)
    d. Left upper quadrant (LUQ)

63. During a focused assessment of the abdomen, which examination technique should the medical-surgical nurse perform second?
    a. Percussion
    b. Palpation
    c. Auscultation
    d. Inspection

64. The medical-surgical nurse discovers a change in their 81-year-old patient's level of consciousness and notes increased confusion, agitation, and poor motor skills. Which diagnosis does the nurse suspect may be responsible for these findings and warrants further examination?
    a. Urinary tract infection
    b. Diverticulitis
    c. Rectal polyps
    d. Benign prostatic hypertrophy

65. After attempting to support and deescalate an aggressive patient with a comorbid diagnosis of schizophrenia, the medical-surgical nurse calls the provider and discusses the situation using the SBAR technique. How should the nurse communicate their report?
    a. "I think we should provide the patient a sedative."
    b. "Should we call a behavioral code?"
    c. "Please share what you already know of this patient's background."
    d. "How should we proceed with the patient's care?"

66. Which type of angina does the medical-surgical nurse attribute the patient's chest pain from coronary vasospasms to?
    a. Chronic stable angina
    b. Unstable angina
    c. Prinzmetal angina
    d. Variant angina

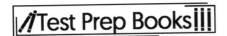

67. The nurse is preparing a teaching plan for a patient with diabetes. Which of the following teaching points would the nurse include when teaching about the causes of hyperglycemia?
   a. Hyperglycemia may be caused by administering too much insulin.
   b. Skipping a meal can cause hyperglycemia.
   c. Taking too much anti-diabetic medication can cause hyperglycemia.
   d. Illness can lead to the development of hyperglycemia.

68. The nurse is assessing a 22-year-old patient with asthma. Which manifestation would alert the nurse of impending respiratory failure?
   a. Tachycardia
   b. Cyanosis
   c. No audible wheezes
   d. Hypoxemia

69. Which of the following is a contraindication for thrombolytic therapy?
   a. Current anticoagulant therapy
   b. Over age seventy-five
   c. Severe hepatic disease
   d. INR of 3.5

70. After delivering unexpected news, the nurse states, "Don't worry, everyone feels that way." Which block to communication is the nurse committing during this engagement?
   a. Judging
   b. Falsely reassuring
   c. Defending
   d. Belittling

71. Which precautions should the medical-surgical nurse engage in while caring for a patient with pertussis?
   a. Standard
   b. Contact
   c. Droplet
   d. Airborne

72. The nurse is developing a teaching plan for a patient newly diagnosed with myasthenia gravis. To prevent relapses, which of the following instructions would NOT be included in the teaching plan?
   a. Stay away from people who are sick.
   b. Take hot baths when feeling stressed.
   c. Consider a yoga class to reduce stress.
   d. Stay in air conditioning when the weather is hot.

73. When must the discharge planning process start for each patient?
   a. The day before discharge is scheduled to occur
   b. The morning of the planned discharge
   c. After the discharge order has been written
   d. As soon as admission begins

344

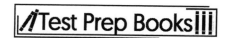
74. Which form of consent for treatment does the patient give by presenting for care and voluntarily moving forward with admission?
    a. Explicit
    b. Implied
    c. Expressed
    d. Surrogate

75. The outgoing nurse is providing a report to the oncoming nurse regarding a patient fall during the shift. What information collected using the PQRST method of pain assessment should the nurse include in their report of a 42-year-old patient with vertigo who fell in the shower?
    a. Pain, Quadrant, Radiate, Sensation, Timing
    b. Provoke, Quality, Region, Severity, Timing
    c. Pain, Quality, Radiate, Severity, Task
    d. Provoke, Quadrant, Region, Sensation, Tension

76. Which statement by a patient going home on warfarin (Coumadin) for treatment of a pulmonary embolism alerts the nurse that more teaching is needed?
    a. "I will take this medication orally."
    b. "Any bleeding or bruising needs to be reported to my doctor right away."
    c. "I will seek medical attention if I develop chest pain or shortness of breath."
    d. "Blood monitoring is not needed."

77. The medical-surgical nurse is reviewing dietary orders prior to breakfast. Which diet should be implemented for a patient with gout?
    a. Low-purine
    b. High-fructose
    c. Low-caffeine
    d. High-fat

78. Which of the following is/are true regarding advance directives?
    a. They are an expression of the patient's preferences.
    b. They are based on a person's values and beliefs.
    c. They include identification of a surrogate.
    d. All of the above

79. The medical-surgical nurse becomes concerned after witnessing the provider use language that negatively impacts a patient's ability to make their own decision regarding their care without provider influence. Which ethical principle may the provider be violating at this time?
    a. Nonmaleficence
    b. Veracity
    c. Beneficence
    d. Autonomy

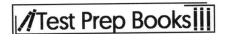

80. The nurse is caring for a 30-year-old male patient with a ventriculoperitoneal shunt who is being assessed for shunt failure. The shunt was inserted four years ago when the patient developed hydrocephalus after a severe closed-head injury, and the patient has exhibited satisfactory control of ICP until twelve hours ago, when the patient complained of a headache, nausea, and tiredness. The patient's vital signs are BP 130/70, HR 82, RR 24, T 98.6°F, PaO_2 97 percent. Which of the following complications is most likely responsible for the patient's condition?
   a. Choroid ingrowth of the proximal catheter
   b. Migration of the distal catheter to an area that impedes absorption of the CSF
   c. Disconnection of the distal reservoir from the distal catheter tip
   d. Infection of the proximal catheter

81. While using the SBAR method of communication, which term aligns with the patient's laboratory findings?
   a. Situation
   b. Background
   c. Assessment
   d. Recommendations

82. The medical-surgical nurse is establishing patient-centered goals in the nursing care plan. What do these measurable targets reflect?
   a. Greatest improvement in individual health outcome
   b. Interest in specific nursing interventions
   c. Aims for care designated by the provider
   d. Normalized behavior for specified illness

83. Which imbalance does the nurse expect to observe as a complication of total parenteral nutrition (TPN)?
   a. Metabolic acidosis
   b. Respiratory acidosis
   c. Metabolic alkalosis
   d. Respiratory alkalosis

84. While caring for a 52-year-old patient with Broca's aphasia, which action should the medical-surgical nurse implement during verbal communication?
   a. Request assistance from a linguistic interpreter
   b. Speak loudly
   c. Use typical verbal expression, without significant change
   d. Provide only short, simple sentences of 3-4 words

85. The medical-surgical nurse ensures the patient is fully supported to make their own decisions, without coercion, regarding their care. What ethical principle guides this practice?
   a. Autonomy
   b. Utility
   c. Fidelity
   d. Conflict of interest

86. During medication reconciliation, the medical-surgical nurse notes that a patient with dementia is struggling to recall how many times per day their gabapentin is ordered for. Which action should the medical-surgical nurse take next to best support a thorough history collection of patient data?
   a. Obtain a release of information to contact the outpatient pharmacy.
   b. Wait to complete the medication reconciliation until the patient's son arrives.
   c. Delegate completion of the medication reconciliation to the patient's physician.
   d. Check the discharge paperwork from last admission and record the finding.

346

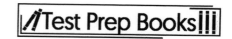

87. While receiving nurse-to-nurse report from the emergency department on a pending transfer, the medical-surgical nurse learns that an incoming 43-year-old patient is struggling with delusional thinking. What understanding is necessary to ensure effective communication is used upon receiving this patient?
    a. The patient experiences insistent false beliefs despite invalidating evidence.
    b. The patient experiences perceptions irrelevant to actual external stimuli.
    c. The patient experiences acute, short-lasting confusion and disorientation.
    d. The patient experiences a gradual impairment in cognitive functioning.

88. Which action does the medical-surgical nurse engage in during the assessment phase of the nursing process?
    a. Perform nursing intervention
    b. Obtain a nursing health history
    c. Develop nursing care plan
    d. Establish physical and psychosocial outcomes

89. In planning care for a patient with acute glomerulonephritis, what should be the main goal for treatment?
    a. Maintain fluid balance
    b. Raise blood pressure
    c. Elevate serum potassium levels
    d. Increase consumption of protein

90. What risk does high blood pressure pose in the postoperative period following an endarterectomy?
    a. Bleeding
    b. Infection
    c. Pulmonary edema
    d. Stroke

91. Mr. Jones is scheduled for an abdominal aortic aneurysm repair. Which surgical position does the nurse anticipate for Mr. Jones?
    a. Lithotomy
    b. Left lateral
    c. Supine
    d. Kraske

92. The surgical time out is documented by which member of the surgical team?
    a. Perioperative nurse
    b. Anesthesiologist
    c. Surgeon
    d. Surgical technologist

93. What solutions should be used to keep instruments free of bioburdens?
    a. Saline
    b. Sterile water
    c. Tap water
    d. Lactated Ringer's solution

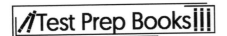

94. What information is usually discussed during a pre-operative interview?
    a. What the patient is most nervous about and the lifestyle behaviors that contributed to the operation
    b. The patient's demographic information, medical history, review of the procedure, pre-operation requirements, discharge and post-operative requirements, and any last-minute questions the patient might have
    c. Detailed discussions of case studies relating to the procedure and the different outcomes that can result in order to prepare the patient for all outcomes
    d. The patient's financial status, the type of insurance coverage they carry, the patient's financial responsibility at check-in and discharge, and where to get financial assistance if needed

95. If dopamine does not do an adequate job of maintaining blood pressure in a patient experiencing cardiogenic shock, which potent vasoconstrictor will be considered to raise the blood pressure?
    a. Dobutamine
    b. Norepinephrine
    c. Milrinone
    d. Nitroglycerin

96. The nurse is working with a patient before a scheduled surgical procedure and administers the preoperative sedative medication ordered in the patient's chart. After administering the medication, the nurse notices that the patient has not signed the surgical consent form. What should the nurse do first?
    a. Call the nursing supervisor
    b. Page the surgeon
    c. Ask the health care proxy to sign for consent
    d. Initiate a code

97. The medical-surgical nurse is preparing written patient education for a patient with chronic otitis media. Which surgical treatment does the nurse print patient education on to include in their teaching?
    a. Tympanoplasty
    b. Septoplasty
    c. Rhinoplasty
    d. Myringoplasty

98. Which of the following is a concern that a nurse would escalate to the surgeon?
    a. Normal laboratory values
    b. Patient not understanding postoperative care needs
    c. Pain management plan and schedule
    d. Family care plan for patient after discharge

99. During a level of consciousness assessment, the nurse finds no articulated verbal response with limited moaning, accompanied by arousal only after vigorous stimulation. How should the nurse document these findings?
    a. "The patient is lethargic."
    b. "The patient is obtunded."
    c. "The patient is stuporous."
    d. "The patient is comatose."

100. What is one benefit of electronic health records?
    a. They can be accessed across multiple medical facilities.
    b. They can be accessed internationally, as many countries have adopted the same system.
    c. They require minimal training to adopt.
    d. They can be easily accessed in areas with limited internet service, such as rural areas.

101. The Five Rights of Delegation include all of the following EXCEPT:
  a. Person
  b. Task
  c. Narrative
  d. Direction

102. The nurse notices a decreased level of consciousness in a patient. During the assessment, the nurse observes mottled extremities and distant heart sounds. The nurse demonstrates an understanding of the physician's diagnosis of cardiogenic shock by anticipating which of the following?
  a. Arterial blood gas (ABG)
  b. Chest x-ray
  c. Angiogram
  d. Doppler study of the lower extremities

103. The emergency care of the patient with temporal arteritis is complex due to the wide range of possible complications that are associated with this condition. Which of the following complications requires immediate intervention to prevent irreversible damage?
  a. Lower extremity claudication
  b. Vertebral body fracture
  c. Early onset of blindness
  d. Infection related to immunosuppression

104. Which of the following nursing interventions is most consistent with the competencies of caring practices, advocacy, and moral agency?
  a. Developing cultural awareness of care team members
  b. Mentoring novice nurses in the use of research findings
  c. Facilitating the patient's transition from one level of care to another on the health continuum
  d. Refining educational programs for patients and families

105. The nurse is caring for a post-op patient with a history of prescription drug abuse who is having difficulty managing their pain. Which of the following actions will help the nurse manage this patient's pain appropriately?
  a. Assess pain at least twice in a 12-hour shift.
  b. Provide care in the least invasive ways possible.
  c. Refuse pain management due to history of drug abuse.
  d. Offer pain medication after patient has finished ambulating and dressing changes.

106. Which of the following communication techniques represents good therapeutic communication for the nurse to use with a patient?
  a. Asking simple yes or no questions
  b. Using silence when appropriate
  c. Using clichés to establish rapport
  d. Asking patients to explain their behavior

107. A nurse is reading a research article on new treatments for patients with COPD. In order to critically read, the nurse should actively try to determine all of the following aspects of the article EXCEPT:
  a. Thesis
  b. Process
  c. Outcomes
  d. Funding

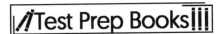
108. When creating a lesson plan to teach a new topic to a patient and their family, which of the following components would NOT help create and foster a comprehensive lesson plan?
   a. Set goals.
   b. Create open-ended objectives.
   c. Focus on one or two topics.
   d. Assess the patient's understanding.

109. A nurse is managing the care for three patients on a fully staffed unit with a certified nursing assistant (CNA). During the morning care, the nurse has to pass medications for all of their patients, complete two dressing changes, and give a bed bath to two incontinent patients. The nurse attempts to independently complete all these tasks and is unable to do so. As a result, two of their patients do not receive their morning medications on schedule. What is this consequence most likely a result of?
   a. Poor staffing ratios
   b. Disorganization
   c. Failure to delegate
   d. Inappropriate patient assignment

110. Regulatory bodies such as TJC and CMS clearly identify which need as one that must be fulfilled in order to promote optimal patient outcomes?
   a. Holistic care model
   b. Discharge planning
   c. Culturally based care
   d. Patient education

111. Public libraries and government offices are examples of which type of community resources?
   a. Local
   b. Demographical
   c. Institutional
   d. Geographical

112. A hospital located on the Florida panhandle reviews evacuation protocol at the beginning and middle of every hurricane season. What document does this hospital likely review with its staff members?
   a. Hospital flood insurance policies
   b. A published disaster plan
   c. Fire drill safety locations
   d. How to receive free ride-sharing credits to use in the event of a hurricane

113. When should adverse events that occur at the end of the nurse's shift be reported?
   a. The following day
   b. As soon as reasonably possible
   c. Only if there is litigation
   d. Only if it was a never event and in full detail in the patient's medical record

114. Which of the following is a framework in continuous quality improvement that can be used by frontline workers to test changes in the nursing environment?
   a. PDSA cycle
   b. DMAIC method
   c. Value-stream mapping
   d. Lean

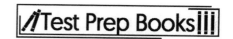

115. An English-speaking medical-surgical nurse is completing a history and physical on a newly admitted patient. How should the nurse communicate with a Spanish-speaking patient?
    a. Speak loud and slowly
    b. Use a monotone voice to avoid inflection
    c. Phone the interpreter line for assistance
    d. Request that a family member translate the discussion

116. Being under obligation to provide safe patient care refers to what legal domain?
    a. Negligence
    b. Liability
    c. Standard of care
    d. Nurse Practice Act

117. What is the purpose of the World Health Organization's (WHO's) Surgical Safety Checklist? Select the BEST answer.
    a. Increase patient safety throughout the perioperative spectrum.
    b. Reduce preoperative surgical risks.
    c. Reduce postoperative surgical risks.
    d. Replace perioperative checklists currently in place in surgical centers.

118. The nursing assistant is performing post-mortem care. While repositioning the body to place in the body bag, the body lets out a sound that sounds like a gasp. The medical-surgical nurse assures the aide that this a natural body process where air is released from the lungs after death and that death has been verified. What are some other possible characteristics a deceased body may display?

    I. Twitching of muscles
    II. Release of bowel and bladder
    III. Deep tendon reflexes
    IV. Eyes remain open

    a. All of the above
    b. Choices I, II, and III
    c. Choices II and IV
    d. Choices I, II, and IV

119. The nurse is caring for a 68-year-old patient who has been recently diagnosed with hypercholesterolemia and coronary artery disease (CAD). The patient has a family history of heart disease, and they currently smoke and live a sedentary lifestyle. Their BMI is 32, and their lipid profile shows a total cholesterol level of 240 mg/dL, LDL cholesterol level of 160 mg/dL, and HDL cholesterol level of 40 mg/dL. They are motivated to make lifestyle changes to improve their health. What is the most appropriate health promotion goal based on this patient's condition?
    a. Increasing HDL cholesterol level to >60 mg/dL
    b. Achieving a BMI of <30
    c. Quitting smoking within 3 months
    d. Reducing LDL cholesterol level to <100 mg/dL

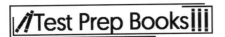
120. The nurse is caring for a 44-year-old patient that has been recently diagnosed with type 2 diabetes, and their family wants to learn more about the condition and how to manage it. Which of the following resources should the nurse recommend for this patient's family?

   a. Internet search engines
   b. Patient support groups
   c. Healthcare provider's office
   d. Social media websites

121. A 75-year-old patient who has recently been discharged from the hospital is now at home recovering. However, the patient is having difficulty managing their medications and is feeling overwhelmed. The nurse who was previously in charge of their care is now visiting the patient in their home to check in and provide support. What is the nurse's main priority in this scenario as a patient advocate?

   a. Ensuring the patient is taking their medications correctly
   b. Making sure the patient is comfortable in their home
   c. Representing the patient's needs and ensuring their voice is heard
   d. Providing information about additional resources that are available to them

122. A 50-year-old patient recently diagnosed with type 2 diabetes has been admitted for uncontrolled hyperglycemia. The patient has an insulin pump and reports to the nurse that they have been experiencing high blood sugar levels despite following the instructions given by their provider. What action should the nurse take in response to the patient's report of high blood sugar levels despite following the instructions provided for the insulin pump?

   a. Perform a blood glucose test and assessing the patient's technique for using the insulin pump
   b. Increase the insulin dose as prescribed by the healthcare provider
   c. Advise the patient to stop using the insulin pump
   d. Contact the manufacturer of the insulin pump for technical support

123. A 70-year-old patient who has been diagnosed with congestive heart failure (CHF) has been admitted to the hospital several times in the past year for CHF exacerbations. Which of the following interventions is most effective in reducing the risk of readmission for CHF patients with readmission history?

   a. Discharging the patient as soon as possible to avoid hospital-associated infections
   b. Ensuring that the patient has transportation to follow-up appointments with healthcare providers
   c. Providing the patient with written and verbal education on managing symptoms, adhering to medication regimens, and making lifestyle modifications
   d. Administering medications to the patient via IV at home

124. A 35-year-old patient who has been recently diagnosed with type 2 diabetes lives in a low-income community and has limited access to education. How does having a limited education affect this patient's ability to manage their diabetes, and what nursing intervention would be most appropriate to address this concern?

   a. Limited education can make it difficult for this patient to understand how to manage their diabetes, and providing the patient with written instructions for diabetes management is the most appropriate nursing intervention.
   b. Limited education can make it difficult for this patient to understand how to manage their diabetes, and referring the patient to a diabetes educator is the most appropriate nursing intervention.
   c. Limited education is not likely to affect this patient's ability to manage their diabetes. Prescribing medications to help control the patient's blood sugar levels is the most appropriate nursing intervention.
   d. Limited education is not likely to affect this patient's ability to manage their diabetes. Providing the patient with a list of community resources, such as food banks and transportation services, is the most appropriate nursing intervention.

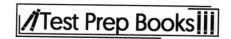

125. A 60-year-old patient who has been hospitalized for an exacerbation of heart failure has a history of hypertension and takes multiple medications, including a diuretic and an ACE inhibitor. The patient also has a history of peripheral vascular disease and diabetes and requires daily blood glucose monitoring and insulin injections. Which of the following tasks related to this patient's care can be delegated by the medical-surgical nurse to the nursing assistive personnel (NAP)?
   a. Administering the patient's medications
   b. Assessing and interpreting the patient's blood pressure and heart rate
   c. Measuring the patient's blood glucose using a glucometer
   d. Providing education to the patient about their conditions

126. A 60-year-old female patient who has been diagnosed with breast cancer and is undergoing chemotherapy is experiencing side effects such as nausea, fatigue, and hair loss. The patient has two adult children who are actively involved in providing care and emotional support. Which of the following actions best demonstrates patient and family-centered care for this patient?
   a. Providing the patient with a pamphlet about chemotherapy and its side effects and encouraging her to read it
   b. Asking the patient's children to leave the room during her physical examination to maintain patient privacy
   c. Encouraging the patient's children to participate in care, such as accompanying her to chemotherapy appointments
   d. Deciding on the patient's chemotherapy regimen without involving her or her family in the decision-making process

127. A 65-year-old patient with a history of diabetes and hypertension has been seeing their primary care physician for several years to manage their chronic conditions. Recently, the patient was diagnosed with prostate cancer and was referred to an oncologist for further management. They are concerned about how their care will be coordinated between their primary care physician and oncologist. Which of the following actions best ensures continuity of care for this patient in the management of their chronic conditions and prostate cancer?
   a. Referring the patient to a new primary care physician who specializes in both chronic conditions and cancer care
   b. Encouraging the patient to manage their conditions with the primary care physician and oncologist separately
   c. Establishing a care coordination plan between the patient's primary care physician and oncologist
   d. Encouraging the patient to manage care coordination independently

128. A new graduate nurse who just started working in a busy hospital setting has been struggling with documenting patient care effectively and efficiently. Their manager has recommended coaching to help improve their documentation skills. Which of the following coaching techniques would be most effective for the new graduate nurse?
   a. Telling the graduate nurse what to document and how to document it
   b. Providing the graduate nurse with feedback on their documentation and offering suggestions for improvement
   c. Asking the graduate nurse to read policy and procedure manuals related to documentation
   d. Assigning the graduate nurse to shadow experienced nurses to learn how to document patient care

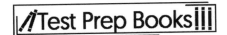

129. A 70-year-old patient has been admitted to the hospital for heart failure. The patient reports to the nurse that they have never had any heart problems in the past. However, when the nurse talks to the patient's daughter, they report that the patient has had multiple heart attacks in the past. What is the most appropriate action for the nurse to take when there are discrepancies in a patient's reported health history and information provided by family members?

    a. Documenting both the patient's reported health history and the family member's information

    b. Disregarding the patient's reported health history and only relying on the family member's information

    c. Assuming that the family member is incorrect and only relying on the patient's reported health history

    d. Ignoring the discrepancies and continuing with the patient's care plan as originally planned

130. A hospital is experiencing low employee engagement among its nursing staff. The hospital administration is exploring several strategies to improve engagement among nursing staff and, in turn, improve patient outcomes. Which of the following is an example of how low employee engagement among nursing staff can directly impact patient outcomes?

    a. Decreased patient satisfaction scores

    b. Increased adverse events

    c. Increased hospital-acquired infections

    d. Decreased patient safety scores

131. A nurse is working in a hospital where staffing levels have been significantly reduced due to budget cuts. As a result, the nurse is frequently asked to work overtime and take on additional patients, which is impacting their ability to provide safe and effective care. The nurse raises concerns with management about the unsafe working conditions, but management has not taken any action to address the issue. What is an appropriate action for the nurse to take to advocate for safe working conditions?

    a. Continuing to work overtime and taking on additional patients to meet staffing demands

    b. Refusing to work overtime or take on additional patients, even if it means facing disciplinary action

    c. Documenting the unsafe working conditions and filing a complaint with the state nursing board

    d. Discussing the issue with colleagues and encouraging them to also raise concerns with management

132. A nurse is caring for a patient who has been admitted with CHF exacerbation. The nurse notices that the patient's family members are constantly arguing and disagreeing with each other about the patient's care. One family member insists that the patient should receive alternative therapies, while another insists on strictly adhering to conventional medical treatments. The family members are causing disruption and tension in the unit, and it is difficult for the nurse to provide optimal care in this environment. What is the best approach for the nurse to manage the conflict between the patient's family members in this scenario?

    a. Avoiding the conflict and focusing on providing optimal care to the patient

    b. Encouraging the family members to discuss their concerns with the healthcare team and involving a professional mediator if necessary

    c. Taking sides and supporting the family member who has the most reasonable argument

    d. Limiting the family members' visits to the patient to reduce the potential for conflict

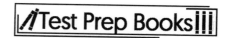

133. A nurse is caring for a patient who is uninsured and has limited resources to pay for their care. The patient requires a surgical procedure that will be costly and there are concerns about how the patient will be able to afford the bill. The patient has expressed fear and anxiety about the financial burden of the procedure and its potential impact on their quality of life. What is the most appropriate action for the nurse to take to address the financial concerns of an uninsured patient who requires a costly surgical procedure?

    a. Informing the patient that they will need to pay for the procedure out of pocket and providing them with resources to apply for financial assistance

    b. Suggesting that the patient delay the procedure until they can secure the necessary funds

    c. Consulting with the healthcare team to explore alternative treatment options that are less expensive and discussing these options with the patient

    d. Advise the patient to take out a loan or use a credit card to pay for the procedure.

134. A nurse has been assigned to care for several patients with a variety of complex medical conditions. As the nurse is performing their rounds, they receive an urgent call from the laboratory reporting that one of their patients has critical lab values that require immediate attention. The nurse is also due to administer medications to another patient who is in severe pain and has been waiting for over an hour for relief. What is the most appropriate action for the nurse to take in this scenario to ensure proper prioritization of patient care?

    a. Attending to the patient with critical lab values first since this is an urgent situation

    b. Attending to the patient in severe pain first since relieving pain is a basic human need

    c. Attending to the patient with the highest acuity level first since they require the most attention

    d. Delaying care for both patients until a backup nurse arrives to assist

135. A nurse manager has been tasked with managing the supply inventory to ensure that the unit stays within the allocated budget. The manager notices that one of the staff nurses is using an excessive amount of disposable supplies, which are costly and may lead to shortages and increased expenses. The staff nurse insists that using these supplies is necessary to ensure patient safety and comfort. What is the most appropriate action for the nurse manager to take to address the excessive use of disposable supplies?

    a. Allowing the nurse to continue using the disposable supplies to ensure patient safety and comfort

    b. Confronting the nurse about their excessive use of disposable supplies and demanding that they use them more sparingly

    c. Collaborating with the nurse to identify alternatives to the disposable supplies that are cost-effective and safe for the patient

    d. Reporting the nurse's excessive use of disposable supplies to the hospital's administration to ensure compliance with budgetary considerations

136. A nurse working in the medical-surgical unit has recently established a unit council. The council is designed to promote shared governance and collaboration among staff nurses, management, and other healthcare professionals in the unit. The council has been meeting regularly to discuss issues related to patient care, quality improvement, and professional development. One of the nurse's colleagues is not interested in participating in the council's activities and has expressed skepticism about the value of the council. The colleague is also disengaged during meetings and does not contribute to discussions. What is the most appropriate action for the nurse to take to promote professional engagement in the unit council?

    a. Confronting the colleague about their disengagement and demanding that they participate in the council's activities

    b. Ignoring the colleague's disengagement and focusing on their own participation in the council

    c. Discussing the value of the council with the colleague and encouraging them to share their concerns and ideas during meetings

    d. Reporting the colleague's disengagement to the council's leadership and requesting disciplinary action

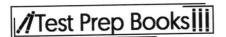

137. A newly hired registered nurse on a medical-surgical unit has been assigned a preceptor to help them with their orientation and training. However, the new nurse notices that the preceptor is frequently absent from work and does not provide them with adequate guidance and support. They also observe that the preceptor is often critical and belittling when giving feedback and does not encourage questions or open communication. What is the most appropriate action for the newly hired nurse to take to address the conflict with the preceptor?
    a. Ignoring the preceptor's behavior and trying to adapt to the situation
    b. Reporting the preceptor's behavior to the unit manager and requesting a new preceptor
    c. Confronting the preceptor about their behavior and requesting a change in their approach to the orientation process
    d. Seeking feedback and guidance from other nurses and healthcare professionals in the unit

138. A nurse has been assigned to care for a patient who has a history of drug abuse and is being treated for a leg infection. The patient refuses to take medications, eat, or cooperate with the care plan. The patient's family is unresponsive and does not provide any assistance. The nurse is struggling with how to provide effective care for this patient. Which of the following is the most appropriate action for the nurse to take?
    a. Refusing to care for the patient and asking for reassignment to another patient
    b. Continuing to provide care as usual, even if the patient is uncooperative
    c. Engaging in reflective practice to evaluate the situation and considering new strategies for care
    d. Reporting the patient to the hospital's administration for non-compliance

139. A nurse is participating in an interprofessional rounding session on a 45-year-old patient who was admitted with a complicated urinary tract infection. The healthcare team includes the patient's primary care physician, the hospitalist, the case manager, the pharmacist, and a social worker. What is the role of the nurse during interprofessional rounding?
    a. To lead the rounding session and provide updates on the patient's condition and care plan
    b. To advocate for the patient's needs and preferences and provide input on the care plan
    c. To observe the rounding session and take notes for later review
    d. To administer medications and carry out interventions as ordered by the healthcare team

140. A new nurse is struggling to manage their workload and is having difficulty with time management and prioritization. The new nurse expresses to their preceptor that they are feeling overwhelmed and are worried about making mistakes that could negatively impact patient care. Which of the following coaching strategies is most appropriate for the preceptor to use to support the new nurse's learning?
    a. Giving direct instruction and demonstration of nursing skills
    b. Facilitating self-reflection and problem-solving through questioning
    c. Providing written resources and materials for the new nurse to review
    d. Assigning the new nurse to work with an experienced nurse to observe and learn

141. A nurse manager has noticed that many of the nurses on the unit are feeling burned out and disengaged. The nurses are struggling to manage their workload and are feeling unsupported by the healthcare organization. The nursing team is experiencing high turnover rates, which is impacting the quality of care provided to patients. Which of the following professional empowerment strategies is most appropriate for the nurse manager to use to support the nursing team?
    a. Developing a reward and recognition program for staff nurses who demonstrate exceptional performance
    b. Implementing shared governance structures that allow staff nurses to have a greater voice in decision-making
    c. Assigning a mentor to each staff nurse to provide ongoing support and guidance
    d. Providing additional training and education opportunities for staff nurses to enhance their skills and knowledge

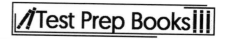

142. A newly hired nurse in the medical-surgical unit has been struggling to adjust to the work environment. The orientation process they were given was disorganized and rushed, and they were not given enough time to learn the policies and procedures of the unit. They are feeling frustrated and unsupported, and they are worried that their inexperience may negatively impact patient care. What is the most appropriate action for the nurse to take?

   a. Seeking additional training and education opportunities outside of work to improve their skills and knowledge
   b. Communicating their concerns to their preceptor and nurse manager and working together to develop a new orientation plan
   c. Continuing to work without addressing the issue, hoping to eventually adjust to the work environment
   d. Quitting the job and looking for a new position in a more supportive environment

143. A medical-surgical nurse who has been feeling stagnant in their career is interested in pursuing additional training and education opportunities to enhance their skills. What is the most appropriate action for the nurse to take to support their career development?

   a. Seeking advice from a mentor who can provide support and guidance in career development
   b. Researching external training and education opportunities to gain additional knowledge and skills
   c. Meeting with the hospital's human resources department to discuss career goals and identify potential resources within the hospital
   d. Working with a career coach to identify career goals and develop a career development plan

144. A nurse who has been feeling isolated in their practice is interested in connecting with other nurses and staying current with the latest developments in nursing practice. What is the most appropriate action for the nurse to take?

   a. Attending a nursing conference to learn about the latest developments in nursing practice
   b. Starting a nursing journal club with other nurses to share knowledge and discuss best practices
   c. Participating in an online nursing forum to connect with other nurses and exchange information
   d. Joining a professional nursing organization to network with other nurses and stay current with nursing practice

145. A nurse has noticed that some of their colleagues are engaging in improper peer review methods. They are not providing constructive feedback, but instead are making personal attacks and engaging in behaviors that could be considered bullying. This behavior is impacting the work environment and may be contributing to poor job satisfaction and morale among nursing staff. What is the most appropriate action for the nurse to take?

   a. Ignoring the behavior and focusing on their own work to avoid being implicated
   b. Talking to the colleagues who are engaging in improper peer review methods and encouraging them to use constructive feedback
   c. Bringing the issue to the attention of the nurse manager and suggesting a more formal approach to peer review
   d. Filing a formal complaint with the human resources department against the colleagues

146. A new graduate nurse is assigned to a patient who requires a blood transfusion. The nurse has some concerns about the transfusion, as they are not sure what the regulatory and compliance standards are for administering blood transfusions in the hospital. What is the most appropriate action for the nurse to take?

   a. Administering the blood transfusion according to their best judgment and experience
   b. Asking another nurse for advice on how to administer the blood transfusion
   c. Consulting the hospital's policies and procedures on blood transfusions before administering the transfusion
   d. Calling the physician to ask for clarification on the blood transfusion order

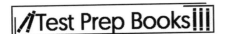

147. A nurse manager working in the medical-surgical unit has been tasked with improving retention rates and employee morale. The nurse manager decides not to communicate with the staff nurses to determine the root cause of these issues, but rather implement a solution that they personally feel will work best. What is the disadvantage of having an organizational structure that is based on a top-down leadership style?
    a. It can increase staff workload and lead to burnout.
    b. It can decrease accountability and create an unstructured work environment.
    c. It can lead to poor communication and collaboration among team members.
    d. It can promote inflexibility and discourage innovation.

148. A nurse is caring for a patient who has been recently diagnosed with late-stage breast cancer. The patient is struggling to understand their treatment options and is looking to the nurse for guidance. What is the most appropriate action for the nurse to take?
    a. Providing the patient with a detailed explanation of their treatment options and making a recommendation based on their medical history
    b. Encouraging the patient to make their own decision and providing support and resources to help them make an informed choice
    c. Contacting the patient's family members to discuss the treatment options and make a joint decision
    d. Referring the patient to a physician to make the treatment decision on their behalf

149. A nurse has been assigned to care for a patient whose cultural beliefs and values are different from their own. The patient has expressed a desire for a particular type of treatment that is not commonly practiced in the hospital, but that aligns with their cultural traditions. What is the most appropriate action for the nurse to take?
    a. Explaining to the patient that the treatment they desire is not commonly practiced in the hospital and encouraging them to try the hospital's standard treatment
    b. Respecting the patient's cultural beliefs and values and working with the healthcare team to provide the treatment that the patient desires
    c. Consulting with the hospital's ethics committee to determine the best course of action
    d. Referring the patient to a different hospital or healthcare provider that is better equipped to meet their cultural needs

150. A nurse is caring for a patient who is upset about the care that they have received so far. The patient reports that they have completed multiple surveys about their experience, but their concerns have not been addressed. They express dissatisfaction and threaten to leave the hospital against medical advice. What is the most appropriate action for the nurse to take in this scenario to address the patient's concerns and improve the customer experience?
    a. Apologizing to the patient and providing them with a detailed explanation of the care they have received so far
    b. Informing the patient that their complaints will be reviewed and addressed at a later time
    c. Listening to the patient's concerns and working with them to develop a plan to address their specific needs
    d. Dismissing the patient's concerns as unfounded and focusing on providing standard care to them

Answer Explanations #2

1. A: Choice A represents the type of leadership style that involves the nurse taking on an informal leadership role by functioning as a resource to meet the needs of the team. Servant leadership also involves leading by example, focusing on values and ethics, and continuously using foresight and empathy to advance the team. While often engaged by informal leaders, formal leaders may also adopt this style. Choice B involves ensuring team members follow direction precisely, with little to no support of innovation or creativity. Choice C indicates leadership that involves tremendous leeway in work specifics with greater focus on the end-result rather than the process, while lending support only when requested. Choice D indicates leadership that involves expected output with reward and consequence.

2. D: A pregnancy test is performed first to determine if the patient is pregnant. A Pap smear, uterine biopsy, and pelvic ultrasound may be performed, based on the patient's history and physical findings, but they would not be the first test performed, making A, B, and C incorrect answers.

3. C: Choice C represents a hindrance to the development of a therapeutic nurse-to-patient discussion and should be avoided. Choice A displays understanding, Choice B encourages deeper dialogue, and Choice D shows comprehension of what the patient communicated.

4. B: Diabetic ketoacidosis is an acidotic metabolic state that can be caused by poor diabetic management, leading to hyperglycemia. Diabetic management involves regular visits to the healthcare provider, taking insulin or oral anti-diabetic agents as ordered, following a healthy diet, exercising regularly, and monitoring blood glucose levels at home. Hyperglycemia can occur when the patient does not have enough insulin in the body. Since ingesting high glucose levels leads to hyperglycemia, not reduced glucose levels, Choice C is not the correct answer. It can also occur when the oral anti-diabetic management is not sufficient to control high blood glucose levels.

5. B: Choice B involves the nurse revising the plan as needed to meet individualized patient-centered goals of treatment. The evaluation phase also involves comparing actual outcomes with expected outcomes. Choice A should be avoided, as the patient should be assessed in relation to established goals. Choice C should be avoided, as the goals should be modified as care priorities change. Choice D should be avoided, as the nurse should maintain flexibility, not rigid control.

6. B: Choice B is a common symptom found within uremic syndrome post systemic infection. Choices A, C, and D do not correlate with uremic syndrome and would not relate to a clinical presentation of this condition.

7. D: Choice D should be omitted from the plan of care for a patient struggling with hemorrhoids because this patient would benefit from a high fiber diet. Choices A, B, and C all provide symptom relief and encourage the management or resolution of hemorrhoids; therefore, these measures should be included in the treatment plan.

8. C: Understanding the patient concerns validates the patient's viewpoint, which can enhance the patient's self-image. A positive self-image can increase self-efficacy, which is the patient's perception of the ability to succeed. Choice A engages the patient with an open-ended question; therefore, Choice A is incorrect. Choice B asks for clarification, but it will not enhance self-efficacy, so Choice B is incorrect. Choice D is part of a summary statement that is giving the patient the opportunity to contribute more information, so Choice D is incorrect.

9. C: Injuries above the T6 level are associated with neurogenic shock, due to alterations of the autonomic nervous system, resulting in the loss of vagal tone. This manifests as decreased vascular resistance and vasodilation. Injury at this level is also associated with alterations in respiratory function, which results in symptoms such as decreased vital capacity and the presence of adventitious breath sounds. In addition, hypothermia is common; therefore, Choice C is correct. A vital capacity level that equals 45 percent of normal is associated with injuries at the T1 level

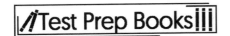

or below and is an indication of hemorrhagic shock rather than neurogenic shock. A hemoglobin level of 10.4 g/dL in a male patient is also associated with acute or occult blood loss rather than loss of vagal tone and is indicative of hemorrhagic shock. The patient's level of injury is consistent with neurogenic shock, which is manifested by bradycardia, not tachycardia; therefore, Choice *A* is incorrect. Loss of somatic and reflex function is associated with spinal shock, and hypertension and an effective cough effort are inconsistent with the level of the patient's injury; therefore, Choice *B* is incorrect. The collective manifestations of hypotension, oliguria, and tachycardia are associated with hypovolemic shock rather than neurogenic shock; therefore, Choice *D* is incorrect.

10. C: Choice *C* would provide the least support for the patient's iron deficiency anemia. Choices *A*, *B*, and *D* are all supportive of improved nutritional status regarding iron and should be encouraged via dietary intake.

11. C: Choice *C* indicates a delegated role outside of the scope of the unlicensed assistive personnel (UAP), which alerts the registered nurse (RN) to provide education to the licensed practical nurse (LPN) regarding safe delegation. UAPs cannot administer medication of any kind, including over-the-counter medicated creams. Choices *A*, *B*, and *D* represent appropriate delegation, as all actions are within the scope of the UAP.

12. B: Diabetic ketoacidosis is an acute complication of type I diabetes due to a lack of adequate insulin. When this occurs, there is not enough insulin to break down nutrients into glucose. The body begins to break down fatty acids into ketones for energy, leading to ketones in the blood and an acidic body pH level; therefore, Choice *A* is not the correct response. Choices *C* and *D* are not correct since clinical manifestations include dehydration, hyperglycemia, nausea, sweet-smelling breath, confusion, and fatigue.

13. B: Choice *B* is a cause for concern regarding the patient's knowledge deficit on medication storage. The patient should not store reconstituted amoxicillin on the bedroom dresser. While this location would be appropriate prior to reconstituting, this medication must be stored in the refrigerator once reconstituted. Choices *A*, *C*, and *D* demonstrate proper storage of the medications and do not need to be addressed by the nurse at this time.

14. B: The nurse suspects that the IV has infiltrated, meaning the catheter tip has become dislodged and IV medication and/or fluids are leaking into the surrounding tissues. The nurse should stop the infusion, remove the IV, and dress the site. An allergic reaction or infection would be warm, not cold, due to the inflammatory response present in such conditions. This is not a normal assessment of a peripheral IV.

15. A: Crohn's disease is recurrent. Surgery may be necessary to excise a segment of the intestine that has been damaged by the transmural effects of the disease process; however, progression to additional areas is common because Crohn's disease can affect the entire length of the GI tract. This is in contrast to ulcerative colitis, which may be cured by a total colectomy because the disease can only affect the colon. Therefore, Choice *A* reflects the need for additional teaching and is the correct answer. Crohn's disease is an autoimmune-mediated disease and is associated with an increased risk for other immune diseases such as arthritis; therefore, Choice *B* does not reflect the need for additional teaching. Crohn's disease commonly affects the terminal ileum, which is the site of vitamin B-12 absorption. Deficiency of this vitamin can result in decreased red cell production and anemia; therefore, Choice *C* does not reflect the need for additional teaching. Crohn's disease is often complicated by fistulae formation between bowel segments, which results in localized pain in the right lower quadrant of the abdomen. Early recognition and treatment are necessary to prevent systemic effects including sepsis; therefore, Choice *D* does not reflect the need for additional teaching.

16. B: Unstable angina, caused by an unstable atherosclerotic plaque, is not predictable and may occur at rest. The pain may worsen over a brief time period, last up to 20 minutes, and is not responsive to nitroglycerine. Choices *A*, *C*, and *D* are descriptive of stable angina.

17. B: The patient is in hepatic (liver) failure based on the symptomology and the presentation. Kidney failure would present with electrolyte and fluid abnormalities and their symptoms. Diseases of the stomach would present with GI

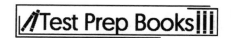

symptoms such as nausea, vomiting, and abdominal pain in the left upper quadrant. Diseases of the spleen would manifest as blood disorders and would not be similar to symptoms of liver failure.

18. B: Choice *B* is an appropriate length of time prior to surgery to discontinue the patient's heparin drip. Choice *A* is too close to surgery, which poses a risk for bleeding complications. Choices *C* and *D* would discontinue a needed therapy too far in advance of the scheduled surgery time and should be avoided.

19. A: Choice *A* is the appropriate length of time for the patient to be total npo, which involves nothing by mouth, before their scheduled colonoscopy. Choice *B* represents the length of time before a procedure where the patient is supported to continue consuming clear liquids. Choices *C* and *D* represent times that are too early prior to procedure to encourage the patient to refrain from all food and drink.

20. C: This scenario is an example of a high-stress and potentially dangerous situation, which can have a significant impact on the nurse's resiliency and well-being. In this situation, it is important for the nurse to prioritize their own safety and well-being, rather than trying to engage with the patient or respond with force, as in Choices *A* and *B*. Continuing to engage with the patient or responding with force can put the nurse at further risk of harm and increase the potential for emotional trauma. Choice *D* can be helpful, but it is important to prioritize the nurse's safety first.

21. C: Since chemotherapy may affect the bone marrow, the patient receiving chemotherapy may have low red blood cell, white blood cell, and platelet counts. This patient has a low neutrophil count, which means the patient does not have enough white blood cells in her body. Since white blood cells help the body fight infection, the patient is at risk for infection and should avoid being in crowds, especially during influenza season. Choice *A* is not correct; using a safety razor reduces the risk of bleeding due to a low platelet count. Choice *B* is not correct; iron supplements help in the production of red blood cells, not white blood cells. Although the patient may benefit from drinking fluids, this instruction will not reduce the risk of infection.

22. D: Cardiac output is the volume of blood that the heart pumps in one minute. It is measured by multiplying the heart rate by stroke volume. Choice *A* is the incorrect choice since it describes pulmonary vascular resistance. Choice *B* is not the answer since it describes preload. Choice *C* is incorrect because it describes afterload.

23. C: Choice *C* describes the chief reason for conducting a 5 Whys Analysis, which is to understand the root cause of an incident. Choices *A* and *D* represent potential gains from conducting this analysis but not the main purpose. Choice *B* may be deduced from this analysis but is not the main goal. The focus is on understanding and planning rather than on punitive consequences.

24. B: Choice *B* requires the medical-surgical nurse to don a surgical mask while interacting with the patient. Choice *A* requires the nurse to don an N95 respirator while working with the patient. Choices *C* and *D* do not require respiratory shielding.

25. A: Beck's triad of muffled heart sounds, distended neck veins, and hypotension are cardinal signs of cardiac tamponade. Chest pain and back pain are the most common presenting symptoms with the AAA. Heart function, breathing, and consciousness are not evident in cardiopulmonary arrest. Cardiogenic shock includes ashen, cyanotic, or mottled extremities; distant heart sounds; and rapid and faint peripheral pulses.

26. C: Choice *C* represents the member of the interdisciplinary team that the nurse should consult with regarding patient dressing and hygiene aids, as such aids are required for daily functioning and within the role of the occupational therapist. Choice *A* supports strength in movement. Choice *B* aligns services for quality of life and overall functioning. Choice *D* manages care coordination between disciplines.

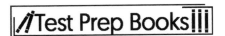

27. D: Choice *D* indicates an emergent concern post furosemide administration. The medical-surgical nurse is aware that this patient is suffering from a significantly reduced white blood cell count and likely from a critically low neutrophil count in the blood. Choices *A*, *B*, and *C*, while potentially uncomfortable side effects of furosemide administration, are all expected and not emergent concerns at this time.

28. B: Phenytoin is FDA approved for most types of seizures. Memantine is a neurological drug used to treat dementia. Pregabalin is a drug used to treat diabetic neuropathy. Rifaximin is a drug used to treat hepatic encephalopathy.

29. D: Choice *D* indicates a food item that is risky for the patient with acquired immunodeficiency syndrome (AIDS) to consume. Blue cheese is an unpasteurized food item and should be omitted from the therapeutic diet, along with unpasteurized drinks, meats, and raw or undercooked animal products. Choices *A*, *B*, and *C* are considered safe to consume as they do not pose any direct risks to the health of a patient with AIDS.

30. C: Choice *C* is an intervention that is appropriate for the nurse to engage in to support the patient with early dumping syndrome. Choice *A* should be avoided; fluids should be consumed outside of mealtimes. Choice *B* should be avoided, as the patient should consume several small meals per day. Choice *D* should be avoided; the patient should increase fiber intake.

31. D: Troponin is a muscle cell protein that is released when cardiac tissue is broken down during an ischemic event. Elevated levels of troponin in the bloodstream indicate cardiac muscle damage. Creatinine and BUN are waste products of the body, and higher levels of these in the bloodstream indicate kidney failure or damage, not heart damage. Creatine kinase is an enzyme found in muscle tissue. One form of the enzyme, CK-MB, is a cardiac enzyme, but its structure is similar to creatine kinase found in skeletal muscle. Therefore, it's a less specific indicator of cardiac muscle damage.

32. B: Choice *B* should be avoided in the plan of care for a patient with acute Deep Vein Thrombosis (DVT) as spontaneous compression devices may dislodge a preexisting thrombus and lead to a pulmonary embolism, a blockage in a lung artery. Choice *A* is an appropriate intervention as this medication is an anticoagulant. Choice *C* should be included in the plan of care to characterize the coagulation of blood. Choice *D* is necessary to monitor for irregular heartbeat including preventricular contractions that the patient may feel as palpitations, along with other cardiac signs and symptoms that may come from a dislodged blood clot.

33. A: Choice *A* is correct as the dysphagia diet places this food item at a level 3, proving challenging for a patient with difficulty swallowing to consume. Choice *B* is considered a level-2 item and is appropriate for this patient. Choices *C* and *D* are considered level-1 food items and are appropriate for this patient to consume. Soft solid foods should be avoided for this patient, while they are struggling to move food and liquid from their mouth to their stomach. The consumption of beets poses a safety risk.

34. D: A fracture to the eighth rib on the right side of the chest may cause injury to the liver, which lies beneath this rib. Choices *A* and *B* are not correct since injury to the bronchus or trachea is likely to be caused by fractures to the first or second ribs. Choice *C* is incorrect since the spleen is likely to be injured with a fracture to the eighth rib or greater on the left side of the chest.

35. B: Choice *B* influences ketone bodies, which provide some symptom relief regarding cognition and memory for the patient with Alzheimer's disease. Choices *A*, *C*, and *D* should be avoided with this patient, as symptoms tend to be aggravated by these actions.

36. A: The patient utilizing oxygen for respiratory management should switch from aerosol to stick deodorant, as aerosol cans present a fire risk. To promote safe discharge, the nurse must assess for understanding of proper use of new equipment in the home. Choices *B*, *C*, and *D* do not show safe handling to prevent fire.

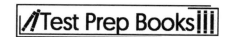

37. B: Constant clearing of the throat is a sign that a patient is silently aspirating. Integument symptoms such as rash are not associated with this condition. Swollen lymph nodes on the neck indicate possible upper respiratory infection. Neurological deficits such as memory and orientation loss are not associated with silent aspiration, but may occur because of stroke, which is a precursor to difficulty swallowing in some cases.

38. C: Choice C represents a risk to infection control and warrants further education. The unlicensed assistive personnel (UAP) should wash their hands with soap and water after caring for a patient with *Clostridium difficile* because hand sanitizers kill bacteria but do not kill the spores. Choice A is within the scope of the UAP and does not warrant education. Choice B is an appropriate care measure and does not warrant education. Choice D represents the correct placement of the Foley catheter bag to avoid urine collection in the bladder.

39. B: Cushing's disease is caused by a dysfunction of the adrenal glands, which are on top of the kidneys, leading to excess glucocorticoid production. As a result, Choices A, C, and D are incorrect.

40. C: Pregnant women with gestational diabetes need to exercise regularly, avoid excessive weight gain, and monitor food intake. They also need to seek regular prenatal care since gestational diabetes can affect fetal growth and increase the baby's risk of obesity. Therefore, Choices A, B, and D are not correct.

41. A: Choice A indicates a post-renal cause of acute renal failure. Sources of obstruction include stones, strictures, and tumors. Choices B and C are direct renal causes, while Choice D is a prerenal cause of acute renal failure.

42. C: Acute bronchitis, an inflammation of the bronchial tubes, can cause wheezing, coughing, fever, myalgia, and chest pain. Other manifestations include sore throat, headache, nasal congestion, rhinorrhea, dyspnea, and fatigue. While treatment is generally supportive, a beta-2 agonist, such as albuterol, may be administered to reduce wheezing. Since this medication does not act as a cough suppressant, fever-reducing agent, or analgesic, A, B, and D are incorrect.

43. C: This scenario depicts a case of community-acquired pneumonia (CAP), specifically pneumococcal pneumonia. The most common cause of CAP is Streptococcus pneumoniae, or pneumococcus. It's a gram-positive bacterium, usually occurring in pairs (diplococci). The other bacteria (Haemophilus influenzae, Moraxella catarrhalis, and Staphylococcus aureus) are less common causes of CAP.

44. A: A laparoscopic procedure is minimally invasive and makes very small incisions for the surgeon to enter the abdominal cavity and remove the gall bladder. Laparotomy involves the surgeon making a large incision to completely open up the abdominal cavity. Bronchoscopy is a scope of the airways and lungs. Endoscopy is a scope of the upper GI tract.

45. D: The patient with an upper gastrointestinal bleed may be covertly bleeding superiorly to the junction of the duodenum and jejunum. Because the nurse cannot directly observe the bleeding, the amount of blood loss must be estimated. A patient with a gastrointestinal bleed who experiences a 10-millimeter drop in diastolic blood pressure when moving from a lying to a standing position is estimated to have lost 1,000 milliliters of blood.

46. B: Choice B is correct, as a normal prothrombin time test (PTT) falls within a 10-14 second range. Choice A is below normal. Choices C and D are both above the normal range. The medical-surgical nurse is responsible for reviewing this laboratory result to ensure proper clotting ability prior to surgery.

47. C: Choice C represents a patient condition that is in direct conflict with the administration of antimuscarinic medications; therefore, the patient with this condition is unable to receive this treatment. Antimuscarinics can lead to pupillary blockage due to their effect on nerve impulses. Choices A, B, and D do not pose risks for contraindication and do not prevent the patient from engaging in this treatment option.

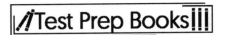

48. C: This scenario depicts the diagnosis of a right-sided tension pneumothorax. The triad of tracheal deviation (to opposite side), mediastinal shift (to opposite side), and depression of the hemidiaphragm (on affected side) is pathognomonic for tension pneumothorax. Medical professionals must be quick and decisive in their treatment of tension pneumothorax. The condition is life-threatening and valuable time is often wasted waiting around for the results of imaging studies. Definitive treatment of a tension pneumothorax is emergent needle thoracostomy.

49. A: Patients with Barrett's esophagus are at an increased risk for developing esophageal adenocarcinoma. When a patient has reflux disease, the cells of the esophagus become irritated and go through a metastatic transformation, thus increasing the risk for cancer. Therefore, the statement that the patient is not at an increased risk for cancer needs to be corrected by the nurse. Choice *B* is not correct since corticosteroids are used to treat Barrett's esophagus. Choice *C* is not the correct answer since the patient does need to make healthy lifestyle choices to reduce the risk of reflux disease. Choice *D* is not correct since the patient should be taught signs and symptoms of reflux disease to report to the physician, including heartburn and difficulty swallowing.

50. C: Cushing's triad of manifestations are late signs of increased ICP. Choice *C* is an example of widening pulse pressure. Normal pulse pressure = 40 mmHg. Choice *C* pulse pressure = 130 mmHg. Choices *A, B,* and *D* are all early signs of increased ICP, and therefore are incorrect.

51. D: Choice *D* represents an infection of the tissue lining the inner abdominal wall. Choice *A* manifests as inflammation of the iris of the eye. Choice *B* involves an inflammation and the potential for infection of the skin. Choice *C* aligns with inflammation and the potential of infection of the bladder.

52. B: In glycogenosis, the patient's body is not able to convert stored glycogen to glucose when the body needs glucose. In severe cases, the patient can experience chronic gout, seizures, coma, intestinal sores, and kidney failure. Choices *A, C,* and *D* are not correct since liver failure, respiratory failure, and congestive heart failure are not common findings in severe glycogenosis.

53. B: Both the patient's symptoms and blood glucose level indicate that the patient is experiencing hypoglycemia. Manifestations of hypoglycemia include a decreased level of consciousness, tremors, fatigue, excessive sweating, dizziness, and syncope. A blood glucose level below 70 milligrams per deciliter confirms this diagnosis. Insulin would not be given to a patient with hypoglycemia, as this would further lower the blood glucose level. Choices *A, C,* and *D* are incorrect because it would be appropriate to administer oral glucose, IV dextrose, or parenteral glucagon to the patient with hypoglycemia.

54. D: Endoscopic band ligation should be implemented for all varices that are 5 millimeters or more in diameter and/or associated with red wales, because these characteristics are associated with a greater risk for hemorrhage. Band ligation decreases this potential but may be associated with stricture formation and obstruction of the esophageal lumen. This procedure may need to be repeated as the liver failure progresses. Therefore, Choice *D* is correct. Sclerotherapy of the esophageal veins is considered as a form of secondary prevention by many because beta-blocker therapy is readily available, well tolerated, and equally effective as compared to sclerotherapy. In the event of hemorrhage due to ruptured esophageal varices, sclerotherapy can be used to decrease the blood loss; therefore, Choice *A* is incorrect.

55. A: Nausea, Choice *A*, is not a typical finding, as a key assessment notation for this diagnosis is vomiting in the absence of nausea. Choices *B, C,* and *D* all represent early warning signs of increased intracranial pressure which could be found in a patient suffering from a head injury.

56. C: Urinary retention occurs when a patient has cessation of urination or incomplete emptying of the bladder. This may lead to overflow incontinence as the bladder becomes overfilled with urine, which then is involuntarily released from the overfull bladder. Therefore, *A, B,* and *D* are not correct.

57. D: Choice *D* is the priority action for the nurse to rank in the plan of care for a patient with a history of aggressive behavior. Choices *A*, *B*, and *C* are not yet necessary; these actions represent potential interventions that may come later in the treatment plan if warranted. The nurse should focus on the least restrictive measures first.

58. A: The patient's manifestations are consistent with a diagnosis of hemorrhagic stroke. Although there is no single therapeutic agent that is specific to the treatment of hemorrhagic stroke, aggressive treatment of hypertension and the use of agents to counteract the anticoagulative effect of warfarin are common interventions. Mannitol is an osmotic diuretic used to decrease intracranial pressure that results from the hematoma formation at the hemorrhagic site. Vitamin K is used to counteract warfarin therapy, and the dose will be titrated to the results of the coagulation studies; therefore, Choice *A* is correct. Warfarin is an anticoagulant that is not recommended for use in hemorrhagic stroke. Labetalol is an antihypertensive agent that might be used for hemorrhagic stroke. However, it would not be ordered with warfarin therapy; therefore, Choice *B* is incorrect. Alteplase is a fibrinolytic agent, and nitroprusside is a potent vasoconstricting agent. Neither of these medications is appropriate in the care of hemorrhagic stroke; therefore, Choice *C* is incorrect. Enalapril is an antihypertensive agent that might be used for hemorrhagic stroke. However, it would not be ordered with ASA, which is an antiplatelet agent; therefore, Choice *D* is incorrect.

59. B: Choice *B* represents the nurse's focus while discussing the professional role and function of the registered professional nurse with an interdisciplinary colleague. Choices *A*, *C*, and *D* do not rely on state law to define the description of scope witnessed in this engagement.

60. A: Choice *A* is a significant outcome focus for a patient with Marfan syndrome as this genetic disorder affects the cardiac system and leads to challenges with maintaining adequate tissue perfusion. Choices *B*, *C*, and *D* are not concerns associated with this disorder.

61. A: Choice *A* is a concerning response by the patient regarding their daily levothyroxine administration. This medication should be taken once daily on an empty stomach, at least 30 minutes before and four hours after meals. Choices *B*, *C*, and *D* all meet these administration guidelines and do not necessitate patient education at this time.

62. A: Choice *A* involves the quadrant where the appendix is located and where pain is typically felt. The nurse should ask the patient to rate their pain level in the right lower quadrant in order to provide effective pain management at this time. Choices *B*, *C*, and *D* represent quadrants outside of the appendix location.

63. C: Choice *C* should be performed second when completing a focused abdominal assessment. Choice *A* should be third; Choice *B* should be fourth, while Choice *D* happens first when engaging in a focused abdominal assessment. Other body systems retain the typical order of inspection, percussion, palpation, and auscultation, however with the abdomen, the medical-surgical nurse must auscultate prior to percussion to avoid altering the bowel sounds.

64. A: Choice *A* is often the cause of increased confusion, agitation, and poor motor skills in the geriatric patient population. These symptoms can present suddenly and alert the medical-surgical nurse to a notable change in the patient's level of consciousness. Further assessment is warranted. Choices *B*, *C*, and *D* are not associated with this symptom presentation and should not be considered for further assessment at this time.

65. A: Choice *A* includes language that aligns with the SBAR format of communication. This statement provides a direct recommendation. The SBAR technique calls for a report that includes situation, background, assessment, and recommendation. Choices *B*, *C*, and *D* request information or direction from the provider rather than offering a clear recommendation for treatment.

66. C: Choice *C* represents a type of angina that is instigated by coronary vasospasms. Choice *A* occurs when the heart is chronically working harder than usual due to a lack of oxygen. Choice *B* is due to a lack of blood flow and oxygen from a blood clot, potentially leading to a myocardial infarction. Choice *D* is due to coronary artery spasms.

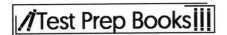

67. D: Hyperglycemia may occur in a patient who does not have enough insulin or anti-diabetic medication, ingests too much glucose, experiences an illness that disrupts the normal routine, or experiences a crisis that causes emotional stress.

68. C: The typical manifestations of status asthmaticus are wheezing, coughing, and dyspnea. With severe airway obstruction, auscultation of the chest may reveal a "silent chest" and a lack of audible wheezing. Tachycardia, cyanosis, and hypoxemia are all manifestations of the patient with status asthmaticus but are not signs of impending respiratory failure; therefore, Choices A, B, and D are incorrect.

69. D: An INR of 3.5 is elevated and will cause bleeding complications if thrombolytic therapy is initiated before the INR returns to the normal level of less than or equal to 1.1.

70. D: Choice D aligns with the nurse's statement, "Don't worry, everyone feels that way," and demonstrates a poor example of therapeutic communication, which hinders the nurse-patient relationship. Choice A projects the nurse's opinion. Choice B provides comfort in a misleading outcome. Choice C guards a party, such as a provider. All communication blocks reviewed in this question encourage misunderstandings and failure to listen, which should be avoided in patient care environments.

71. C: Choice C involves appropriate precautions for the management of infection control in the patient with pertussis. This illness, also known as whooping cough, produces droplets that can spread when talking, coughing, and sneezing. Choice A and Choice B would provide inadequate protection with vulnerabilities in disease transmission. Choice D represents a higher level of precaution, which is not required for this patient at this time.

72. B: Relapses are common in the patient with myasthenia gravis. To reduce the risk of relapse, the nurse should teach the patient to avoid infection, increases in body temperature, stress, and pregnancy. Therefore, Choices A, C, and D should be included in the plan of care.

73. D: The discharge planning process starts right away at admission for every patient. Each aspect of care is provided with an end-goal in mind. When the patient comes into the care of a healthcare organization, the treatment plan involves interventions with an ultimate anticipated outcome of safe discharge.

74. B: Choice B represents the form of consent for treatment that the patient gives by presenting for care and voluntarily moving forward with admission; implied consent is inferred from the patient's actions. Choices A and C involve the patient's direct agreement to move forward with treatment by giving either verbal or written permission to receive care. Choice D involves consent given by a third party acting on behalf of the patient's interest.

75. B: Choice B sets forth that when using the PQRST method the nurse should include information regarding the patient's pain that includes the following characteristics: provoke, quality, region, severity, and timing. Choices A, C, and D are incorrect as they do not provide accurate details of a PQRST method pain assessment for a nurse-to-nurse report. This method is exclusive to a focused pain assessment and includes specific characteristics.

76. D: The patient who has had a pulmonary embolism may require warfarin (Coumadin) after discharge from the hospital to prevent blood clot formation leading to pulmonary embolism. With warfarin, frequent blood monitoring is needed to maintain INR between 2-3. Choice A does not require more teaching since warfarin is taken orally. Choice B does not require more teaching since bleeding is a risk with this drug and should be reported to the physician, if it occurs. Choice C does not require more teaching since chest pain and shortness of breath are possible manifestations of pulmonary embolism.

77. A: Choice A represents the diet that should be implemented for the patient with gout. Choices B and C should be avoided as they may exacerbate symptoms. Choice D is not necessary for this patient at this time. Purines can cause gout attacks and should be avoided. Some examples of high-purine foods include red meat, seafood, organ meat, and alcohol.

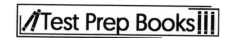

78. D: The patient's preferences, values, and beliefs, as well as indication of a surrogate decision maker, are all included in advance directives.

79. D: Choice *D* supports the patient's right to engage in independent, self-directed decision-making. The provider must avoid language that impedes this right. Choice *A* involves avoiding patient harm. Choice *B* represents truthfulness. Choice *C* includes the moral imperative to do right by the patient.

80. A: The most common complication associated with shunts is the obstruction of the proximal catheter. Over a period, the proximal tip of the catheter can become embedded in the choroid, obstructing the catheter and delaying the drainage of the CSF. The shunt valve on the proximal end can also become obstructed with blood cells and other cellular debris. Obstruction of the distal catheter is less common than proximal obstruction but occurs more frequently than infection or dislocation. Migration of the catheter tip is most commonly related to the growth of the patient, which means that this complication occurs in younger children most often. The patient referenced in this scenario was an adult at the time of insertion of the catheter; therefore, this is not a likely cause for his current problem, and Choice *B* is incorrect. Disconnection of the segments of the shunt system is a rare occurrence that is due to a manufacturer's defect or improper installation of the device. When this malfunction does occur, it is readily discovered in the postoperative period; therefore, Choice *C* is incorrect. Infection most commonly occurs during the initial two to four months after the catheter is inserted. Infection is most often associated with overt signs of infection such as erythema, purulent drainage, peritonitis, and abdominal pain; however, fever may or may not be present. The patient included in the scenario has had the shunt in place for four years, which exceeds the common timeline for site infection, and the assessment does not provide any support for a diagnosis of infection; therefore, Choice *D* is incorrect.

81. C: Choice *C* aligns with the patient's laboratory findings when utilizing the SBAR as a method of communication. SBAR stands for situation, background, assessment, and recommendations. Laboratory findings are a form of assessment data; therefore, they align with the assessment aspect of reports. Choice *A* includes the current condition. Choice *B* includes the context of the circumstance. Choice *D* includes the nurse's suggestions to respond to the situation.

82. A: Choice *A* reflects patient-centered goals to be included in the nursing care plan. These goals encourage the greatest improvement in individual health outcomes, encompassing physical and mental wellbeing and the ability to care for self. Choice *B* does not align, as patient-centered goals do not revolve around the interest of any specific nursing interventions. Choice *C* is provider-centered, not patient-centered. Choice *D* is not appropriate, as "normalized" is subjective and does not focus on this specific patient's individualized health improvement.

83. A: Choice *A* is correct because the patient is at risk for developing metabolic acidosis while on total parenteral nutrition (TPN). The medical-surgical nurse should be aware of this risk and routinely assess for the development of this complication. Choices *B*, *C*, and *D*, while all significant imbalances that would profoundly affect the patient's health status, are not typically observed with this treatment and not expected responses at this time.

84. C: Choice *C* indicates the action that the nurse should implement at this time. The nurse understands that Broca's aphasia influences the patient's ability to produce verbal expression but does not limit their ability to understand incoming verbal responses. Choices *A*, *B*, and *D* are unnecessary as these actions would not provide care that is diagnosis-specific and supportive. Multiple types of aphasia exist; knowing the differences between them promotes sensitive care.

85. A: Choice *A* involves the patient's determination to self-directed decisions that are free from coercion. Choice *B* sets forth that actions are right or wrong depending on the level of pleasure they promote. Choice *C* endorses that the nurse will remain true to their professional commitments. Choice *D* involves conflicting concerns of multiple parties.

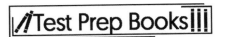

86. A: Choice *A* is the appropriate response by the nurse because it supports accurate medication reconciliation with continued management of care. Choices *B*, *C*, and *D* should all be avoided, as they would delay treatment and potentially provide inaccurate information. The medical-surgical nurse should obtain a written release of information from the patient, and then proceed to contact the outpatient pharmacy to discuss the patient's current prescription for gabapentin. If the patient is prescribed additional medication by other outpatient providers, it would also be appropriate for the nurse to gather that data as well to support a thorough medication reconciliation process.

87. A: Choice *A* describes the patient's thought process when experiencing delusional thinking. The medical-surgical nurse must understand how delusional thinking impairs beliefs, as well as understanding and cooperation, to ensure the establishment of effective communication and a holistic plan of care. Choice *B* describes hallucinations. Choice *C* describes delirium. Choice *D* describes dementia.

88. B: Choice *B* is an activity that takes place during the assessment phase of the nursing process. Choice *A* aligns with the implementation phase. Choice *C* correlates with the planning phase. Choice *D* represents an activity in the evaluation phase.

89. A: Choice *A* is significant, as a patient with acute glomerulonephritis struggles to maintain fluid balance and requires substantial assistance with this process. The medical-surgical nurse should monitor this balance and intervene as necessary. Choices *B*, *C*, and *D* are not goals for treatment. On the contrary, the patient should be supported to lower blood pressure, reduce serum potassium levels, and decrease consumption of protein in the diet.

90. D: A stroke is a potential complication of hypertension in a patient post-endarterectomy. The nurse must carefully monitor and treat high blood pressure should it occur. Bleeding would be marked by low blood pressure. Infection is a noncardiac issue; thus, it is unrelated to blood pressure in this instance. Pulmonary edema can occur as a result of heart failure and is not pertinent to the monitoring for high blood pressure.

91. C: In the supine position, the patient lies on their back with legs on the bed. This is the routine position for most abdominal, open heart, and lower extremity procedures. In lithotomy position, the patient's legs are in stirrups; this is indicated for gynecological, urology, and colorectal procedures. In left lateral position, the patient lies on their left side with right side up.

92. A: The perioperative nurse documents the surgery record, perioperative medication administration record, surgical time out, and nursing pathway. The surgical time out is not documented by the surgeon, anesthesiologist, or surgical technologist.

93. B: Sterile water should be used to irrigate channels and flush debris from instruments. Saline should not be utilized for this process because it can cause mineral deposits to form. Tap water can cause contamination, and lactated Ringer's solution is not commonly used to keep instruments moist.

94. B: The pre-operative interview allows the nurse to discuss the patient's medical and health history (to prepare necessary equipment, medication, and personnel for the procedure) and the operative procedure in depth with the patient. Patient finances, case studies, and behaviors that contributed to the need for the procedure aren't usually discussed during the pre-operative process, as this can cause anxiety, guilt, shame, and other negative feelings for the patient. The pre-operative interview is meant to be an informative and soothing process.

95. B: Norepinephrine is a potent vasoconstrictor that may be used if dopamine is inadequate in maintaining normal blood pressure in a patient experiencing cardiogenic shock. Dobutamine is an option but is used for systemic vasodilation with stronger beta effects than the others mentioned here. Milrinone causes vasodilation and positive inotropic effects. Nitroglycerin is a potent vasodilator that would lower blood pressure rather than raise it.

368

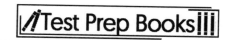

96. A: The nurse should report this issue to the nursing supervisor. This action promotes the elevation of a concern up the discipline (nursing) chain of command. In this specific case, the nursing supervisor may opt to connect with the surgeon (Choice *B*) to formulate a plan for next steps, including consent (Choice *C*). Choice *D*, a code team, is not necessary to determine how to proceed at this time.

97. A: Choice *A* is a surgical procedure highly associated with chronic otitis media. This procedure, also known as eardrum repair, provides needed reconstruction. Choices *B*, *C*, and *D* represent Ear, Nose, and Throat (ENT) surgical procedures that are not typically associated with this diagnosis. The nurse would not need to print and share patient education on these options at this time.

98. B: Patients or families who do not understand postoperative care needs for the patient may create an atmosphere of risk for poor patient outcomes. The patient or family needs to have a strong understanding of postoperative care needs prior to surgery and again prior to discharge. While the other answers are "good-to-know" information, the surgeon has to be made aware of details that indicate risk for the patient.

99. C: Choice *C* identifies a stuporous patient exhibiting no articulated verbal response with limited moaning, accompanied by arousal only after vigorous stimulation. Lethargic, Choice *A*, describes a patient who appears drowsy and arouses with gentle stimulation. Obtunded, Choice *B*, describes a patient who responds to repeated external stimulation to maintain attention. A patient that is comatose, Choice *D*, indicates they have no discernible response to stimulation. The levels of consciousness proceed with increasing severity from confused, to lethargic, to obtunded, to stuporous, and finally to comatose.

100. A: A major benefit of an electronic health record is that it can be easily accessed by multiple providers, which increases access to coordinated, interdisciplinary care for patients, improves quality of care, and reduces medical errors. Additionally, patients can access their medical records easily, which can improve patient satisfaction. At this time, types of health records used vary by country, and accessing one's record in a different country will likely require additional steps. Therefore, Choice *B* can be eliminated. Training is extensive, as users need to be trained on data input, data management, security, and other administrative protocols, so Choice *C* can be eliminated. Rural facilities have had a harder time with the implementation and adoption of electronic health record systems, due to lower tech literacy in patient populations and limited tech and internet availability, therefore, Choice *D* can be eliminated.

101. C: Choice *C* is not involved in the Five Rights of Delegation, which include the right person, task, circumstance, direction, and supervision. Choices *A*, *B*, and *D* are all components of the Five Rights of Delegation and used by the medical-surgical nurse when assigning patient care.

102. C: An angiogram to restore coronary blood flow is the priority treatment for cardiogenic shock. ABGs, a chest x-ray, and a Doppler study are not treatments; they are diagnostic tools.

103. C: If complete or partial blindness develops in a patient with temporal arteritis prior to therapeutic intervention, the deficit may progress and become irreversible, which constitutes an ophthalmologic emergency. Lower limb claudication due to vasculitis and ischemic changes may occur as the result of the inflammatory process, and the condition does require assessment and monitoring; however, visual alterations remain a higher priority for emergency care. Vertebral body fractures and infection are related to steroid therapy, which may occur during therapy, and both conditions will require assessment and intervention; however, the need to prevent irreversible blindness is a more urgent priority.

104. C: Facilitating a patient's transition from one point on the health continuum to another requires caring practices in addition to advocacy and moral agency. Moral agency may be employed to ensure that the patient's wishes are considered, especially those wishes associated with end-of-life concerns. Developing cultural awareness is an example of a response to diversity, and the remaining two choices refer to the facilitation of learning.

369

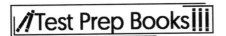

105. B: To help manage and minimize pain, care should be provided in the least invasive and painful ways possible. Choice *A* is incorrect because pain should be assessed at least every two to four hours, depending on a patient's needs. Choice *C* is incorrect because all patients have the right to pain management, regardless of histories of drug abuse. Patients with history of drug abuse may need to have their pain management regimen reviewed and more closely monitored, but their pain is still real and must be addressed. Choice *D* is incorrect because the nurse should identify ambulation and dressing changes as times that may cause increased pain and consider managing pain before these events take place. Additional means to help provide supportive pain management include emotional support, open communication, creating a pain control plan, and working with an interdisciplinary team to address pain concerns.

106. B: When indicated and appropriate, using silence allows time for the patient to reflect on how they are feeling and may allow them to process their thoughts and come up with their own solutions. Choice *A* is incorrect because yes or no questions can be limiting; instead, open-ended questions should be used to garner more information from the patient and allow for better communication. Choice *C* is incorrect because clichés can come across as insincere and may add little meaning to the conversation. Choice *D* is incorrect because asking patients to explain their behavior may come across as accusatory and cause a patient to close off their communication.

107. D: When critically reading a new research article, it is not imperative that the nurse sees where funding comes from for the research. While funding can have some influence over research and should be examined when appraising research, it is not necessary when trying to critically read and understand new research information. Choices *A, B,* and *C* are incorrect because the nurse should determine the thesis, process, and outcomes when critically reading research.

108. B: When creating a lesson plan, the nurse should create definite and measurable goals and objectives. Creating open-ended objectives makes it more difficult to create a structured lesson and assess if the learner gained the knowledge that the goal set. Choices *A, C,* and *D* are incorrect because these are all accurate and important components to include in a lesson plan when educating a patient. Additionally, the material in the lesson should relate to and cover both the goals and objectives of the teaching.

109. C: This nurse exhibited a failure to delegate appropriate tasks and therefore fell behind schedule. They had multiple time-heavy tasks to complete in the morning that were difficult to carry out independently. Since the nurse is on a fully staffed floor that includes nursing assistants, the nurse should delegate the tasks of completing bed baths because this task is within the scope of practice for the nursing assistant to complete. This would allow the nurse to complete the other tasks that require nursing-level competency. Choice *A* is incorrect because the nurse is working on a fully staffed unit, so it is unlikely that staffing ratios would be the cause of this delayed care. Choice *B* is incorrect because regardless of organization and planning, the nurse may still not be able to complete all these tasks independently in a certain amount of time. Instead, tasks should be delegated appropriately. Choice *D* is incorrect because a nurse working in a critical care setting may have patients that have very involved care. Delegating tasks helps the nurse complete all their care in the appropriate time.

110. D: Regulatory bodies such as TJC and CMS clearly identify patient education as a need that must be fulfilled in order to promote optimal patient outcomes. While holistic care, discharge planning, and culturally based care are important aspects of nursing, these are not identified by TJC and CMS as ones that must be fulfilled in order to promote optimal patient outcomes.

111. D: Geographical community resources include public libraries and government offices. Institutional resources include tuition reimbursement, employee assistance programs (EAPs), and other health care professionals. Local and demographical resources are not specific types of resources for patient/family education.

112. B: All medical facilities should have written, comprehensive disaster plans that can be consulted to adequately prepare and implement procedures in the event of a natural disaster or environmental threat. In this case,

370

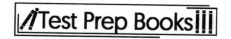

reviewing the hospital's flood insurance policy isn't necessary for the staff, and a fire drill is unlikely to occur during a hurricane. Ride-sharing credits aren't relevant to this case.

113. B: All types of adverse events should be reported as soon as reasonably possible, even if the nurse's shift extends into overtime. Timely reporting of events ensures that necessary details are not omitted or forgotten. The nurse should follow the facility's policies and procedures for event reporting, which may include documentation in an internal tracking system. The nurse should document the appropriate information in the patient's medical record, but there may be potentially causative details that are not appropriate in the patient's medical record. The nurse should review the report and documentation with their supervisor or manager.

114. A: The Plan-Do-Study-Act (PDSA) cycle is recommended by the Institute of Healthcare Improvement and the Agency for Healthcare Research and Quality as a simple framework for healthcare providers and administrators to continuously improve processes. A change is selected to test, and the participant or team who is testing the change will plan for the change, do the change, study successes and obstacles related to the change, and act to adopt, abandon, or anchor the change. The DMAIC method (Define, Measure, Analyze, Improve, Control) is similarly used to improve processes, but is more common in manufacturing and business contexts; therefore, Choice *B* can be eliminated. Value-Stream Mapping is another tool for quality improvement, used to show what steps of a process add value to the customer or organization. While it can gather valuable information to determine what kinds of changes could be tested, it does not provide a framework for testing a process change itself, so Choice *C* is incorrect. Lean is a methodology for analyzing how best to maintain or create value while using the least number of resources. It is not related to tests of change, so Choice *D* can be eliminated.

115. C: Choice *C* indicates the appropriate professional response by the nurse to address the present language barrier. Choices *A* and *B* would not directly support communication that is free from misunderstanding and should be omitted. Choice *D* would not rely on a professional, non-biased party for translation and should be avoided if possible.

116. B: Liability means to be responsible to or under obligation, and negligence is defined as the failure to exercise the standard of care that a reasonably prudent person would exercise under similar conditions. Each state board of nursing has a Nursing Practice Act that sets the standards of care a nurse is expected to maintain in practice.

117. A: The World Health Organization (WHO) created the Surgical Safety Checklist with the intention to promote patient safety and to improve documentation standards. The remaining answers are partially correct. The checklists aim to reduce the risk for complications before, during, and after surgery.

118. D: The patient may display all of these examples of the body shutting down. Deep tendon reflexes are present in a person who is alive.

119. D: Elevated LDL cholesterol levels are a major risk factor for CAD, and reducing LDL cholesterol levels has been shown to reduce the risk of cardiovascular events. While Choice *A* is a desirable outcome, as a higher HDL cholesterol level is associated with a lower risk of cardiovascular disease, there is no evidence to suggest that increasing HDL cholesterol levels alone is an effective strategy for reducing the risk of cardiovascular events. While Choice *B* is also a desirable outcome, weight loss may be a challenging goal for this patient to achieve, particularly if they have a sedentary lifestyle and do not engage in regular physical activity. Choice *C* can be difficult and may take longer than three months, particularly if the patient has been a smoker for many years.

120. B: Patient support groups can provide a supportive and educational environment for patients and their families. They can connect with others who have similar experiences and receive practical tips, resources, and emotional support. Choice *A* can provide a large amount of information, but not all of it may be reliable or relevant. Choice *C* can provide specific information about the patient's condition, but may not address the needs of the entire family. Choice *D* can be a source of misinformation.

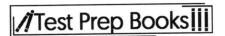

121. C: While choices *A*, *B*, and *D* are all important for the nurse to address, the primary focus should be on the patient's individual needs. In this scenario, the nurse should work to address the concerns and difficulties that the patient is currently facing. In doing so, the nurse is advocating for the patient and making sure their voice is being heard.

122. A: The nurse should assess the patient's technique for using the insulin pump to ensure that they are using it correctly. The nurse should also perform a blood glucose test to evaluate the patient's current blood sugar level. If the test indicates that the blood sugar level is elevated, the nurse can then work with the healthcare provider to adjust the insulin dose as needed; therefore, Choice *B* would be a premature action for the nurse to take. Choice *C* is not appropriate without first assessing the underlying issue. Contacting the manufacturer for technical support, Choice *D*, may be helpful, but it is not the most appropriate initial action in this scenario.

123. C: Congestive heart failure is a chronic condition that requires ongoing management to prevent exacerbations and hospital readmissions. Education is a crucial component of managing CHF, as it empowers patients to take an active role in their own care. Choice *A* may not be appropriate if the patient requires additional care or education before being discharged. Choice *B* is important but does not address the underlying issue of managing the patient's CHF. Choice *D* may be helpful in certain situations, but it is not the most effective intervention for reducing the risk of readmission for a patient with CHF.

124. B: Limited education is a social determinant of health (SDOH) that can have a significant impact on a patient's ability to manage their health conditions. In this patient's case, limited education is likely to affect their ability to understand how to manage their diabetes and adhere to their medication regimen. Referring this patient to a diabetes educator can help them receive a tailored education to better manage their condition. Providing written instructions, Choice *A*, may be helpful but may not be sufficient given this patient's limited education. Choices *C* and *D* are both incorrect because they disregard education as an important SDOH.

125. C: Nursing assistive personnel (NAP) are commonly delegated the task of blood glucose readings in the hospital setting. Other tasks that may be delegated to the NAP include feeding meals, assisting with hygiene, or changing bed linens for patients. These tasks do not require nursing judgment, clinical expertise, or critical decision-making. Choice *A* is a task that cannot be delegated by the RN to the NAP, as medication administration is within the RN's scope of practice. Choice *B* is a task that requires critical thinking and clinical judgment and should not be delegated to the NAP. Choice *D* is also within the RN's scope of practice and should not be delegated to the NAP.

126. C: Patient and family-centered care (PFCC) is an approach to healthcare that involves collaboration among healthcare providers, patients, and their families to meet the patient's physical, emotional, and psychological needs. It recognizes the importance of involving patients and their families in the care and decision-making process. Choices *A*, *B*, and *D* do not demonstrate PFCC.

127. C: This is the best option, as it addresses the need for communication and collaboration between providers. While Choice *A* may be a viable option, it does not address the need for continuity of care between the patient's primary care physician and oncologist. Choices *B* and *D* may lead to fragmented care and poor communication between providers.

128. B: This is the best option, as it provides the graduate nurse with specific feedback on how to improve their documentation skills. Choice *A* is not effective, as it does not allow the graduate nurse to develop their own documentation strategies. While Choices *C* and *D* may be helpful, they do not provide the graduate nurse with personalized feedback on their documentation skills.

129. A: It is not uncommon for patients and family members to have differing recollections of a patient's health history. When there are discrepancies in the information provided, it is important for the nurse to clarify the information with the patient and family members. Documenting both the patient's reported health history and the

372

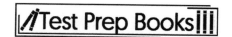

information provided by family members ensures that all relevant information is documented in the patient's medical record. Disregarding one source of information over another, as in Choices B and C, can lead to incomplete or inaccurate information in the medical record. The nurse should never ignore discrepancies in a patient's health history, as in Choice D.

130. B: Low employee engagement among nursing staff can have a significant impact on patient outcomes, as disengaged nurses may be less likely to provide high-quality care or catch potential errors. While Choices A, C, and D can also be caused by low employee engagement, they may not have as direct a link to nursing staff as adverse events.

131. B: Advocating for safe working conditions is an important responsibility of nurses, and refusing to work under unsafe conditions is one way to demonstrate staff advocacy. Nurses should not compromise their own safety or the safety of their patients by taking on too much work or working under conditions that are unsafe. Choice A may be seen as accepting the unsafe working conditions, which is not demonstrating staff advocacy. Choice C is a potential option, but it may not address the immediate safety concerns for the nurse and their patients. Choice D is a good way to build support for the issue, but it may not lead to immediate action to address the unsafe working conditions.

132. B: Conflict management is an important skill for nurses to possess, and it involves being able to recognize, address, and resolve conflicts that arise in the patient care setting. Encouraging the family members to discuss their concerns with the healthcare team is the best approach in this scenario. Avoiding the conflict or taking sides, as in Choices A and C, may exacerbate the situation and lead to further tension and disagreements. Choice D may be necessary in some cases, but it is not the best approach in this scenario.

133. C: Financial stewardship is an important principle in nursing that involves using healthcare resources efficiently and effectively to provide high-quality care while being mindful of costs. In this scenario, the patient is uninsured and cannot afford a costly surgical procedure. The nurse should work with the healthcare team to explore alternative treatment options that are less expensive and discuss these options with the patient. Choices A and D are not appropriate solutions for this patient. Choice B may not be a viable option if the patient's condition requires immediate treatment.

134. A: Attending to the patient with critical lab values first is the most appropriate action for the nurse to take to prevent further complications. While relieving pain is a basic human need, as in Choice B, the patient's pain is not immediately life-threatening and can be addressed after the patient with critical lab values has been stabilized. While prioritization based on acuity level may be a useful strategy, as in Choice C, the patient with critical lab values requires immediate attention regardless of their acuity level. Choice D is not recommended, as it may further compromise the patients' conditions.

135. C: Managing the supply inventory requires balancing the need for adequate resources with the need to stay within budget constraints. The most appropriate approach is to collaborate with the nurse to identify alternatives to the disposable supplies that are cost-effective and safe for the patient. This approach takes into consideration the need to ensure patient safety and comfort while being mindful of budgetary constraints. Choice A is incorrect, as it does not address the issue. Choice B may be inappropriate and confrontational. Choice D may not be necessary at this stage.

136. C: Professional engagement in unit councils is a key aspect of shared governance and collaborative practice in nursing. The most appropriate approach is to discuss the value of the council with the colleague and encourage them to share their concerns and ideas during meetings. By promoting open communication and respect for diverse perspectives, the nurse can facilitate active engagement in the council and enhance the quality of patient care and

373

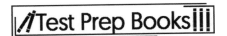

professional development. Choices A and D may create tension and resistance to the council's activities and may lead to further disengagement. Choice B may also compromise the effectiveness of the council.

137. B: Preceptor conflicts can be a common challenge for newly hired nurses. By reporting the preceptor's behavior to the unit manager and requesting a new preceptor, the newly hired nurse can ensure that their orientation and training are of high quality and that their professional development is supported. The unit manager can work with the nurse to identify a new preceptor who is supportive, knowledgeable, and experienced in providing guidance and support to newly hired nurses. Choices A and D may not be the most effective approaches, as the nurse may not have access to the necessary resources or support to address the conflict. Choice C may be a viable option, but it may not always lead to a resolution of the conflict.

138. C: Reflective practice is a process of self-assessment, evaluation, and problem-solving that allows nurses to examine their own beliefs, attitudes, and assumptions about patient care. By engaging in reflective practice, the nurse can consider alternative approaches to care that may be more effective for this particular patient. Choice A does not address the patient's needs and does not reflect the professional responsibility of a nurse to provide care. Continuing to provide care as usual without considering alternative approaches, as in Choice B, may not be effective for this patient. Choice D does not reflect a patient-centered approach to care and may worsen the situation.

139. B: The nurse is a crucial member of the healthcare team and has extensive knowledge of the patient's condition, as well as their preferences and concerns. During interprofessional rounding, the nurse can provide valuable input on the care plan, share updates on the patient's progress, and identify potential issues that may impact the patient's care. Choice A is incorrect because the nurse does not lead the rounding session, but rather participates as a member of the healthcare team. Choice C is incorrect because the nurse's role during interprofessional rounding is not merely to observe and take notes, but rather to actively participate in the discussion and contribute to the care plan. While Choice D is part of the nurse's routine responsibilities, it is not specifically related to interprofessional rounding.

140. B: By facilitating self-reflection and problem-solving through questioning, the preceptor can help the new nurse identify their strengths and areas for improvement and develop strategies for improving their time management and prioritization skills. This approach also helps to build the new nurse's confidence and critical thinking skills, which are essential for effective nursing practice. Choice A may be appropriate in certain situations, but in this case, it is not the best answer because the new nurse is not struggling with nursing skills, but rather with time management and prioritization. Choice C may be helpful for some learners, but this may not be the best approach for a nurse who may benefit from more interactive coaching strategies. Choice D may also be appropriate in some cases, but it is not the best answer in this scenario because the new nurse may benefit more from individualized coaching and problem-solving.

141. B: Shared governance is an organizational structure that empowers nurses to participate in decision-making and take ownership of their practice. It is based on the principles of equity, accountability, and partnership and can help to improve job satisfaction, engagement, and retention among nursing staff. By implementing shared governance structures, the nurse manager can help to create a more collaborative and supportive work environment that values the input of nursing staff and allows them to contribute to the development of policies and procedures, thus positively impacting professional empowerment. Choice A may not address the underlying causes of burnout and disengagement among nursing staff. Choices C and D are more individual-focused and may not address the broader organizational issues that are contributing to the nursing team's burnout and disengagement.

142. B: Effective orientation is essential to the success of new nurses, and if the orientation process is rushed or disorganized, it can negatively impact job satisfaction, performance, and patient care. By communicating their concerns to their preceptor and nurse manager, the nurse can work collaboratively to identify areas of improvement and develop a new orientation plan that addresses their needs and concerns. Choice A may not address the underlying issues with the orientation process. Choice C can lead to further frustration and burnout and

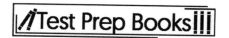

potentially impact patient care. Choice *D* does not reflect a problem-solving approach and may not resolve the underlying issues of poor orientation planning.

143. C: The human resources department is typically responsible for overseeing career development programs within the hospital and can provide valuable guidance and support to employees who are interested in pursuing additional training and education opportunities. By meeting with the human resources department, the nurse can discuss their career goals, learn about available resources within the hospital, and develop a plan to achieve their career objectives. Choice *A* may be appropriate in some situations, but a mentor may not have access to all the available resources within the hospital. External training and education opportunities, as in Choice *B*, may not be tailored to the specific needs and objectives of the nurse. Choice *D* may be a more expensive and time-consuming option than simply meeting with the human resources department.

144. D: Professional nursing organizations provide valuable networking opportunities, access to the latest research and developments in nursing practice, and resources for continuing education and professional development. By joining a professional nursing organization, the nurse can connect with other nurses who share their interests and goals and gain access to a wealth of information and resources to support their practice. Choices *A*, *B*, and *C* may not provide the same ongoing networking and professional development opportunities as a professional nursing organization.

145. C: Improper peer review methods, such as personal attacks and bullying, can be detrimental to the work environment and can negatively impact job satisfaction and morale among nursing staff. By bringing the issue to the attention of the nurse manager, the nurse can help to promote a more professional and constructive approach to peer review. This approach can help to ensure that feedback is given in a way that is constructive, respectful, and focused on improving patient care and nursing practice. Choice *A* can perpetuate the issue and may not be an effective solution. Choice *B* may be appropriate in some situations, but it is not the best answer in this scenario because the colleagues may not be receptive to feedback. Choice *D* should be considered a last resort after all other attempts to resolve the issue have been exhausted.

146. C: Blood transfusions come with many potential risks and complications, and it is essential to follow regulatory and compliance standards to ensure the safety and well-being of the patient. By consulting the hospital's policies and procedures, the nurse can ensure that they are following the correct process for administering the blood transfusion. Choice *A* may not take into account the regulatory and compliance standards that are necessary to ensure patient safety. Choice *B* is not the best answer in this scenario because it relies on the experience and knowledge of another nurse rather than the hospital's policies and procedures. Choice *D* may cause unnecessary delay in administering the blood transfusion, which can be critical in some situations.

147. D: A top-down approach can be effective in certain situations, but it can also create a rigid hierarchical structure that may stifle creativity and innovation. It is important for leaders to consider alternative approaches that foster creativity, innovation, and teamwork. Choice *A* is incorrect because while a top-down approach can be demanding, it is not necessarily the cause of burnout. Choice *B* is incorrect because a top-down approach may lead to increased accountability and a more structured work environment, although a rigid one. Choice *C* is incorrect because a top-down approach can increase communication and collaboration but only in a hierarchical way.

148. B: Shared decision making involves the patient, their family, and the healthcare team collaborating together to make treatment decisions that are in the best interests of the patient. By encouraging the patient to make their own decisions, the nurse can help to empower the patient and promote their autonomy in the decision-making process. Choice *A* does not take into account the patient's preferences, values, and goals for care. Choice *C* does not guarantee that the patient's preferences and values will be taken into account. Choice *D* does not promote the patient's autonomy and may not lead to the best outcome for the patient.

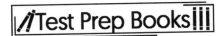

149. B: A core part of nursing philosophy is providing patient-centered care that respects the dignity, worth, and rights of every patient regardless of their cultural background. By respecting the patient's cultural beliefs and values, the nurse can help to establish trust and build a therapeutic relationship with the patient. Choice A does not respect the patient's cultural beliefs and values and does not align with the nursing philosophy of patient-centered care. Choice C may cause unnecessary delay in providing care to the patient. Choice D also does not reflect patient-centered care.

150. C: In healthcare, customer experience is becoming increasingly important, with value-based purchasing programs tying payment to patient satisfaction scores. Data results, such as surveys, are used to measure patient experience and provide feedback to healthcare providers. In this scenario, it is important for the nurse to acknowledge the patient's concerns and work with them to develop a plan to address their specific needs. This can include listening actively to their complaints, empathizing with their concerns, and working collaboratively with them to find a solution. Choice A does not necessarily address the patient's specific needs or concerns. Choice B dismisses the patient's concerns and may result in further dissatisfaction. Choice D focuses solely on providing standard care, without addressing the patient's unique needs or concerns.

Practice Test #3

To keep the size of this book manageable, save paper, and provide a digital test-taking experience, the 3rd practice test can be found online. Scan the QR code or go to this link to access it:

testprepbooks.com/bonus/medsurg

The first time you access the tests, you will need to register as a "new user" and verify your email address.

If you have any issues, please email support@testprepbooks.com.

Dear Medical Surgical Nurse Test Taker,

Thank you again for purchasing this study guide for your Medical Surgical Nurse exam. We hope that we exceeded your expectations.

Our goal in creating this study guide was to cover all of the topics that you will see on the test. We also strove to make our practice questions as similar as possible to what you will encounter on test day. With that being said, if you found something that you feel was not up to your standards, please send us an email and let us know.

We would also like to let you know about other books in our catalog that may interest you.

CCRN

This can be found on Amazon: amazon.com/dp/1637753454

PCCN

amazon.com/dp/1628458909

We have study guides in a wide variety of fields. If the one you are looking for isn't listed above, then try searching for it on Amazon or send us an email.

Thanks Again and Happy Testing!
Product Development Team
info@studyguideteam.com

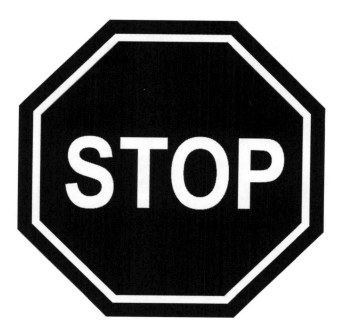

FREE Test Taking Tips Video/DVD Offer

To better serve you, we created videos covering test taking tips that we want to give you for FREE. **These videos cover world-class tips that will help you succeed on your test.**

We just ask that you send us feedback about this product. Please let us know what you thought about it—whether good, bad, or indifferent.

To get your **FREE videos**, you can use the QR code below or email freevideos@studyguideteam.com with "Free Videos" in the subject line and the following information in the body of the email:

    a. The title of your product

    b. Your product rating on a scale of 1-5, with 5 being the highest

    c. Your feedback about the product

If you have any questions or concerns, please don't hesitate to contact us at info@studyguideteam.com.

Thank you!

Made in the USA
Columbia, SC
24 January 2024

30868178R00213